AF566976

1998
YEAR BOOK OF
NEPHROLOGY, HYPERTENSION, AND MINERAL METABOLISM

Statement of Purpose

The YEAR BOOK Service

The YEAR BOOK series was devised in 1901 by practicing health professionals who observed that the literature of medicine and related disciplines had become so voluminous that no one individual could read and place in perspective every potential advance in a major specialty. In the final decade of the 20th century, this recognition is more acutely true than it was in 1901.

More than merely a series of books, YEAR BOOK volumes are the tangible results of a unique service designed to accomplish the following:

- to *survey* a wide range of journals of proven value
- to *select* from those journals papers representing significant advances and statements of important clinical principles
- to provide *abstracts* of those articles that are readable, convenient summaries of their key points
- to provide *commentary* about those articles to place them in perspective

These publications grow out of a unique process that calls on the talents of outstanding authorities in clinical and fundamental disciplines, trained literature specialists, and professional writers, all supported by the resources of Mosby, the world's preeminent publisher for the health professions.

The Literature Base

Mosby and its editors survey more than 1,000 journals published worldwide, covering the full range of the health professions. On an annual basis, the publisher examines usage patterns and polls its expert authorities to add new journals to the literature base and to delete journals that are no longer useful as potential YEAR BOOK sources.

The Literature Survey

The publisher's team of literature specialists, all of whom are trained and experienced health professionals, examines every original, peer-reviewed article in each journal issue. More than 250,000 articles per year are scanned systematically, including title, text, illustrations, tables, and references. Each scan is compared, article by article, to the search strategies that the publisher has developed in consultation with the 270 outside experts who form the pool of YEAR BOOK editors. A given article may be reviewed by any number of editors, from one to a dozen or more, regardless of the discipline for which the paper was originally published. In turn, each editor who receives the article reviews it to determine whether the article should be included in the YEAR BOOK. This decision is based on the article's inherent quality, its probable usefulness to readers of that YEAR BOOK, and the editor's goal to represent a balanced picture of a given field in each volume of the YEAR BOOK. In addition, the editor indicates when to include figures and tables from the article to help the YEAR BOOK reader better understand the information.

Of the quarter million articles scanned each year, only 5% are selected for detailed analysis within the YEAR BOOK series, thereby assuring readers of the high value of every selection.

The Abstract

The publisher's abstracting staff is headed by a seasoned medical professional and includes individuals with training in the life sciences, medicine, and other areas, plus extensive experience in writing for the health professions and related industries. Each selected article is assigned to a specific writer on this abstracting staff. The abstracter, guided in many cases by notations supplied by the expert editor, writes a structured, condensed summary designed so that the reader can rapidly acquire the essential information contained in the article.

The Commentary

The YEAR BOOK editorial boards, sometimes assisted by guest commentators, write comments that place each article in perspective for the reader. This provides the reader with the equivalent of a personal consultation with a leading international authority—an opportunity to better understand the value of the article and to benefit from the authority's thought processes in assessing the article.

Additional Editorial Features

The editorial boards of each YEAR BOOK organize the abstracts and comments to provide a logical and satisfying sequence of information. To enhance the organization, editors also provide introductions to sections or individual chapters, comments linking a number of abstracts, citations to additional literature, and other features.

The published YEAR BOOK contains enhanced bibliographic citations for each selected article, including extended listings of multiple authors and identification of author affiliations. Each YEAR BOOK contains a Table of Contents specific to that year's volume. From year to year, the Table of Contents for a given YEAR BOOK will vary depending on developments within the field.

Every YEAR BOOK contains a list of the journals from which papers have been selected. This list represents a subset of the more than 1,000 journals surveyed by the publisher and occasionally reflects a particularly pertinent article from a journal that is not surveyed on a routine basis.

Finally, each volume contains a comprehensive subject index and an index to authors of each selected paper.

The 1998 Year Book Series

Year Book of Allergy, Asthma, and Clinical Immunology: Drs. Rosenwasser, Borish, Boguniewicz, Nelson, Routes, and Spahn

Year Book of Anesthesiology and Pain Management®: Drs. Tinker, Abram, Chestnut, Roizen, Rothenberg, and Wood

Year Book of Cardiology®: Drs. Schlant, Collins, Gersh, Graham, Kaplan, and Waldo

Year Book of Chiropractic®: Dr. Lawrence

Year Book of Critical Care Medicine®: Drs. Parrillo, Balk, Calvin, Franklin, and Shapiro

Year Book of Dentistry®: Drs. Meskin, Berry, Jeffcoat, Leinfelder, Roser, Summitt, and Zakariasen

Year Book of Dermatologic Surgery®: Drs. Greenway, Barrett, Papadopoulos, and Whitaker

Year Book of Dermatology®: Dr. Thiers

Year Book of Diagnostic Radiology®: Drs. Osborn, Groskin, Dalinka, Maynard, Pentecost, Rebner, Ros, Smirniotopoulos, and Young

Year Book of Drug Therapy®: Drs. Lasagna and Weintraub

Year Book of Emergency Medicine®: Drs. Wagner, Dronen, Davidson, King, Niemann, and Roberts

Year Book of Endocrinology®: Drs. Bagdade, Braverman, Horton, Kannan, Landsberg, Molitch, Morley, Nathan, Odell, Poehlman, Rogol, and Ryan

Year Book of Family Practice®: Drs. Berg, Bowman, Davidson, Dexter, and Scherger

Year Book of Gastroenterology®: Drs. Aliperti and Fleshman

Year Book of Geriatrics and Gerontology®: Drs. Burton, Beck, Ostwald, Rabins, Reuben, Roth, Shapiro, and Whitehouse

Year Book of Hand Surgery®: Drs. Amadio and Hentz

Year Book of Hematology®: Drs. Spivak, Bell, Ness, Quesenberry, Wiernik, and Horowitz

Year Book of Infectious Diseases: Drs. Keusch, Barza, Bennish, Poutsiaka, Skolnik, and Snydman

Year Book of Medicine®: Drs. Cline, Frishman, Jett, Klahr, Malawista, Mandell, McCallum, and Utiger

Year Book of Neonatal and Perinatal Medicine®: Drs. Fanaroff, Maisels, and Stevenson

Year Book of Nephrology, Hypertension, and Mineral Metabolism: Drs. Schwab, Bennett, Emmett, Hostetter, Kumar, and Toto

Year Book of Neurology and Neurosurgery®: Drs. Bradley and Gibbs

Year Book of Nuclear Medicine®: Drs. Gottschalk, Blaufox, Neumann, Strauss, and Zubal

Year Book of Obstetrics, Gynecology, and Women's Health: Drs. Mishell, Herbst, and Kirschbaum

Year Book of Occupational and Environmental Medicine®: Drs. Emmett, Frank, Gochfeld, and Hessl

Year Book of Oncology®: Drs. Ozols, Eisenberg, Glatstein, Loehrer, and Tallman

Year Book of Ophthalmology®: Drs. Wilson, Augsburger, Cohen, Eagle, Grossman, Laibson, Maguire, Nelson, Penne, Rapuano, Sergott, Spaeth, Tipperman, Ms. Gosfield, and Ms. Salmon

Year Book of Orthopedics®: Drs. Morrey, Beauchamp, Currier, Tolo, Trigg, and Swiontkowski

Year Book of Otolaryngology–Head and Neck Surgery®: Drs. Paparella and Holt

Year Book of Pathology and Laboratory Medicine®: Drs. Raab, Cohen, Olson, Sirgi, and Stanley

Year Book of Pediatrics®: Dr. Stockman

Year Book of Plastic, Reconstructive, and Aesthetic Surgery®: Drs. Miller, Bartlett, Garner, McKinney, Ruberg, Salisbury, and Smith

Year Book of Psychiatry and Applied Mental Health®: Drs. Talbott, Ballenger, Frances, Lydiard, Meltzer, Schowalter, and Tasman

Year Book of Pulmonary Disease®: Drs. Jett, Maurer, Ryu, Strollo, and Wenzel

Year Book of Rheumatology®: Drs. Panush, Hadler, LeRoy, Liang, Reichlin, Simon, and Weinblatt

Year Book of Sports Medicine®: Drs. Shephard, Drinkwater, Eichner, Torg, Alexander, and Mr. George

Year Book of Surgery®: Drs. Copeland, Bland, Deitch, Eberlein, Howard, Luce, Seeger, Souba, and Sugarbaker

Year Book of Thoracic and Cardiovascular Surgery®: Drs. Ginsberg, Wechsler, and Williams

Year Book of Urology®: Drs. Andriole and Coplen

Year Book of Vascular Surgery®: Dr. Porter

1998
The Year Book of NEPHROLOGY, HYPERTENSION, AND MINERAL METABOLISM

Editor-in-Chief
Steve J. Schwab, M.D.

Associate Editors
William Bennett, M.D.
Michael Emmett, M.D.
Thomas H. Hostetter, M.D.
Rajiv Kumar, M.B.B.S.
Robert D. Toto, M.D.

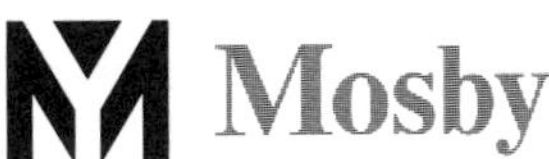

St. Louis Baltimore Boston Carlsbad Naples New York Philadelphia Portland London
Madrid Mexico City Singapore Sydney Tokyo Toronto Wiesbaden

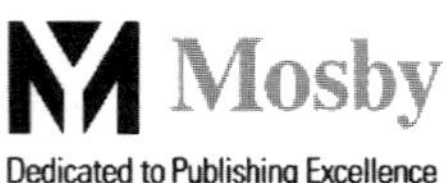

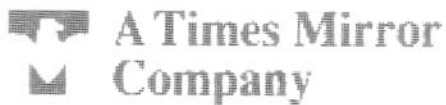

Associate Publisher: Gretchen C. Murphy
Developmental Editor: Jacquelyn M. Leonard
Manager, Periodical Editing: Kirk Swearingen
Manuscript Editor: Amanda Maguire
Project Supervisor, Production: Joy Moore
Production Assistant: Laura Bayless
Manager, Literature Services: Idelle L. Winer
Illustrations and Permissions Specialist: Steve Ramay

1998 EDITION

Printed in the United States of America
Composition by Reed Technology and Information Services, Inc.
Printing/binding by Maple-Vail

Editorial Office:
Mosby, Inc.
11830 Westline Industrial Drive
St. Louis, MO 63146
Customer Service: customer.support@mosby.com
www.mosby.com/Mosby/CustomerSupport/index.html

International Standard Serial Number: 1046-6266
International Standard Book Number: 0-8151-9646-6

Editorial Board

Table of Contents

Journals Represented

Mosby and its editors survey more than 1,000 journals for its abstract and commentary publications. From these journals, the Editors select the articles to be abstracted. Journals represented in this YEAR BOOK are listed below.

American Journal of Gastroenterology
American Journal of Kidney Diseases
American Journal of Nephrology
American Journal of Surgery
Annals of Internal Medicine
Archives of Surgery
British Medical Journal
Cell
Circulation
Clinical Nephrology
Critical Care Medicine
Diabetes
Diabetes Care
Diabetic Medicine
Diabetologia
Hypertension
Infection Control and Hospital Epidemiology
Intensive Care Medicine
Journal of Bone and Mineral Research
Journal of Clinical Endocrinology and Metabolism
Journal of Clinical Investigation
Journal of Clinical Pathology
Journal of Nuclear Medicine
Journal of Surgical Research
Journal of Urology
Journal of Vascular Surgery
Journal of the American Academy of Dermatology
Journal of the American College of Surgeons
Journal of the American Medical Association
Journal of the American Society of Nephrology
Kidney International
Lancet
Medicine
Nature Genetics
Nephrology, Dialysis, Transplantation
Nephron
New England Journal of Medicine
Pediatric Nephrology
Proceedings of the National Academy of Sciences
Quarterly Journal of Medicine
Radiology
Surgery
Transplantation

Standard Abbreviations

The following terms are abbreviated in this edition: acquired immunodeficiency syndrome (AIDS), cardiopulmonary resuscitation (CPR), central nervous system (CNS), cerebrospinal fluid (CSF), computed tomography (CT), deoxyribonucleic acid (DNA), electrocardiography (ECG), health maintenance organization (HMO), human immunodeficiency virus (HIV), intensive care unit (ICU), intramuscular (IM), intravenous (IV), magnetic resonance (MR) imaging (MRI), ribonucleic acid (RNA), and ultrasound (US).

Note

The Year Book of Nephrology, Hypertension, and Mineral Metabolism is a literature survey service providing abstracts of articles published in the professional literature. Every effort is made to assure the accuracy of the information presented in these pages. Neither the editors nor the publisher of the Year Book of Nephrology, Hypertension, and Mineral Metabolism can be responsible for errors in the original materials. The editors' comments are their own opinions. Mention of specific products within this publication does not constitute endorsement.

To facilitate the use of the Year Book of Nephrology, Hypertension, and Mineral Metabolism as a reference tool, all illustrations and tables included in this publication are now identified as they appear in the original article. This change is meant to help the reader recognize that any illustration or table appearing in the Year Book of Nephrology, Hypertension, and Mineral Metabolism may be only one of many in the original article. For this reason, figure and table numbers will often appear to be out of sequence within the Year Book of Nephrology, Hypertension, and Mineral Metabolism.

Introduction

The 1998 YEAR BOOK OF NEPHROLOGY, HYPERTENSION, AND MINERAL METABOLISM reviews the literature in renal investigation and clinical nephrology for 1998. The YEAR BOOK editors review and present studies that have significant clinical importance. While the majority of these observations will be patient based, some basic science observations have sufficient clinical implications to warrant presentation in this year's edition. The selections for 1998 are characterized by a steady increase in our knowledge about the science and clinical practice of nephrology. Blockbuster multicenter trials that change the face of the practice of nephrology have not characterized 1998. However, 1998 is characterized by the initiation and continuation of a series of large prospective trials that may shed significant light on our current practice patterns. In the area of dialysis, national and international multicenter trials dealing with the effect of hematocrit on morbidity and mortality as well as the effect of dialysis dose on morbidity and mortality are underway or have been recently completed. In the era of transplanation, multiple new therapeutic agents are undergoing prospective clinical trials. In the area of renal injury, prospective studies directed at focal glomerular sclerosis, IgA nephropathy, and membranous nephropathy are underway. We look forward to reporting the results of these recently initiated or recently completed studies to you in subsequent issues.

This is a year characterized by an emphasis on evidence-based medicine. The National Kidney Foundation's DOQI (Dialysis Outcome Quality Initiative) has identified key areas where evidence-based practice guidelines may improve dialysis patient care. The four areas selected—anemia management, adequacy of hemodialysis, adequacy of peritoneal dialysis, and vascular access management—are emphasized throughout the dialysis section. In addition, a series of significant new observations have occurred, such as those of Marr and colleagues (Abstract 1–9), who defined the incidence of catheter-mediated bacteremia in patients dialyzing with silastic cuffed catheters. In calcium phosphorus, new vitamin D analogs and new noncalcium, nonaluminum phosphate binders have come to clinical trials. In transplantation, new data on the use of mycophenolate, tacrolimus, and cyclosporine is emerging. In the renal and electrolytes chapters, there is new data showing advances in our understanding of genetic-derived electrolyte disorders such as Bartter's syndrome.

Nineteen ninety-eight also marks the final year for Dr. Rajiv Kumar from the Mayo Clinic who served as our editor for mineral metabolism. Dr. Sharon Moe from Indiana University has agreed to accept the challenge of the mineral metabolism section for the 1999 edition.

It is with pleasure that we present the 1998 edition.

Steve J. Schwab, M.D.
Editor-in-Chief

1 Dialysis

Introduction

The articles selected for this year's YEAR BOOK OF NEPHROLOGY, HYPERTENSION, AND MINERAL METABOLISM encompass a wide range of prospective and retrospective studies dealing with issues in patients with end-state renal disease. This points out that both types of studies have significant value. Large retrospective analyses of databases, such as those of the United States Renal Data System (USRDS), the large dialysis chains, and the end-stage renal disease networks provide an important glimpse into practice patterns. These retrospective observations identify key issues that require further evaluation in order to determine what we are doing wrong or doing right. The weaknesses of these studies are that selection bias is not evaluated and there is no control of the observed variables. Multiple selections this year come from these retrospective databases. A good example of this class of retrospective observations are those of Held and associates from the USRDS examining their large database for the the effect of dose of dialysis on patient mortality (Abstract 1–19). The weaknesses of this study are large patient selection biases and no control over the manner by which dose of dialysis was measured.

Prospective studies seek to conclusively resolve issues by eliminating bias in a clear-cut patient enrollment format. An example of propsective studies are the observation of Marr and colleagues (Abstract 1–9) who define the likelihood of catheter-mediated bacteremia in a large hemodialysis population and defined unequivocally the very limited likelihood of antibiotic therapy alone as a curative therapy without catheter exchange or removal. The prospective study defines limited issues in a specific and formal fashion, whereas the retrospective observation defines problems, identifies issues for investigation, and often asks more questions than it answers. Both types of observations are crucial to the advancement of our understanding of dialytic therapy.

While not included in this year's YEAR BOOK OF NEPHROLOGY, HYPERTENSION, AND MINERAL METABOLISM because it does not reflect an original observation, the National Kidney Foundation's Dialysis Outcomes Quality Initiative (DOQI) performed the single largest analysis of the literature in four key areas (*American Journal of Kidney Diseases*, special supplements, September and October, 1997). These 4 were areas where major improvements were needed in the practice of end-stage renal disease. They included: (1) hemodialysis vascular access, (2) adequacy of hemodialysis, (3) adequacy of peritoneal dialysis, and (4) management of anemia of end-stage renal disease. These evidence-based practice guidelines provide a basis for practice, and I refer to them throughout my comments when we come to manuscripts on which the DOQI based some of its guidelines. The concept of evidence-based medicine, based on prospective and retrospective observation, is actively gaining ground. Thoughtful practice guidelines derived from this evidence-based review of the available literature continues to advance our practice. I hope you enjoy this year's selections.

Steve J. Schwab, M.D.

Vascular Access

Introduction

Hemodialysis vascular access continues to be a major problem for nephrologists providing care for patients with end-stage renal disease. Recent investigators estimate the costs of vascular access exceeds $1 billion annually in the United States. Many managed care organizations have assumed that almost one third of the total end-stage renal disease budget is devoted to the placement, maintenance, and salvage of hemodialysis access. Thus, it is appropriate to begin the hemodialysis section with this year's selections of studies focusing on hemodialysis vascular access.

The initial paper (Abstract 1–1), a retrospective observation published in the *Journal of the American College of Surgeons*, confirms multiple previous observations that prospective detection of outflow stenoses improves the outcome of vascular access grafts. The second selection (Abstract 1–2) shows the steady advance of technology in prospective access screening. These investigators validate that US velocity dilution technique for measuring access graft flow is indeed accurate and reproducible. Thus, as suggested in the Dialysis Outcome Quality Initiative guidelines, access flow technology has been shown to be reliable and may in the near future supplant all other vascular access prospective screening techniques.

In Abstract 1–3, the mechanism by which vascular stenosis occurs is explored by Windus and associates. These investigators have previously documented the locations of platelet deposition following and during hemodialysis. It has been proposed that platelet-derived cytokines, such as platelet-derived growth factors that are released when platelet deposition occurs, stimulate the progressive fibromuscular and endothelial hyperplasia that leads to access stenoses. In the study featured in this year's selection, these investigators studied the role of ticlodipine and aspirin on platelet deposition in hemodialysis grafts. Abstract 1–4 addresses the issue of the role of erythropoietin (EPO) as the facilitator of access thrombosis. Investigators have previously speculated that EPO may act as a mitogen stimulating endothelial and fibromuscular hyperplasia. In this study however, long-term EPO therapy did not appear to increase the risk of progressive stenosis in native arteriovenous fistulas. This study did not deal with the effect of EPO on hemodialysis arteriovenous access grafts, which remains to be investigated. In Abstract 1–5, Schuman and associates evaluated the role of reinforced versus nonreinforced polytetrafluroethylene (PTFE) grafts for hemodialysis access. They conclude that nonreinforced PTFE grafts are better for long-term patency than reinforced PTFE. Although this is interesting, what is even more striking from this study is the effect of the surgeon placing the access on primary patency.

The final 2 selections dealing with permanent vascular access seek to deal with treatment strategies once an access stenosis is detected. In Abstract 1–6, Lumsden and associates from Emory, in a retrospective evaluation of their data, suggest that transluminal angioplasty is an ineffective therapy for prolonging access patency. This is in contrast to multiple other studies that found many access stenoses responded satisfactorily to angioplasty and increased access patency. One of the reasons for these differences is that the retrospective nature of the observation may have led to higher grade stenoses selected for angioplasty. In a similar vein, Marston and associates evaluate transluminal angioplasty and surgical revision in the treatment of vascular access stenoses detected post thrombosis (Abstract 1–7). These authors also conclude that surgical revision is superior to transluminal angioplasty. My opinion, as outlined in my comments on these articles, is that both papers are probably correct. Higher grade stenoses, those greater than 70%, probably do not respond as favorably to transluminal angioplasty as do stenoses of 50% to 60%. Most prospectively detected stenoses are of the 50% to 60% lumen diameter category and have been shown to respond well to angioplasty. Ideal treatment strategy for detected stenoses is emerging and will be reported here as it occurs.

Steve J. Schwab, M.D.

Graft Surveillance and Angioplasty Prolongs Dialysis Graft Patency

Roberts AB, Kahn MB, Bradford S, et al (Allegheny Univ, Philadelphia; Thomas Jefferson Univ, Philadelphia; Temple Univ, Philadelphia)

J Am Coll Surg 183:486–492, 1996 1–1

Background.—For American patients with end-stage renal disease (ESRD), the most common cause of death is vascular access complications. For those with prosthetic graft fistulas, thrombosis is the major complication. At the authors' dialysis unit, graft surveillance is carried out by measuring venous resistance, early fistulagram, and percutaneous dilation of identified fistulas greater than 50%. The impact of this graft surveillance policy on graft life and patency was analyzed.

Methods.—The retrospective study examined the outcomes of 2 groups of patients receiving dialysis with upper-extremity angio-access grafts. Two hundred ten patients were treated in the 2 years before adoption of the new graft surveillance policy (control group), and 260 patients were treated in the 3 years afterward (study group). Patients requiring more than 1 intervention over a 12-month period were considered "complicated" cases. Twenty-four percent of patients in the control group and 27% of those in the study group fell into this category. The graft history of the 2 groups of patients was compared.

Results.—There were 50 patients with complications in the control group, who had a total of 104 operations for treatment of thrombosis. The rate of thrombotic episodes and operations was thus 1.04/patient/year. There were 70 new grafts placed in these patients, with a mean survival of 6.3 months. In the study group, there were 71 patients with complications who had a total of 11 fistulagrams and 80 angioplasties. A total of 110 operations were performed in this group, which had a rate of thrombotic episodes and operations of 0.52/patient/year. The patients received a total of 45 new grafts, which had a primary patency of 11.5 months and a mean graft survival of 15.8 months.

Conclusions.—Graft surveillance can improve graft survival in dialysis patients with upper-arm prosthetic grafts. Potentially compromised grafts can be identified by measuring venous dialysis pressures. Stenoses can be effectively identified by fistulagram and treated by percutaneous angioplasty. The surveillance policy used in this study can reduce the occurrence of graft thrombosis and surgery while prolonging graft longevity.

▶ This retrospective surgical study lends further support for the role of careful prospective screening of atrioventricular (AV) grafts. When combined with therapeutic intervention, access patency was significantly improved. The arguments are no longer whether screening is useful but rather which technique of screening and what method of stenosis correction are best to improve AV graft patency.

S.J. Schwab, M.D.

Validation in the Sheep of an Ultrasound Velocity Dilution Technique for Haemodialysis Graft Flow

Gleed RD, Harvey HJ, Dobson A (Cornell Univ, Ithaca, NY)

Nephrol Dial Transplant 12:1464–1467, 1997 1–2

Introduction.—A recently developed flowmeter based on the dilution principle can be used easily to measure access flow during routine hemodialysis. This minimally invasive method depends on perturbations of the velocity of sound in the blood passing through the dialysis circuit. Injection of a small bolus of isotonic NaCl dilutes the hemoglobin and plasma proteins, thus transiently perturbing the US velocity. An animal study was designed to validate the US velocity dilution technique.

Methods.—The US velocity dilution technique was compared with the graft flow measured by the transit-time flowmeter, a method that is reliable but requires surgical implantation. Two adult ewes were anesthetized and equipped with a perivascular flow probe on the right carotid artery. A 4–7 mm PTFE graft was introduced between the same carotid artery and the

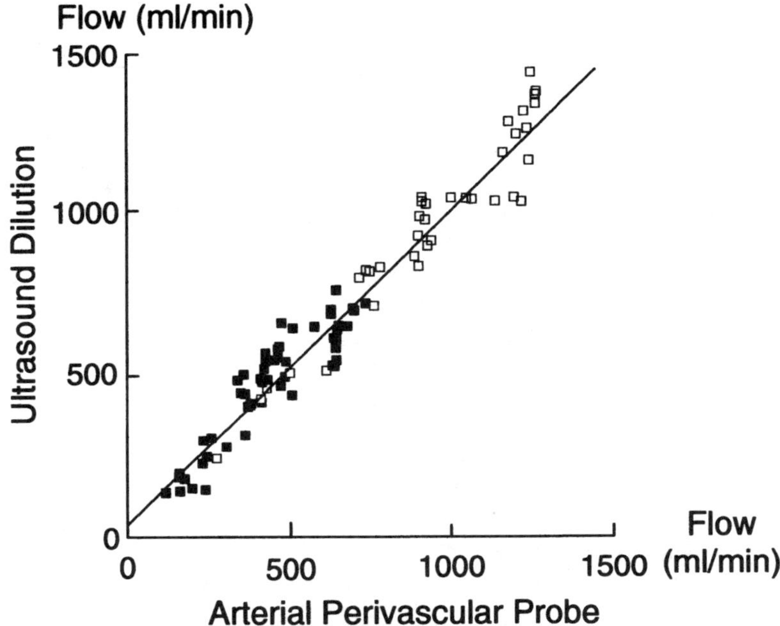

FIGURE 2.—Relationship between access blood flow measured by both an ultrasound dilution method and a perivascular flow probe. ■Sheep 1; □Sheep 2. (Courtesy of Gleed RD, Harvey HJ, Dobson A: Validation in the sheep of an ultrasound velocity dilution technique for hemodialysis graft flow. *Nephrol Dial Transplant* 12:1464–1467, 1997. Reprinted by permission of Oxford University Press.)

jugular vein. With the animals under general anesthesia and on a hemodialysis circuit, a 5–10 ml bolus of isotonic NaCl was injected. A transit-time blood flow meter was used to measure the pump tubing flow. To estimate graft flow, this flow was combined with the areas of perturbation generated by the injection before and after mixing in the access flow.

Results.—Fifty-four comparisons of flow were made on the first sheep over 3 sessions. In the second sheep, 36 comparisons of flow were made during 2 sessions. Data from the 2 animals were combined to give 90 comparisons of access flow measured directly by perivascular probe and indirectly by US dilution. Over a 10-fold range (120–1,260 mL/min), access graft flow measured by the 2 techniques (Fig 2) agreed well with a scatter of 76 mL/min about the regression line.

Discussion.—The most accurate measurement of access flow is provided by a calibrated perivascular probe directly on the arterial supply of this access flow. Graft flow measured by US velocity dilution closely followed that of the invasive method. Ultrasound dilution appears to be a feasible method for measuring flow in the graft and is accurate enough for the clinical evaluation of patients on dialysis.

▶ This article compares hemodialysis graft flow in a group of experimental sheep and compares direct measurement of flow with a velocity probe and compares that to US dilution technique with a transonic flowmeter. The result (Fig 2) shows a remarkable degree of correlation. Thus, US dilution using the device tested here should provide a very accurate measure of graft flow. This supports the use of this device as a prospective measure of impending access dysfunction.

S.J. Schwab, M.D.

Effects of Antiplatelet Drugs on Dialysis-associated Platelet Deposition in Polytetrafluoroethylene Grafts

Windus DW, Santoro SA, Atkinson R, et al (Washington Univ, St Louis; Mallinkrodt Inst of Radiology, St Louis)

Am J Kidney Dis 29:560–564, 1997 1–3

Background.—Platelet deposition in polytetrafluoroethylene (PTFE) graft fistulas have been associated with hemodialysis. The potential of aspirin or ticlopidine to modify this response was determined.

Methods.—Indium-111–labeled platelets were injected into patients with forearm loop PTFE fistulas, and a baseline scan of the fistula arm was obtained. These scans were repeated after a routine dialysis treatment. Four weeks later, the labeled platelet study was repeated after the patients ingested aspirin, 325 mg/day, or ticlopidine, 250 mg/day, orally for 7 days.

Findings.—In the 6 patients assessed before and after aspirin ingestion, uptakes greater than 1.5-fold compared with the predialysis images occurred in 12 of 40 image regions. These uptakes were 292% of predialysis values before and 193% after aspirin treatment. In the remaining regions, the uptakes were 107% before and 115% after aspirin ingestion. In the 5 patients assessed before and after ticlopidine therapy, uptakes increased by more than 1.5 times that of the predialysis images in 19 of 30 regions, with a median increase of 286% before and 160% after drug treatment. In the remaining regions, uptakes were 116% before and 134% after drug treatment.

Conclusion.—Aspirin and ticlopidine partially inhibit hemodialysis-induced platelet deposition. Newer antiplatelet agents now merit investigation.

► These investigators studied the effect of either aspirin or ticlopidine on platelet aggregation after dialysis in dialysis grafts. The authors' previous observations have shown that platelets do not deposit at the vein graft anastomosis but deposit at other areas along the graft. This study shows that these agents may have some effect on at least the quantitative nature of platelet deposition. Thus, the cause of endothelial fibromuscular hyperplasia at the vein graft anastomosis in PTFE grafts remains unknown. The role of antiplatelet agents also remains unknown, but this and other studies are moving toward determining what role these agents have and the pathophysiologic impact.

S.J. Schwab, M.D.

Long-term Effects of Erythropoietin Therapy on Fistula Stenosis and Plasma Concentrations of PDGF and MCP-1 Hemodialysis Patients

De Marchi S, Cecchin E, Falleti E, et al (Univ of Udine, Italy; Gen Hosp, Cividale del Friuli, Italy)

J Am Soc Nephrol 8:1147–1156, 1997 1–4

Introduction.—Erythropoietin (EPO) therapy appears to be associated with a risk for thrombosis of the vascular access in patients with chronic renal failure. Most vascular access thromboses are the result of stenotic lesions in the venous outflow system, but the effect of EPO therapy on fistula stenosis has not been determined. A cross-sectional, prospective pilot study examined the long-term effects of EPO on progressive fistula stenosis and the plasma concentrations of platelet-derived growth factor (PDGF) and monocyte chemoattractant protein-1 (MCP-1), potential mediators of neointimal hyperplasia.

Methods.—Patients selected for the study had clinically stable end-stage renal disease, were undergoing maintenance dialysis, had a native arteriovenous fistula that had been functioning well for at least 6 months, and had never been treated with EPO. Sixteen patients who received EPO and 14 who received a placebo were monitored for 3 years. Sixty healthy age- and sex-matched individuals served as a control group.

Results.—The EPO and placebo groups were similar in predialysis systolic and diastolic blood pressure values and in blood flow rate at baseline. All patients receiving EPO reached a target hemoglobin level of 10–11 g/dL within 4–12 weeks, and this value was maintained throughout the study. Withdrawal of EPO reduced hemoglobin to pretreatment levels over a 1-month period. Patients on hemodialysis differed from healthy controls in a number of measured variables. Patients on hemodialysis had elevated levels of PDGF, MCP-1, and interleukin-6, proteins that might be involved in the neointima formation regulating proliferation of vascular smooth muscle cells. They also exhibited endothelial and hemostatic abnormalities indicative of a thrombophilic state. A progressive stenosis in the venous circuit of the fistula developed in 6 (37.5%) patients receiving EPO and in 5 (35.7%) taking placebo, which was not a significant difference. The 2 groups also were similar in vascular access, event-free survival over 36 months of follow-up.

Conclusion.—Long-term EPO therapy did not increase the risk of progressive stenosis of native arteriovenous fistula in this series of patients on maintenance dialysis. During EPO therapy, patients exhibited a significant decrease in plasma values of PDGF and vascular cell adhesion molecule-1 and an increase of MCP-1.

► The role of erythropoietin as a potential mitogen stimulating fibromuscular and endothelial hyperplasia leading to vascular access stenosis has been debated for some time. This reflects the first serious clinical trial to come to grips with this issue. In this study, 60 hemodialysis patients were randomized to either receive human synthetic erythropoietin or placebo during a

3-year prospective pilot trial. All patients had native arteriovenous (AV) fistula. These patients were carefully monitored for the development of stenosis with Doppler ultrasonography, as well as with other screening techniques. The authors report that there was no significant difference in the development of stenoses, nor was there a significant difference in the incidence of access thrombosis over the treatment period. Thus, in this small trial, moderate doses of intravenous EPO do not appear to result in additional stenoses in hemodialysis patients. I am impressed by the level of hemoglobin that was achieved in the absence of EPO therapy in the control group. Thus, this study, which has been conducted in primary AV fistulas, now needs to be conducted in a substantial number of patients with AV grafts to clinically confirm the hypothesis. The problem with undertaking such a trial is maintaining a suitable level of hemoglobin in those patients who do not receive erythropoietin. How the authors managed to achieve this is not reported in the article.

S.J. Schwab, M.D.

Reinforced Versus Nonreinforced Polytetrafluoroethylene Grafts for Hemodialysis Access

Schuman ES, Standage BA, Ragsdale JW, et al (Legacy Good Samaritan Hosp, Portland, Ore)

Am J Surg 173:407–410, 1997 1–5

Background.—Over the past 2 decades, the 2 major types of polytetrafluoroethylene (PTFE) graft material have been Gore-Tex, which is reinforced, and Impra, which is nonreinforced. There is research evidence to suggest that Impra gives better performance as a hemodialysis conduit. The authors have used both types of graft material since 1976. This study, using concurrently collected retrospective data, compared the performance of Gore-Tex and Impra PTFE grafts for hemodialysis access.

Methods.—The analysis included 632 patients receiving a new Gore-Tex or Impra graft between 1987 and 1995. Half of the patients had diabetes. The patients were followed up until death, successful renal transplantation, transfer to another mode of dialysis, return of renal function, transfer to another dialysis unit, or graft failure. All data were entered into a database for analysis by a biostatistician. The performance of the 2 graft types was compared.

Results.—Every category and subgroup showed better performance with Impra (nonreinforced PTFE) than with Gore-Tex (reinforced PTFE) grafts (Table 2). Impra had a significant advantage in terms of mean duration and on life-table analysis. There was no significant difference in secondary patency: at 1 year, 80% of Impra and 77% of Gore-Tex grafts were functioning. In the overall experience, median duration for secondary patency was 1,554 days.

Conclusions.—Used as a hemodialysis conduit, Impra (nonreinforced) PTFE offers better performance than Gore-Tex (reinforced) PTFE. Pending

TABLE 2.—Reinforced Versus Nonreinforced PTFE Grafts

		Comparison of Surgeons		
Surgeons	% Gore-Tex	% Diabetic Patients	Primary Patency	Secondary Patency
Surgeon 1	68	55	190	534
Surgeon 2	55	52	248	495
Surgeon 3	77	47	211	421
Surgeon 4	88	55	141	270

(Reprinted with permission from Excerpta Medica Inc. from Shuman ES, Standage BA, Ragsdale JW, et al: Reinforced versus nonreinforced polytetrafluoroethylene grafts for hemodialysis access. *American Journal of Surgery* 173:407–410, 1997.)

the results of a multicenter, prospective, randomized trial, nonreinforced PTFE should be considered the graft material of choice for hemodialysis access.

▶ This retrospective study examines data for reinforced and nonreinforced PTFE grafts. The authors then argue that their retrospective observation supports the use of nonreinforced PTFE hemodialysis grafts. The authors may be correct, but there were enough selection biases in this study to expect that a randomized prospective trial be done to resolve the issue. What I found striking, however, is the effect of surgeon on primary patency [Table 2]. Although the authors argue this did not reach statistical significance and does not account for other factors such as graft location, the differences in primary patency range from a high of 248 to a low of 141 days. Although many things such as patient selection and graft location could explain these differences, this looks like even more fertile ground for a prospective trial.

S.J. Schwab, M.D.

Hemodialysis Access Graft Stenosis: Percutaneous Transluminal Angioplasty

Lumsden AB, MacDonald MJ, Kikeri DK, et al (Veteran Affairs Med Ctr, Decatur, Ga; Emory Univ, Atlanta, Ga)

J Surg Res 68:181–185, 1997 1–6

Objective.—The subcutaneous arteriovenous fistula remains the pathway of choice for dialysis access, although thrombosis and stenosis remain a problem. The utility of percutaneous transluminal angioplasty (PTA) for treating vascular access graft stenosis is retrospectively reviewed.

Methods.—Between 1987 and 1993, 47 PTA procedures were performed on 40 patients (17 females), average age 48 years, receiving hemodialysis using arteriovenous grafts. Graft types were 35 expanded polytetrafluoroethylene, 3 bovine, and 2 unknown. Percent stenosis was determined by fistulography. Patency was measured from angioplasty to failure and was determined using the Kaplan-Meier life table method.

Results.—There were 37 venous anastomotic stenoses, 6 arterial anastomotic stenoses, 2 synchronous arterial and venous stenoses, 1 synchronous midgraft arterial and venous anastomotic stenosis, and 1 midgraft alone. The initial success rate was 94%, but complete stenosis was eliminated in only 40% of procedures. Sixty percent of lesions experienced narrowing of as much as 30%. Complications included 2 extravasations and bleeding from the puncture site requiring platelet transfusion in 1 patient. Patency rates were 76% at 1 month, 27% at 6 months, and 10% at 1 year. Average duration of patency was 4.1 months, although arterial anastomotic stenoses had a significantly shorter interval to occlusion. The PTA reduced pressure gradients to 12 mm Hg from 42 mm Hg. Reduction in venous pressure after PTA or improved recirculation was unrelated to duration of patency.

Conclusion.—Percutaneous transluminal angioplasty of stenosed dialysis grafts did not improve medium- or long-term patency. New strategies and technologies need to be tested to provide improved patency for these grafts.

▶ The concept of prospective treatment of outflow stenosis in polytetrafluoroethylene grafts is well established. These authors, in a retrospective evaluation, seek to come to grips with what is the ideal method to treat these lesions once they are detected. These authors show a relatively poor outcome from angioplasty of these lesions. Thus, the role of surgical revascularization vs. transluminal angioplasty needs prospective studies to determine which therapy is preferable. The Dialysis Outcomes Quality Initiative, carefully reviewing the available literature, was unable to come to a conclusion as to whether one therapy was preferred over another. The bias of the study group was that as the stenosis became tighter, angioplasty patency fell dramatically. As the authors so clearly state, prospective studies, looking at therapeutic techniques for venous outflow stenoses, are required to determine what the ideal therapy will become.

S.J. Schwab, M.D.

Prospective Randomized Comparison of Surgical Versus Endovascular Management of Thrombosed Dialysis Access Grafts

Marston WA, Criado E, Jacques PF, et al (Univ of North Carolina, Chapel Hill)

J Vasc Surg 26:373–381, 1997 1–7

Introduction.—The increasing number of patients receiving long-term dialysis has made preservation of thrombosed hemodialysis shunts a more frequently encountered problem. Salvage of the thrombosed shunt can be accomplished by surgical or endovascular means. The efficacy of these 2 methods was compared in a prospective, randomized trial.

Methods.—The 91 patients included in the trial had 115 episodes of polytetrafluoroethylene (PTFE) shunt thrombosis. All shunts were evaluated within 1 week of thrombosis and treated within 48 hours of diagno-

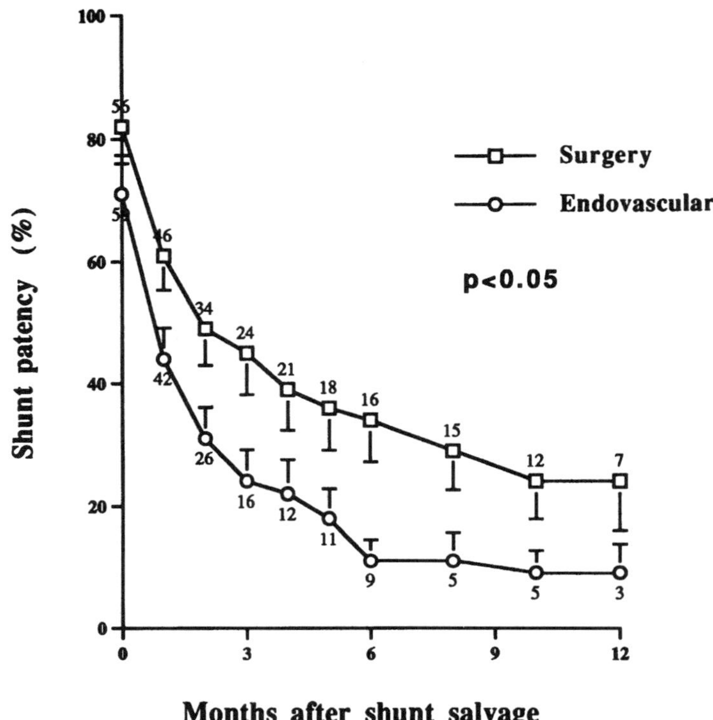

FIGURE 1.—Primary graft patency rate after salvage of thrombosed shunts treated with surgical compared with endovascular techniques. Patency rates are significantly different by log-rank test (*P* less than 0.05). (Courtesy of Marston WA, Criado E, Jacques PF, et al: Prospective randomized comparison of surgical versus endovascular management of thrombosed dialysis access grafts. *J Vasc Surg* 26:373–381, 1997.)

sis. Endovascular salvage was performed in 59 episodes of shunt thrombosis and surgical salvage in 56. The 2 randomized groups were similar in age, sex, and clinical characteristics. Graft function in the endovascular group was restored with mechanical (82%) or thrombolytic (18%) graft thrombectomy followed by percutaneous angioplasty. Surgical salvage was attempted with thrombectomy plus graft revision in 78% of shunts and with thrombectomy alone in 22%. Patients were followed for at least 6 months to compare shunt patency and length of graft function achieved with the 2 methods.

Results.—The initial success rate in restoring graft function was 82% in grafts treated surgically and 71% in those treated with endovascular techniques. In the months after salvage, surgery achieved a significantly better primary graft patency than endovascular therapy (Fig 1). At 12 months, graft patency had been extended in 24% of shunts with surgery, but in only 9% of shunts with endovascular treatment. Patients with venous anastomotic stenosis—the most common cause of shunt thrombosis in both groups (55% overall)—had a significantly better patency rate than those with other causes of graft thrombosis. The patency rate was significantly worse in patients with long-segment venous outflow stenosis or occlusion.

Conclusion.—The primary patency rate after graft salvage was found to be significantly better in the surgical group than in the endovascular group. Patency was greatly reduced in both groups, however, at 6 and 12 months after the salvage procedures.

► The best method for correcting a high-grade stenosis in a dialysis arteriovenous graft after an episode of thrombosis is undetermined. The National Kidney Foundation's practice guidelines on vascular access (the Dialysis Outcome Quality Initiative) were unable to recommend percutaneous angioplasty or surgical revision because the data did not support 1 therapy over another.

This study represents the first prospective attempt to determine whether 1 therapy for this class of lesions is superior to another. The authors found increased patency from surgical correction, compared with percutaneous angioplasty. Both immediate and long-term patency were better with surgical intervention. This observation is beginning to play to the bias of most observers.

Thus, the emerging trend is that prospectively detected lesions using access flows or pressures tend to involve 50% to 60% of the lumen and respond reasonably well to angioplasty with acceptable intermediate term patency. In contrast, grafts that progress to thrombosis tend to have a high-grade 90% or greater outflow stenosis. Percutaneous interventions in this group of patients do not seem to be as successful as surgical revision. This prospective, randomized trial, although small, is the first step in that direction. If additional confirmatory studies become available, there may be sufficient evidence to argue that high-grade stenoses should be treated by surgical revision, whereas those of less severe grade may be amenable to angioplasty.

One criticism of this study is that the overall outcomes, whether by surgical revision or angioplasty, were not that favorable. Thus, it has become increasingly clear that prospective detection and treatment of outflow stenoses is dramatically superior to correction of high-grade lesions after thrombosis.

S.J. Schwab, M.D.

Hemodialysis Access Catheters

Introduction

Hemodialysis vascular access catheters are emerging as a common form of hemodialysis vascular access. In 1987, there was only 1 company engaged in the manufacture of these tunneled catheters, now there are multiple companies manufacturing these devices. Problems associated with these devices are now being carefully studied. Although this is an ideal method of bridge access, most studies find that their role as a kind of permanent vascular access is, as agreed by the Dialysis Outcome Quality Initiative guidelines, considerably inferior to arteriovenous fistulas and grafts. The first manuscript (Abstract 1–8) is a retrospective review of cuffed catheters for hemodialysis. The authors identify that, in carefully selected patients, guidewire exchange of malfunctioning catheters significantly improves technique success. Thus, thrombolytic infusion, catheter guidewire exchange, and catheter fibrin sheath stripping have emerged as ideal means to extend catheter patency when thrombotic dysfunction of these catheters occurs. Infection is now emerging as the overwhelming barrier to the long-term use of these catheters. Abstract 1–9 evaluates the role of catheter-rated bacteremia in a large hemodialysis population. Marr and associates identified a mean of 3.9 episodes of catheter bacteremia per 1,000 catheter days. They found that treating catheter bacteremia without removal or guidewire exchange of the catheter leads to success in only a minority of cases. Interestingly, however, the attempted salvage did not lead to worse clinical outcomes or more metastatic infections than removal of the catheter. In Abstract 1–10, Trerotola, a leader in catheter technology, shows that vascular radiology–inserted catheters perform very well. Abstract 1–11 shows that US-guided cannulation of the femoral vein for acute hemodialysis significantly minimizes access complications. Thus, the addition of technology further improves patient care. Abstract 1–12 looks at the role of elimination of nasal carriage of *Staphylococcus aureus* in preventing bacteremia in hemodialysis patients.

Steve J. Schwab, M.D.

Long-term Vascular Access for Hemodialysis Using Silicon Dual-lumen Catheters With Guidewire Replacement of Catheters for Technique Salvage

McLaughlin K, Jones B, Mactier R, et al (Stobhill Hosp, Glasgow, Scotland)
Am J Kidney Dis 29:553–559, 1997 1–8

Introduction.—Long-term hemodialysis or poor peripheral vasculature at the start of hemodialysis can make it difficult to create long-term "primary" vascular access. Attempts to overcome this problem with "secondary access" surgical procedures have employed polytetrafluoroethylene (PTFE) grafts. Many centers, however, have found silicone-based catheters with a Dacron cuff to be a useful alternative to PTFE grafts. The 3-year experience of 1 center with these catheters was evaluated.

Methods.—Between November 1992 and November 1995, 32 hemodialysis patients with established end-stage renal failure received 54 silicone dual-lumen hemodialysis catheters. One patient chose a catheter to avoid repeated fistula cannulation; in all other cases there was difficulty in identifying a suitable artery or vein to allow creation of a traditional arteriovenous fistula or a secondary access procedure using a PTFE graft. Twenty catheters were placed into subclavian veins by primary insertion and 34 were replaced over a guidewire. Case records of the patients were reviewed for details of catheter insertion, complications, and catheter-technique survival times.

Results.—Catheter survival was 72.7% at 90 days and 48.7% at 1 year. Technique survival was longer: 93.3% for 90 days and 81.8% at 1 year. Mean survival of failed catheters and techniques was 159 days and 217 days, respectively. Overall mean catheter survival time was 387 days and technique survival time was 844 days. Patient mortality for the 3-year study period was 37.5%; no deaths were attributed to the 18 episodes of catheter-related sepsis. Most catheter failures (70.4%) resulted from poor flow. Factors associated with reduced catheter survival were left-sided placement and catheter tip placement in the superior vena cava. Catheters replaced over a guidewire were no more likely to have poor survival or sepsis than those placed by primary insertion.

Conclusion.—In patients undergoing hemodialysis with exhausted vascular access or in whom there is obvious difficulty identifying a suitable peripheral blood vessel, silicone dual-lumen catheters offer a means of long-term vascular access. Guidewire replacement of catheters for technique salvage is feasible, and best results are obtained by right-sided catheter insertion or catheter tip placement in the right atrium.

▶ This retrospective review of silicone dual-lumen catheters for hemodialysis from the United Kingdom has several new observations. The most important observation is that the routine use of guidewire exchange dramatically extends technique survival for catheter use in patients receiving maintenance hemodialysis. The authors' 1-year survival for catheter technique in this patient population of almost 80% is similar to that for well-maintained arteriovenous grafts. Thus, guidewire exchange of hemodialysis catheters dramatically extends technique life. What is very interesting in this observation is that very few catheters were lost secondary to infection. Although stressed in this manuscript, the rate of bacteremia-mediated catheter removal is much smaller than that reported from other centers. Blood flow through these catheters and adequacy of dialysis were not reported, and the reader is cautioned that characteristic catheter flow rates are less than that possible with arteriovenous access. The authors stress that this technique is best used in patients in whom there are no additional access options.

S.J. Schwab, M.D.

Catheter-related Bacteremia and Outcome of Attempted Catheter Salvage in Patients Undergoing Hemodialysis

Marr KA, Sexton DJ, Conlon PJ, et al (Duke Univ, Durham, NC)

Ann Intern Med 127:275–280, 1997 1–9

Introduction.—Dual-lumen cuffed catheters are now used for vascular access in 15% of patients undergoing hemodialysis in the United States. The incidence of bacteremia is said to be lower with cuffed, tunneled catheters than with noncuffed temporary catheters, but the true incidence of bacteremia associated with dual-lumen, tunneled, cuffed catheters is unknown. This question and the appropriate management of catheter-

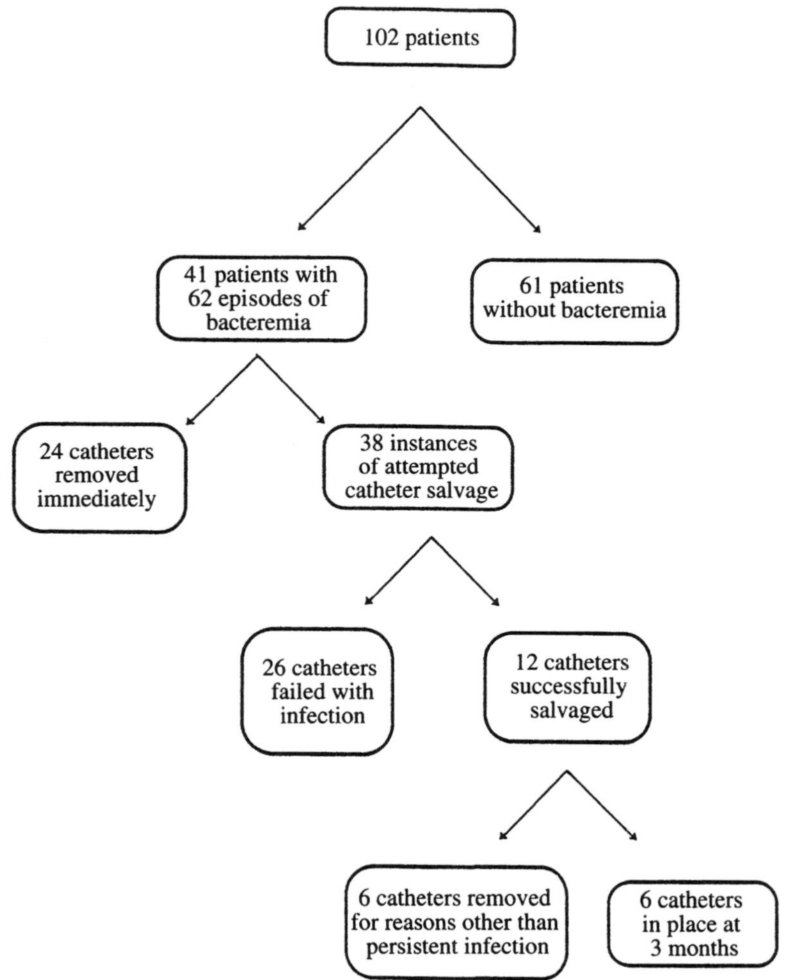

FIGURE.—Diagram of salvage success among patients who underwent dialysis with dual-lumen, tunneled, cuffed catheters between April 1995 and January 1996. (Courtesy of Marr KA, Sexton DJ, Conlon PJ, et al: Catheter-related bacteremia and outcome of attempted catheter salvage in patients undergoing hemodialysis. *Ann Intern Med* 127:275–280, 1997.)

related bacteremia were examined in a prospective study of 102 patients with end-stage renal disease.

Methods.—Enrolled patients were undergoing hemodialysis at 4 centers, with tunneled, cuffed catheters for vascular access. Charts were reviewed for demographic and clinical data. Patients suspected of having catheter-related bacteremia were followed for at least 3 months after the initial episode for clinical response to treatment, complications, and success or failure of catheter salvage with antibiotic therapy.

Results.—The 102 patients had a total of 16,081 catheter days. Sixty-two episodes of bacteremia developed in 41 (40%) patients (mean 3.9

episodes per 1,000 catheter-days). The most common cause of bacteremia was a gram-positive coccus (63%) and the most frequently isolated organism was *Staphylococcus aureus*. Twenty-four catheters were removed immediately and 38 were left in place during antibiotic treatment. Salvage was successful with only 12 of the 38 catheters; 6 were in place at 3 months (Figure). Complications developed in 9 patients with bacteremia (22%). Six patients had osteomyelitis, 4 had infective endocarditis, and 1 had septic arthritis; 2 patients died. Although all complications occurred after an episode of gram-positive bacteremia, none was associated with attempted catheter salvage. Factors such as diabetes mellitus, hypertension, injection drug use, or immunocompromised status did not predispose patients to complications.

Conclusion.—During a 9-month period, 41% of patients undergoing hemodialysis with dual-lumen, tunnelled, cuffed catheters had at least 1 episode of bacteremia. Salvage attempts usually failed but did not appear to increase the incidence of complications; thus, a trial of antibiotics may be warranted in some cases.

► This large, prospective study is the first to document the actual incidence of bacteremia with cuffed catheters in a hemodialysis population. The study documented 3.9 episodes of bacteremia per 1,000 catheter days. Thus, hemodialysis bacteremia is the leading cause of hemodialysis catheter loss and the leading cause of bacteremia in the hemodialysis population. Use of systemic antibiotics to attempt catheter salvage and, thereby, maintain catheter technique was evaluated in detail. The conclusion that only 32% of catheters can be successfully salvaged with long-term antibiotic therapy argues that this technique should be avoided.

The role of catheter exchange, as outlined in some pilot studies, remains to be determined, but attempting to salvage the catheter without catheter exchange clearly is likely to fail. New techniques to minimize this complication need to be developed. The possibility of an implantable port or other technological advances is sorely needed in the field of tunneled hemodialysis catheters.

S.J. Schwab, M.D.

Outcome of Tunneled Hemodialysis Catheters Placed Via the Right Internal Jugular Vein by Interventional Radiologists

Trerotola SO, Johnson MS, Harris VJ, et al (Indiana Univ, Indianapolis)
Radiology 203:489–495, 1997 1–10

Background.—Patients receiving hemodialysis often need tunneled hemodialysis catheters for temporary or permanent access. The outcomes of placing such catheters through the right internal jugular vein by interventional radiologists were reported.

Methods.—Catheters were placed through the right internal jugular vein in 194 patients with no evidence of thrombosis. The radiologists used real-time ultrasound-guided puncture and fluoroscopic guidance to place a total of 250 catheters. The patients were followed until their catheters were removed or until they died.

Findings.—All catheters were placed successfully and functioned immediately after placement. Clinically unimportant air embolus occurred in 2 patients. There were no instances of pneumothorax, hemothorax, or substantial hemorrhage. The median duration of catheterization was 56 days, with no cases of catheter-related symptomatic venous thrombosis or stenosis. The infection rate was 0.08 per 100 catheter days. The rate of malfunctions necessitating removal was 0.22 per 100 catheter days. The rate of definite or possible catheter thrombosis necessitating removal was 0.16 per 100 catheter days.

Conclusion.—The long-term results of interventional radiologic placement of tunneled hemodialysis catheters were at least as good as those of surgical placement. Thus, the radiologic method is preferred.

▶ This large, prospective series shows that interventional radiology placement of dual-lumen cuffed catheters meets or exceeds the standards established by operating room–inserted catheters. It pioneers the use of ultrasound to minimize catheter insertion complications and advocates fluoroscopic placement of the catheter tip to ensure optimal blood flow. The authors not only identify acceptable primary and secondary patencies but report their experience with guidewire exchange of catheters for problems as diffuse as malpositioning and fibrin sheath formation.

S.J. Schwab, M.D.

Ultrasound-guided Cannulation of the Femoral Vein for Acute Haemodialysis Access

Kwon TH, Kim YL, Cho DK (Kyungpook Univ Hosp, Taegu, Korea)

Nephrol Dial Transplant 12:1009–1012, 1997 1–11

Objective.—Femoral vein cannulation is sometimes necessary for hemodialysis. There may be technical difficulties when inserting the catheter using a blind, landmark-guided approach, particularly in patients with coagulopathies, edema, or thrombosed veins or in patients who are obese. Ultrasound-guided cannulation of femoral vein for acute hemodialysis access was studied prospectively.

Methods.—Ultrasound-guided or landmark-guided femoral vein cannulation was performed alternately on a weekly basis for 8 weeks by experienced operators in 28 patients (13 women) and 38 patients (11 women), respectively. The US technique used a 2-dimensional display image; it allowed compressibility of the vein and an increase in vein size with the Valsalva maneuver. Number of complications, femoral nerve irritation, and needle sticks were compared statistically. Patients not cannulated during 2 needle passes were crossed-over to the other method.

Results.—Cannulation was accomplished in 100% of patients with US and in 89.5% of patients with the landmark technique. The US technique was successful the first time in 92.9% of patients, whereas the landmark technique was successful the first time in 55.3% of patients. Because they could not be cannulated in 2 needle passes, 4 patients from the landmark group were crossed-over to the US group. Puncture of the femoral artery occurred in 7.1% of patients undergoing the US procedure with 0% hematoma (odds ratio, 0.44) and in 15.8% of patients undergoing the landmark precedure with 2.6% hematoma (odds ratio, 0.66). Ultrasound procedure time was 45.1 seconds. Landmark procedure time was 79.4%.

Conclusion.—Ultrasound-guided cannulation of the femoral vein for hemodialysis access was faster, required fewer passes, and had fewer complications than landmark cannulation.

▶ These authors evaluate the role of US directed cannulation of the femoral vein for hemodialysis. The authors report that both complications and success rate improved with the use of this machine. We also use the relatively inexpensive US machine used in this study at our center (SITERITE TM, Pittsburgh, Pa) for femoral vein cannulation, but use it primarily to identify the presence of a patent femoral vein before landmark-guided cannulation. Thus, as technology improves, US-directed venous cannulation will probably become the preferred technique. For femoral cannulation, it may well be that real-time cannulation is not necessary if you can verify that the vein is present in the appropriate location to facilitate landmark insertion.

S.J. Schwab, M.D.

Elimination of Nasal Carriage of *Staphylococcus aureus* in Hemodialysis Patients

Kluytmans JAJW, Manders M-J, van Bommel E, et al (Univ Hosp Rotterdam, The Netherlands)

Infect Control Hosp Epidemiol 17:793–797, 1996 1–12

Introduction.—Infection is the second most common cause of death in patients receiving hemodialysis, and *Staphylococcus aureus* is the most frequently isolated pathogen. Because nasal carriage of *S. aureus* increases the risk of infection in patients receiving hemodialysis, the elimination of nasal carriage could decrease morbidity and mortality related to this pathogen. The efficacy of mupirocin in eliminating nasal carriage of *S. aureus* was examined in a prospective study.

Methods.—Study participants were the 226 patients receiving hemodialysis from February 1, 1992, until November 1, 1993. All were screened monthly for nasal carriage of *S. aureus*, and those with positive cultures were treated with mupirocin calcium ointment twice daily for 5 days. Patients whose nasal cultures became positive again were considered to have failed treatment. An historic control group included all patients treated at the hemodialysis unit in 1990 and 1991, a period during which no efforts were made to eliminate nasal carriage. The incidence of *S. aureus* bacteremia was recorded for control and study groups.

Results.—Complete data were available for 172 patients evaluated for nasal carriage and mupirocin efficacy. Sixty-seven were identified as nasal carriers, and 98.5% of these tested negative after 5 days of mupirocin treatment. Cultures remained negative in 94% at 3 months and 91% at 6 months. There were 29 episodes of *S. aureus* bacteremia: 25 in the 273 controls and 4 in the 226 patients in the study group. The rate of bacteremia (number of episodes of *S. aureus* bacteremia per patient-year on hemodialysis) was significantly lower in the study group (0.04) than in the control group (0.25).

Conclusion.—Previous studies have shown that effective elimination of nasal carriage in patients receiving hemodialysis lowers the infection rate with *S. aureus*. Mupirocin nasal ointment was highly effective in this series of patients, significantly reducing the incidence of *S. aureus* bacteremia.

▶ This paper examines the role of *S. aureus* nasal carriage and its prevention with the use of mupirocin in the reduction of *S. aureus* bacteremia. The authors found a significant reduction during the study. Although results appear attractive, resistance over long-term use is probable and has yet to be studied.

S.J. Schwab, M.D.

Indwelling Silicone Femoral Catheters: Experience of Three Haemodialysis Centres

Montagnac R, Bernard Cl, Guillaumie J, et al (Gen Hosp of Troyes, France; Gen Hosp of Montibeliard, France; Gen Hosp of Dole, France)

Nephrol Dial Transplant 12:772–775, 1997 1–13

Objective.—Whereas the rigidity and frequency of reinsertion of femoral vein catheters and the higher rate of local and infectious complications makes them unacceptable for hemodialysis, modern silastic catheters are more flexible and biocompatible. A retrospective analysis of silastic femoral catheters in 3 dialysis centers over 7 months was done.

Methods.—A total of 64 SSL 1220M model (Medcomp, USA) 12F single-lumen silastic catheters were percutaneously inserted into 55 patients (16 females), aged 25–86 years, who were receiving heparin for anticoagulation. The duration of cannulation, the number of catheters used, and the length of dialysis sessions were recorded. The mean blood flow rate was calculated as (arterial blood flow + venus blood flow)/4. Catheter, catheter tip, and exit site samples were cultured on removal. Doppler examination of the iliofemoral veins was performed 1 month after catheter removal.

Results.—The average duration of cannulation was 41.5 days. All but 12 catheters remained in place until renal failure resolved or permanent vascular access was created. On average, each catheter was used for 14.5

sessions that lasted an average of 4 hours. Patient tolerance was good. Two patients had bleeding and 2 patients had lymph leakage. There were no immediate significant complications, but there were significant long-term complications. Blood flow was minimal in 2 patients and inadequate in 2 others. One catheter was replaced on the other side because of continual local bleeding. Three catheters were replaced, 1 because of fissure and 1 because of dislodgment. Clots formed in 29 patients, and were aspirated in 26. The remaining 3 patients received urokinase. Of the 7 catheter thromboses, 3 were treated with urokinase and 4 necessitated catheter removal, 2 of which were replaced. A fibrin sheet developed over 1 catheter tip, necessitating catheter replacement. One patient experienced bilateral phlebitis. Doppler examination in 35 patients showed normal flow in 33 patients and seriously reduced flow in 2. Infection occurred in 14 patients.

Conclusion.—Indwelling silastic femoral catheters inserted in 55 patients undergoing partial or full ambulatory dialysis resulted in low complication rates.

▶ This retrospective observational French study evaluates placing a non-tunnelled, silastic, femorally inserted dialysis catheter for prolonged hospital dialysis. The authors conclude that these femorally inserted catheters were suitable for reasonable periods of use without a high infection risk. Thus, these authors suggest that acute vascular access for hospitalized patients may be obtainable with nontunnelled silastic femoral dialysis catheters that would allow patients some degree of upright posture, rather than being forced to remain bedbound when a femoral catheter is in place. It is an interesting observation that needs a larger prospective trial. Our center's experience with non-cuffed femoral catheters is much less optimistic.

S.J. Schwab, M.D.

Techniques of Dialysis

INTRODUCTION

There are 4 selections in the techniques of dialysis for this year. The first 3 deal with the measurement and understanding of dialysis delivery. In the initial observation, Coyne and associates (Abstract 1–14) compare hemodialysis prescription to delivered dose.They find that impaired dialysis delivery is most commonly either caused by inadequate measurement technique for Kt/V or abnormalities with hemodialysis vascular access. The next 2 papers deal with dialysis measurement technique. Charytan and colleagues (Abstract 1–15) challenge the technique of classic Kt/V urea measurements and argue that techniques for online monitoring will emerge as the preferred method. In the next abstract (1–16), Canaud et al. acknowledge the value of online urea monitoring but argue that simpler techniques may be equally effective without the cost or technology. They argue that the confounding effect of urea rebound in measuring dialysis dose can be avoided by merely measuring a urea value 30 minutes before the termination of dialysis.

In the final paper in this section (Abstract 1–17), the effect of sodium ramping in the dialysate to avoid hemodialysis complications is evaluated by Sang and colleagues. They establish that while higher sodium concentrations minimize symptoms, the sudden decrement in sodium associated with ramping does not avoid the side-effects that are associated with these higher sodium concentrations.

Steve J. Schwab, M.D.

Impaired Delivery of Hemodialysis Prescriptions: An Analysis of Causes and an Approach to Evaluation

Coyne DW, Delmez J, Spence G, et al (Washington Univ, St Louis)
J Am Soc Nephrol 8:1315–1318, 1997 1–14

Introduction.—A number of problems have been identified as contributing to a decline in Kt/V in previously stable hemodialysis patients. Potential causes of a fall in urea kinetic modeling results include noncompliance with the prescribed regimen, vascular access recirculation, dialyzer dysfunction, and laboratory error. A prospective study was designed to identify the relative frequencies of these problems in patients undergoing chronic hemodialysis.

Methods.—The 146 patients included in the study had a mean age of 57.5 years and had been on dialysis for a mean of 4 years. Of these, 66% were women, and 85% were African-American. Urea kinetic modeling was analyzed monthly during the 3-month study period. Baseline Kt/V was defined as the average of each patient's Kt/V values obtained during the previous 4 months. Patients were considered to have a clinically important fall in Kt/V if the decline was at least 0.2 after a baseline Kt/V of at least 1.2, or the decline was at least 0.1 after a baseline Kt/V of less than 1.2.

Results.—Of the 375 modeling sessions done during the study period, 93 met criteria for a significant decline in urea kinetic modeling. In this group, mean baseline Kt/V was 1.33, and the mean abnormal month Kt/V was 1.02. Identified causes for a decline in Kt/V were reduced blood processing (42%), recirculation (25%), and dialyzer dysfunction (1%). No cause was identified in 32% of patients. Reduced blood processing was the result of a lower blood flow or shorter time than prescribed. Most cases of recirculation were attributed to access dysfunction or reversed needles. Subsequent monthly kinetic modeling results returned to baseline in the one third of patients with no cause identified.

Discussion.—At any given kinetic modeling session, approximately 25% of patients undergoing routine hemodialysis will have a decline in urea kinetic modeling results. Even after eliminating patient-requested shortened treatments, 20% of all Kt/V values declined significantly over a 3-month period. A systematic approach to declines of Kt/V found at

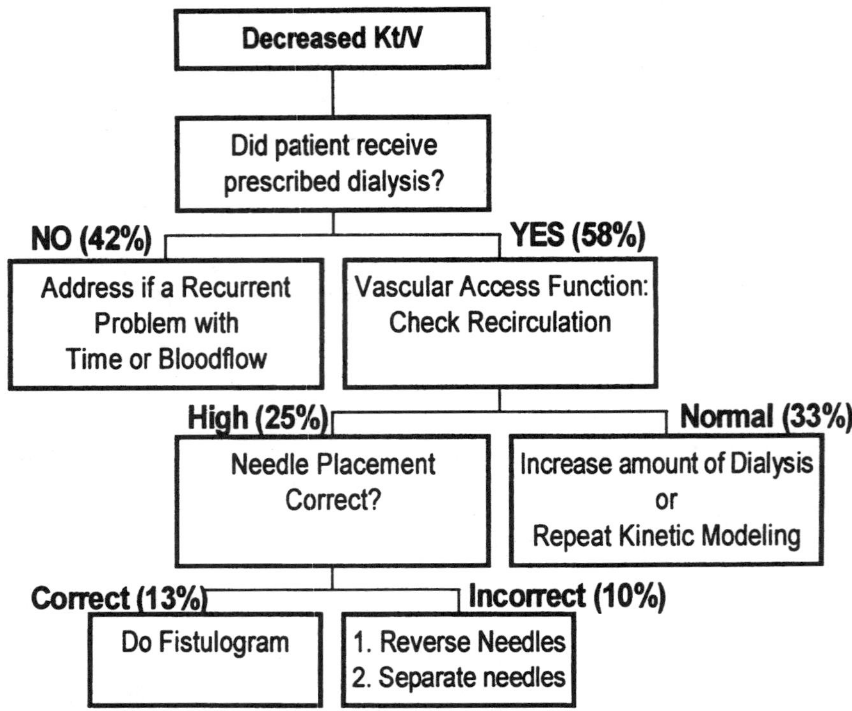

FIGURE 4.—Approach to a low Kt/V and the frequency of problems observed in this study. This figure displays a recommended approach to a decline in Kt/V and our observed frequency of those problems in this study. Two patients with high recirculation were not available for further study. Five patients with high recirculation, which was normal on repeat, were classified as *incorrect needle placement.* (Courtesy of Coyne DW, Delmez J, Spence G, et al: Impaired delivery of hemodialysis prescriptions: An analysis of causes and an approach to evaluation. *J Am Soc Nephrol* 8[8]:1315–1318, 1997.)

routine kinetic modeling is presented in Figure 4. Persistent abnormalities indicate the need for a dialysis prescription change.

▶ This study evaluated the reason for impaired hemodialysis prescription. The authors identified that failure to sit for the appropriate length of dialysis or to achieve the appropriate prescribed blood flow was the reason for 42% of the decrements in delivered dose of dialysis (Fig 4). The remainder were associated with either reversed needles or abnormal access flow. A subset of patients merely had inappropriately drawn samples that were then normal on repeat. The most important issue shown here is that an inappropriately diminished Kt/V on monthly screening requires aggressive prospective intervention. In most instances, a clear-cut cause can be found.

S.J. Schwab, M.D.

Fractional Direct Dialysis Quantification: A New Approach for Prescription and Monitoring Hemodialysis Therapy

Charytan C, Gupta B, Meindel N, et al (New York Hosp Med Ctr of Queens, Flushing, NY)

Kidney Int 50:1845–1849, 1996 1–15

Introduction.—Currently available methods for the quantitative measurement of dialysis adequacy—urea kinetic modeling (UKM) using the Kt/V parameter and direct total dialysate quantification (DDQ)—both have significant flaws. A new approach for the quantitative assessment of hemodialysis, fractional direct dialysis quantification (FDDQ), was described.

Methods.—Study participants were 10 patients who were receiving hemodialysis 3 times a week with a variety of dialyzers, treatment times, and blood flow rates. The dialysate flow rate was maintained at a constant 800 cc/min. Both FDDQ and DDQ were simultaneously performed on 35 treatments. The equipment used for FDDQ is the Fresinius Dialysate Sampling Module, a device electrically and electronically connected to the dialysis machine via a ribbon connector.

Results.—The mean volumes of dialysis effluent collected by DDQ (156.6 L) and calculated by FDDQ (149.56 L) were statistically similar. Total dialysis effluent volume was somewhat greater and solute concentrations minimally lower in DDQ, as compared with FDDQ, but this insignificant difference would not affect the total solute content. Both urea nitrogen and creatinine concentrations were statistically similar in the total DDQ collection (mean, 10.09 mg/dL and 1.17 mg/dL, respectively) and in the FDDQ sample (mean, 10.31 mg/dL and 1.19 mg/dL, respectively). The DDQ measurement and FDDQ calculation of total urea nitrogen and total creatinine removed were statistically equivalent (16.03 g and 15.93 g, respectively, for total urea nitrogen; 1.86 g and 1.85 g, respectively, for total creatinine).

Discussion.—Solute intake and dialytic solute elimination must be measured reliably in patients receiving hemodialysis. The most accurate measure of protein intake and urea nitrogen removal, 2 critical parameters of therapy, is the DDQ. Whereas the DDQ procedure is too cumbersome for routine clinical use and UKM utilizing the Kt/V parameter is dependent on a questionable hypothesis, FDDQ offers the advantages of simplicity and accuracy. In addition, FDDQ permits the use of solutes other than urea and is likely to be inexpensive enough to be performed with each hemodialysis session.

▶ Monitoring of dialysis dose or dose of renal replacement therapy has traditionally been done by measuring substances before and after hemodialysis and extrapolating an appropriate clearance. Traditionally, urea has served as the marker molecule for clearance of all other molecular-weight substances. In an effort to improve measurement of dialysis dose, a series of devices are becoming available to measure urea and other solute generation in the dialysate. Thus, accurate measurement of total removal per unit time and over a given treatment is becoming available.

This paper investigates 1 of these techniques for monitoring online dialysate side urea clearance. It is reasonable to assume that dialysate side measurement will become the standard for measurement of dialysis dose in the future. Ideally, this technique could be performed at each dialysis so that a true measure of monthly dialysis could be calculated. In this manner, the effect of shortened and missed treatments could be evaluated. Using traditional Kt/V measurement, what is actually measured is ideal dialysis capacity, not dialysis dose.

S.J. Schwab, M.D.

A Simple and Accurate Method to Determine Equilibrated Post-dialysis Urea Concentration

Canaud B, Bosc J-Y, Leblanc M, et al (Lapeyronie Univ, Montpellier, France; Lakehead Univ, Thunder Bay, Ont)
Kidney Int 51:2000–2005, 1997 1–16

Introduction.—A 2-point method using predialysis and postdialysis blood urea concentrations is usually used to determine fractional urea clearance, or Kt/V. Immediate postdialysis urea sampling, however, tends to overestimate hemodialysis efficiency. In a previous study, the authors noted that rebound amplitude increased with session efficiency; urea concentration reached a plateau 30 minutes postsession; and intradialytic urea concentration 30 minutes before the end of the session was equivalent to the postdialysis equilibrated value. The latter observation was examined in a study of 10 patients with stable end-stage renal disease.

Methods.—The patient group included 7 men and 3 women with a mean age of 52.7 years. All had arteriovenous fistulas able to deliver blood flows of up to 400 mL/min. Hemodiafiltration was performed 3 times per week over a fixed duration of 180 minutes, followed by 60 minutes of isolated ultrafiltration at a low rate (30 mL/min). At least 3 efficiency regimens were applied for each patient: session 1, low range Kt/V; session 2: medium range Kt/V; session 3, high range Kt/V. Intradialytic and postdialytic urea concentration were monitored continuously with the urea monitoring system placed on the ultrafiltrate outflow of the hemodiafiltration circuit.

Results.—Thirty-eight hemodiafiltration sessions were performed at the various Kt/V levels, and postdialysis urea rebound occurred after all sessions. The amplitude of rebound increased with the efficiency of the session. There was no significant difference in urea concentration at 30 and 60 minutes postdialysis, indicating that rebound was complete at 30 minutes over the entire spectrum of intensity regimens evaluated. There was a highly significant linear correlation between urea concentration 30 minutes before the end of hemodiafiltration and equilibrated urea concentration 30 minutes posthemodiafiltration.

Discussion.—As demonstrated by on-line urea monitoring, equilibrated postdialysis urea concentration accounting for rebound may be accurately predicted by the urea concentration obtained 30 minutes before the end of the session. Only 2 intradialytic blood samples are required with this method, and there is no need to wait an extra 30 minutes after treatment.

► This interesting report seeks a better method for determining dialysis dose. It has been shown previously that urea rebound occurs after all hemodialysis sessions and is most severe in sessions that are shortest and most efficient. By the use of continuous urea monitoring, the authors show that in most sessions, urea rebound is complete 30 minutes after hemodialysis. The authors also show that in aggressively hemodialyzed patients, the rebound can be as great as 25% or as low as 13%. Thus, in high-efficiency, or high-flux, dialysis, measuring the urea sample after dialysis may lead to significant errors of overestimation of dialysis dose. Using continuous urea monitoring, the authors show a strong correlation coefficient with a urea sample obtained 30 minutes before the end of the dialysis session. The authors show that the correlation coefficient between this and a urea sample drawn 30 minutes after the end of dialysis, is very strong. Thus, they argue that a more accurate way than extensive mathematical modeling may be the simple determination of urea 30 minutes before the end of the dialysis session. If found to be true, over a wide range of dialysis times and efficiencies, this would dramatically improve the accuracy and ease the determination of dialysis dose. Although not as elegant as continuously measured urea clearance dialysate, this would reflect a significant improvement in predictive value as well as cost-savings—a novel and intriguing idea that awaits further study.

S.J. Schwab, M.D.

Sodium Ramping in Hemodialysis: A Study of Beneficial and Adverse Effects

Sang GLS, Kovithavongs C, Ulan R, et al (Univ of Alberta, Edmonton, AB, Canada)

Am J Kidney Dis 29:669–677, 1997 1–17

Objective.—The use of osmolal-preserving techniques during hemodialysis has decreased the side effects of treatment but can also result in more thirst and bigger weight gain between sessions. Results of a blinded study comparing standard to continuous to stepwise sodium ramping during dialysis and evaluating the effects and side effects of treatment during, immediately after, and between dialysis sessions were presented.

Methods.—A total of 23 patients requiring dialysis (5 women) underwent random sequencing of 2 weeks of standard hemodialysis with a sodium concentration of 140 mEq/L, 2 weeks with sodium ramped from 155 mEq/L at the beginning of dialysis and continuously lowered to 140 mEq/L at the end of dialysis, and 2 weeks with sodium at 155 mEq/L at the beginning of dialysis for 3 hours and lowered to 140 mEq/L immediately for the remaining hour of dialysis. Blood pressure, pulse rate, and side effects were monitored before, after, and during dialysis. Patients graded each session immediately afterward on a scale of 1 (worst) to 5 (excellent). During a 12-hour period after dialysis, patients rated thirst, cramps, and headaches on a 1 (absent) to 5 (severe) scale. Weight gain and fatigue were recorded. Results for the different treatment arms were compared statistically.

Results.—There were 406 dialysis sessions analyzed. Total symptoms, episodes of hypotension and cramps, and interventions were fewer in the 2 ramping protocols than in the standard dialysis sessions. Patients had no preference among protocols. After standard dialysis, there was much less thirst, fewer symptoms, and less fatigue than after either ramping protocol. Patients were more thirsty after the stepwise protocol and had more symptoms the day after dialysis. Postdialysis sodium was lower for the standard protocol. Patients gained more weight after the ramping protocols and had higher predialysis sodium levels in the next session. Pre- and postdialysis systolic blood pressures were highest for the stepwise ramped protocol. Systolic blood pressure was lowest during and after standard dialysis. Predialysis blood pressure was similar for all protocols. Patients who appear to benefit from ramping are older and gain a lot of weight, have a low albumin level, and experience more than 3 symptoms during dialysis.

Conclusion.—During the ramping protocols, patients had significantly higher systolic blood pressure, more thirst, greater weight gain, but fewer total side effects than during the standard protocol. Older patients who gain a lot of weight, have a low albumin level, and more than 3 symptoms during dialysis appear to benefit from sodium ramping.

▶ The question of the benefits of sodium ramping continue to be hotly debated. Unfortunately very few well-done studies have entered the literature. This, in my judgment, is the best to date. It shows that higher sodium concentrations stabilize blood pressure, as has been previously well established, but that ramping created by a sudden decrease in sodium or by a steady decrease in serum sodium from 155 to 140 mEq/L does not ameliorate the common side effects associated with continuous high-sodium dialysis. Thus, the concept that you can get the benefit and have none of the side efffects, which has been advocated by some, still is not the case. One could argue that just running a moderately higher steady serum sodium would be as beneficial as a ramping protocol.

S.J. Schwab, M.D.

Epidemiology and Outcomes

INTRODUCTION

Three selections from this year's literature are provided here to evaluate epidemiology and outcomes in end-stage renal disease. In Abstract 1–18, Klag et al. evaluate end-stage renal disease in African-American and Caucasian men in the "MRFIT" study. In this provocative retrospective observation, they suggest that, at least to a certain extent, some end-stage renal disease in African-American men may be preventable. Held and associates (Abstract 1–19), using the United States Renal Data System database, evaluate the dose up to a Kt/V of 1.2–1.3. More evidence supporting the recommended dialysis dose.

In the final selection (Abstract 1–20) in this section, Rocco and associates from Winston-Salem, NC conclude that the risk factors for death are very similar to the risk factors for hospital utilization in a large end-stage renal disease database.

Steve J. Schwab, M.D.

End-stage Renal Disease In African-American and White Men: 16-Year MRFIT Findings

Klag MJ, Whelton PK, Randall BL, et al (The Johns Hopkins Univ, Baltimore, Md; Univ of Minnesota, Minneapolis; Northwestern Univ, Chicago)

JAMA 227:1293–1298, 1997 1–18

Background.—African-American men have a four-fold higher incidence of treated end-stage renal disease (ESRD) than white men, a condition linked to 2 factors: the higher prevalence of hypertension in African Americans and their lower socioeconomic status (SES) compared to whites. In a prospective study, the incidence of all-cause and hypertensive ESRD in African-American men was compared with that in white men, with adjustment for blood pressure and income.

Methods.—Participants were members of a large cohort of men screened for the Multiple Risk Factor Intervention Trial (MRFIT) between 1973 and 1975. The trial studied effects on coronary heart disease of interventions to control elevated blood pressure, lower high serum cholesterol level, and achieve smoking cessation. Included in the analysis were 332,544 men aged 35–57 years; 300,645 were white, 20,222 African American, and 11,677 members of other ethnic groups. The incidence of ESRD was assessed through 1990, using a national ESRD treatment registry and data of the National Death Index and Social Security Administration.

Results.—The age-adjusted incidence of all-cause and hypertensive ESRD was 3.2-fold and 5.5-fold higher, respectively, in African Americans than in whites. Asian and Hispanic men had an incidence of all-cause ESRD that was between that of African-American and white men. For both African Americans and whites, higher blood pressure and lower SES were associated with a higher incidence of ESRD. The relative risk of ESRD in African-American men compared to white men was reduced from 3.20 to 1.87 after adjustment for baseline age, systolic blood pressure, cigarettes per day among smokers, previous myocardial infarction, diabetes, income, and serum cholesterol level. Similar results were obtained when hypertensive ESRD was the outcome. The association of systolic blood pressure with hypertensive ESRD was similar in whites and African Americans.

Conclusion.—Although African-American men have a four-fold higher age-adjusted risk of treated ESRD than white men, the relative risk of all-cause ESRD for African-American men is reduced to 1.87 with adjustment for other relevant factors. The excess risk of ESRD in African-American men compared to white men is largely related to disparities in blood pressure and SES between the 2 groups.

▶ The authors of this paper look at the follow-up results of the MRFIT longitudinal study. They identify that the age-adjusted ESRD is substantially higher in African-American men than in white men. When this rate was adjusted for baseline age, systolic blood pressure, number of cigarettes smoked, previous myocardial infarction,diabetes, income, and serum cholesterol, the relative risk in African-American men compared to white men was reduced from 3.20 to 1.87. Thus, at least to a certain extent, underlying disease and behavior characteristics account for a percent of this difference. The authors suggest that treatable factors, such as aggressive control of hypertension, may reduce the incidence of ESRD in African-American men.

S.J. Schwab, M.D.

The Dose of Hemodialysis and Patient Mortality

Held PJ, Port FK, Wolfe RA, et al (Univ of Michigan, Ann Arbor; Univ of Illinois, Chicago; Health Care Financing Administration, Baltimore, Md; et al)

Kidney Int 50:550–556, 1996 1–19

Background.—The association between hemodialysis dose delivered and mortality rate is not clear. Although several observational studies have shown that survival improves with higher doses, other unmeasured variables, changes in patient mix, or medical management may have affected this finding. The relationship of delivered hemodialysis dose and mortality rate was further investigated.

Methods.—Data from a U.S. national sample of 2,311 patients from 347 dialysis units were analyzed. The dose beyond which more dialysis apparently does not reduce the mortality rate was also determined. Patient survival was estimated by proportional hazards regression methods, with adjustment for 21 patient comorbidity/risk factors with stratification for 9 Census regions. The measurement of treatment delivered was based on 2 alternative measures of intradialytic urea reduction—the urea reduction ratio (URR) and Kt/V, with adjustment for urea generation and ultrafiltration.

Findings.—Mortality rate has a strong, robust, inverse association with hemodialysis dose delivered, whether measured by Kt/V or URR. The risk of death was reduced by 7% with each 0.1 increase in delivered Kt/V. At greater than 70% URR or a 1.3 Kt/V, there were no further significant reductions in mortality rate (Fig 2).

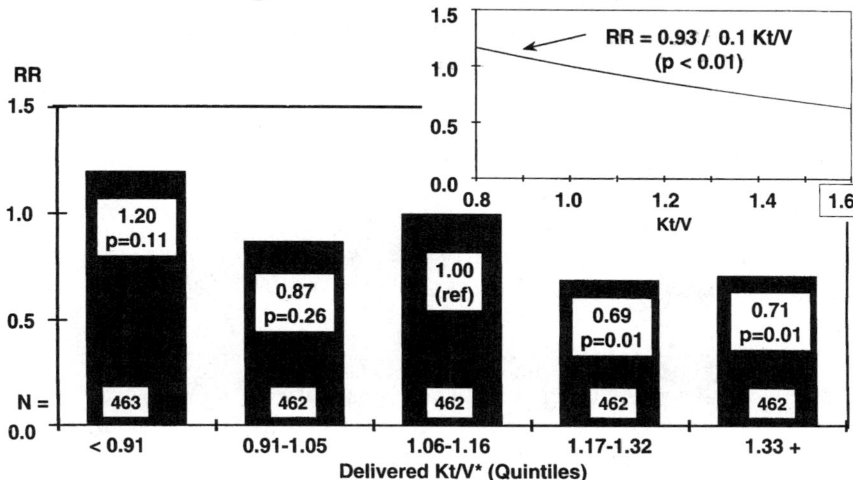

FIGURE 2.—The relative risk of death caused by delivered dose of dialysis (measured as Daugirdas corrected Kt/V) among a random sample of U.S. patients who had been receiving dialysis for more than 1 year on Dec. 31, 1990 (n = 2,311). The *line* represents relationship of delivered Kt/V and mortality risk, with Kt/V as a continuous variable and mean Kt/V (1.10) set as the reference (RR = 1.00). The *thin portion of the line* indicates segment in which correlation may be less steep. *Bars* represent risk of death for different categories of delivered Kt/V, with Kt/V = 1.0–1.2 arbitrarily set as the reference (RR = 1.00). *Asterisk* indicates from (1 − post/pre) blood urea nitrogen. n = 2,311, thrice weekly. (Courtesy of Held PJ, Port FK, Wolfe RA, et al: The dose of hemodialysis and patient mortality. *Kidney Int* 50[2]:550–556, 1996. Reprinted by permission of Blackwell Science, Inc.)

Conclusions.—The hemodialysis dose delivered is an important predictor of mortality rate. Increasing the level of treatment is a practical, efficient means of reducing the mortality rate among patients receiving dialysis.

▶ The effect of hemodialysis dose on the patient mortality rate is a critical issue. It is clear that inadequate hemodialysis increases the patient mortality rate. The issue is what constitutes an adequate hemodialysis dose. This is the latest retrospective analysis of a large database seeking these answers. Figure 2 shows that in this study, a Kt/V above 1.17 was associated with better outcomes than a lower Kt/V. These are more data supporting the national Kt/V goal of at least 1.2. But the real question of what constitutes an adequate dose of hemodialysis remains unanswered. Retrospective studies cannot answer this particular question because Kt/V can be measured with multiple techniques, and the measurement and timing of the postdialysis blood urea nitrogen sample dramatically influence the measurement. Other drawbacks include the fact that Kt/V only measures a single dialysis session and thus may both overestimate and underestimate dialysis dose. Alternately, patients receiving lower doses of dialysis may have more comorbid factors such as angina and hypotension, and this may lead to a lower dose of dialysis prescribed.

Prospective studies that control for all of these variables are needed to determine not only adequate dose of dialysis but also the effect of the dialysis membrane used. The NIH-sponsored HEMO study is such a study. Unfortunately, we must wait an additional 3 to 4 years for the answer. Until then, a dialysis dose greater than 1.2 Kt/V is needed.

S.J. Schwab, M.D.

Risk Factors for Hospital Utilization in Chronic Dialysis Patients

Rocco MV, Soucie JM, Reboussin DM, et al (Wake Forest Univ, Winston-Salem, NC; Emory Univ, Atlanta, Ga)

J Am Soc Nephrol 7:889–896, 1996 1–20

Purpose.—In patients with end-stage renal disease (ESRD), morbidity may result from comorbid medical conditions, as well as from renal failure. It is unknown whether the risk factors for hospital utilization in this group of patients are the same as the risk factors for death; if so, then measures to reduce one outcome should also reduce the other. Risk factors for hospital utilization were investigated in patients receiving long-term dialysis.

Methods.—The study included a cohort of 1,572 patients in 3 southern states who started dialysis in 1989. Fifty-two percent of the patients were women, and 64% were African-American; the mean age was 57 years. The most frequent causes of ESRD were hypertension (39% of patients), diabetes mellitus (33%), and glomerulonephritis (13.5%). The patients were followed up until 1993. Comorbidity and other risk factors for hospitalization were assessed.

Results.—Per year of patient risk, the median number of hospital days per year was 8.8, with a 25th quartile of 3.9 days and a 75th quartile of 20.1 days. A low serum albumin level was the fact most strongly associated with number of hospital days per year of patient risk. This was followed by decreased activity level, diabetes mellitus as the primary cause of ESRD, peripheral vascular disease, Caucasian race, advanced age, absence of hypertension, presence of angina, smoking, and congestive heart failure.

Conclusions.—Risk factors for hospital resource utilization among patients receiving long-term dialysis are identified. The risk factors are similar to those for death. Some are potentially modifiable including serum albumin level, smoking, and activity level. This information will be useful in efforts to reduce morbidity and improve quality of life for patients receiving dialysis.

► The authors, using the Southeastern Kidney Council database, identified that risk factors for death are very similar to the risk factors for hospital utilization. As we proceed to a capitated environment, these observations assume even greater importance.

S.J. Schwab, M.D.

Hepatitis C

INTRODUCTION

The management of hepatitis C continues to be a vexing problem for physicians caring for end-stage renal disease patients. The initial manuscript in this section (Abstract 1–21) selected from the European literature suggests nosocomial transmission of the hepatitis C virus and strongly supports the argument for improved dialysis unit practices. In a second observation (Abstract 1–22), this time from Austria, it is suggested that, at least in a subset of patients, there may be some benefit to α-interferon therapy—especially if viral burden is low at the initiation of therapy.

Steve J. Schwab, M.D.

Incidence and Risk Factors of Hepatitis C Virus Infection in a Haemodialysis Unit

Forns X, Fernández-Llama P, Pons M, et al (Hosp Clínic i Provincial, Barcelona)

Nephrol Dial Transplant 12:736–740, 1997 1–21

Objective.—Patients undergoing hemodialysis are at increased risk of hepatitis C infection (HCV). Although risk factors are known to include blood transfusion and length of time receiving hemodialysis, other risk factors are unknown. The incidence of de novo HCV infection in a hemodialysis unit and the identification of factors involved in the transmission of HCV were prospectively investigated.

Methods.—Routine liver tests and an anti-HCV titer were performed every 6 months in 114 patients (44 women), average age 58 years, who were free of HCV when they entered a long-term hemodialysis program for end-stage renal failure. Predisposing risk factors for HCV were recorded. Blood products were tested for anti-HCV and retested if administered to patients who subsequently became seropositive. The HCV genotype was studied in seroconverters and in patients with previous HCV infection who were treated in the same area.

Results.—Eight patients (7%), 3 treated in the in-hospital area and 5 treated in the out-hospital area, seroconverted to anti-HCV. There were no HCV markers in the blood transfused into seroconverters. There were no non–dialysis-related risk factor differences between seroconverters and nonseroconverters. When HCV genotypes were identified in patients with known HCV infection, similar HCV genotypes were found in 2 seroconverted patients, 2 different genotypes were identified in 2 patients, and 1 partial match was made in 1 patient. No HCV infection was detected in 2 seroconverted patients.

Conclusion.—Because the blood for transfusions was tested and the patients in this group had no outside risk factors for HCV or invasive surgical or diagnostic procedures likely to transmit the virus, evidence suggests nosocomial transmission, probably as a result of poor aseptic practices. Extremely careful and rigorous adherence to aseptic measures is important in a hemodialysis unit.

► The issue of hepatitis C is of increasing importance in in-center hemodialysis populations. Guidelines in the United States from the Centers for Disease Control, other than universal precautions, have not been forthcoming. The importance of this observation is that the authors show nosocomial transmission within the dialysis unit is indeed a major risk that requires our continued vigilance.

S.J. Schwab, M.D.

Patterns of Hepatitis C Viremia in Patients Receiving Hemodialysis

Umlauft F, Gruenwald K, Weiss G, et al (Univ of Innsbruck, Austria; Univ of Graz, Austria; Stanford Univ, Calif)

Am J Gastroenterol 92:73–78, 1997 1–22

Background.—Chronic hepatitis C virus infection is often seen in patients receiving hemodialysis. An infection rate of 10% to 40% in these individuals is often reported. The infection rate in the general population is 0.3% to 1.5%. Immunosuppression after kidney transplantation and resulting changes in immune status may induce inflammatory liver disease. Eradicating hepatitis C virus infection in patients with end-stage renal failure may lower the progression of liver disease after kidney transplantation and the risk of transmission of hepatitis C virus in hemodialysis centers.

Methods.—Serum samples from two groups of patients receiving maintenance hemodialysis who were positive for hepatitis C virus RNA were analyzed. The groups consisted of 33 patients treated with interferon-α and 31 untreated patients.

Results.—In 20 of the 31 untreated patients, serum hepatitis C virus RNA was detected. The other 11 patients had a fluctuating pattern of viremia with virus-free periods of up to 4 weeks. Of the 33 treated patients, 25 became hepatitis C virus RNA negative during treatment. Of these 25 patients, 8 had a breakthrough, which was transient in 7 and persistent in 1. Of the 33 treated patients, 24 had a complete end-of-treatment response, 17 relapsed after completion of therapy, and 7 had a sustained response with undetectable serum hepatitis C virus RNA at 1 year. Significantly lower levels of viremia were seen in patients with a sustained response than in those who relapsed or who did not respond.

Discussion.—In patients receiving hemodialysis, fluctuating hepatitis C viremia with intervals of undetectable hepatitis C virus RNA is common. Low viral load is predictive of a sustained response to interferon therapy.

► Hepatitis C has become an increasingly common problem in patients receiving long-term hemodialysis. The progressive nature of this condition and its effect on the potential for renal transplantation are now acknowledged. This is the first study to suggest that in at least some patients, treatment with interferon-α may be of some long-term benefit. Thus, if the viral burden is low at initiation of therapy, a subset of patients may be persistently cleared of the virus. Unfortunately, in the overall group, only 21% were RNA-negative at 1-year follow-up.

This is a promising research step but is not yet of clinical significance.

S.J. Schwab, M.D.

Peritoneal Dialysis

INTRODUCTION

Peritoneal dialysis, both continuous ambulatory peritoneal dialysis (CAPD) and continuous cyclic peritoneal dialysis (CCPD) accounts for roughly 10% to 12% of end-stage renal disease therapy in the United States. The initial selection in this section is from the CANUSA study (Abstract 1–23). This study shows mortality differences between the United States and Canada for peritoneal dialysis patients.The second selection (Abstract 1–24) deals with the appropriate mechanism of dosing insulin in patients with diabetes mellitus maintained on peritoneal dialysis. Subcutaneous and intraperitoneal insulin have advantages and disadvantages.

The final 3 selections in this section deal with the vexing problem of peritoneal dialysis infection. In the first observation (Abstract 1–25), povidone exit-site therapy is found to prevent peritonitis and other dialysis related infections. In the following selection (Abstract 1–26), simultaneous removal and replacement of infected peritoneal catheters is shown to be a successful strategy in a predominantly pediatric population, thereby avoiding intervening periods of hemodialysis when peritoneal catheters are removed. The next selection (Abstract 1–27) deals with *Xanthomonas maltophilia*, identifying that, unlike most episodes of peritonitis, catheter removal in addition to antibiotic therapy may provide the best outcome for patients with this problem.

Steve J. Schwab, M.D.

Lower Probability of Patient Survival With Continuous Peritoneal Dialysis in the United States Compared With Canada

Churchill DN, for the Canada-USA (CANUSA) Peritoneal Dialysis Study Group (McMaster Univ, Hamilton, Ont et al)

J Am Soc Nephrol 8:965–971, 1997 1–23

Background.—International comparisons of end-stage renal disease (ESRD) patients have indicated that patients requiring dialysis in the United States have worse survival than those treated in other countries. A

North American multicenter prospective cohort study of patients requiring peritoneal dialysis (PD) found that the relative risk (RR) of death was 1.93 for those treated in the United States, compared with those treated in Canada. This study investigates additional factors that might explain this apparent difference in survival, including severity of cardiovascular disease (CVD), residual renal function, race, rates of transfer to hemodialysis or renal transplantation, patient compliance, and dialysis modality selection bias.

Study Design.—A prospective cohort study was performed involving 4 centers in the United States and 10 centers in Canada. The study group consisted of 680 consecutive patients who began continuous ambulatory peritoneal dialysis (CAPD) between September 1990 and December 1992. At enrollment, data on country, age, gender, race, functional status, underlying renal disease, diabetes status, and serum albumin levels were collected. Nutritional status was determined by the subjective global assessment (SGA) of nutrition. The adequacy of dialysis was estimated from total weekly Kt/V for urea and the total weekly creatinine clearance. Clinical outcomes included mortality, technique failure, nonfatal cardiovascular events, and peritonitis.

Findings.—There was no difference in the CVD severity index, residual renal function at the initiation of dialysis, probability of transfer to hemodialysis or transplantation, or time to first peritonitis between the 2 countries. The 2-year survival rate for whites was 77% in Canada and 55% in the United States, so race was not the explanation for the mortality difference. The RR of a nonfatal cardiovascular event was 1.80 for the United States. The observed–predicted creatinine ratio was used to estimate compliance and was 1.13 in Canada and 1.00 in the United States. The prevalence of PD was 48% in Canada and 22% in the United States. The incidence of new dialysis patients was 100 per million population in Canada and 211 per million in the United States.

Conclusions.—The decreased patient survival and increased cardiovascular morbidity for patients undergoing CAPD in the United States, compared with Canada could not be explained by race, age, functional status, initial residual renal function, diabetes, cardiovascular disease, compliance, transfer or transplantation rates, nutritional status, or dialysis adequacy. Although a lower proportion of patients are treated with CAPD in the United States, the direction of this bias is not clear. The much lower acceptance rate for new dialysis patients in Canada may be due to decreased referral of patients with comorbidity, which may explain the better survival and decreased cardiovascular morbidity of Canadian CAPD patients, compared with patients in the United States.

► This is an interesting report from CANUSA investigators group. However, it clearly raises more questions than it answers. The study shows that mortality in the US sectors was higher than that in the Canadian centers for what appears to be a matched patient population. However, the acceptance rate for end-stage renal disease in the United States is more than 2 times that of Canada. In addition, the U.S. centers clearly made up the minority of enrolling sites. There were 10 Canadian and 4 U.S. sites with an expected distribution in the number of enrolled patients. Thus, the relative likelihood of survival for a patient has many interesting questions that were not answered by this study. Specifically, was there a center effect given? There were only 4 U.S. centers. Although aggressively pursuing PD mortality and hemodialysis mortality is useful, I am not certain that cross-national comparisons offer much value.

S.J. Schwab, M.D.

The Influence of Peritoneal Dialysis and the Use of Subcutaneous and Intraperitoneal Insulin on Glucose Metabolism and Serum Lipids in Type 1 Diabetic Patients

Nevalainen P, Lahtela JT, Mustonen J, et al (Tampere Univ, Finland)
Nephrol Dial Transplant 12:145–150, 1997 1–24

Background.—Individuals with diabetes and end-stage renal disease are often treated with continuous ambulatory peritoneal dialysis. This treatment allows intraperitoneal administration of insulin, which may be the closest physiologic insulin replacement method. Because of the advantages in continuous ambulatory peritoneal dialysis, intraperitoneal insulin is a common treatment in patients with insulin-dependent diabetes mellitus. The superiority of intraperitoneal insulin to subcutaneous insulin is unknown.

Methods.—Eleven patients had type 1 diabetes and end-stage renal disease. The mean patient age was 42.9 years. Measurements were made of glycated hemoglobin (HbA_{1c}), euglycemic hyperinsulinemic clamp, serum lipids, and patient well-being. Patients were first treated with subcutaneous insulin, then intraperitoneal insulin.

Results.—After continuous ambulatory peritoneal dialysis was begun, HbA_{1c} increased. After the change to intraperitoneal insulin, HbA_{1c} improved. The insulin dose increased by 15% after continuous ambulatory peritoneal dialysis was begun and by 128% after the change to intraperitoneal insulin. The glucose disposal rate improved by 39% after initiation of continuous ambulatory peritoneal dialysis and by 14% after the change to intraperitoneal insulin. Continuous ambulatory peritoneal dialysis had no significant influence on serum lipids, but intraperitoneal insulin lowered high-density lipoprotein cholesterol and significantly increased the low-density lipoprotein/high-density lipoprotein ratio.

Discussion.—In these patients, continuous ambulatory peritoneal dialysis improved insulin sensitivity, and greater improvement was seen after changing to intraperitoneal administration from subcutaneous administration. Better glycemic control occurred with intraperitoneal insulin. It is unknown whether these improvements affect the long-term survival of such patients.

► These authors are among the first to critically evaluate insulin administration in patients receiving peritoneal dialysis. Unfortunately, the results provide little clinical guidance. This study suggests that intraperitoneal insulin leads to better glycemic control but also leads to decreased HDL levels in these same patients. Longer term studies are now needed to evaluate morbidity before 1 mode of administration is preferred over the other. At least this pilot study sets the stage for larger studies to determine the ideal mechanism of insulin administration.

S.J. Schwab, M.D.

The Efficacy of Exit Site Povidone-Iodine Ointment in the Prevention of Early Peritoneal Dialysis-related Infections

Waite NM, Webster N, Laurel M, et al (St Michael's Hosp, Toronto; Univ of Toronto)

Am J Kidney Dis 29:763–768, 1997 1–25

Objective.—There is no method for preventing infections that commonly occur in patients undergoing peritoneal dialysis. Patients with exit-site or tunnel infections are more likely to get peritonitis. In a prospective, randomized, single-blind study, the effects of povidone-iodine applied topically on incidence of exit-site, tunnel, and peritoneal infections in a peritoneal dialysis population were examined.

Methods.—A total of 117 patients receiving a peritoneal dialysis catheter were treated with povidone-iodine ointment (n = 61) or sterile dressings only (n = 56).

Results.—In the povidone-iodine group, complications included hemorrhage at the catheter site in 2 patients, difficult insertion in 1, and the necessity of catheter manipulation in 2. In the control group, complications included the necessity of catheter manipulation in 3. There were 22 *Staphylococcus aureus* carriers in the povidone-iodine group and 14 in the control group. There were 10 infections in the povidone-iodine group and 14 in the control group. There were significantly fewer *S. aureus* infections in the povidone-iodine group than in the control group (2 vs. 10). There was a reduction in the infection rate of the povidone-iodine group at all time points until 140 days after dialysis when the infection rate increased (Fig 1). Catheters had to be removed in 3 patients because of peritonitis. Ten of 36 *S. aureus* carriers and 14 of 81 noncarriers became infected. Among carriers, 5 of 22 patients in the povidone-iodine group and 5 of 14 in the control group became infected. Among noncarriers, 3 of 39 in the povidone-iodine group and 9 of 42 in the control group became infected. The average time to first infection was 55 days in the povidone-iodine group and 33.2 days in the control group. Povidone-iodine users experienced no adverse effects of treatment.

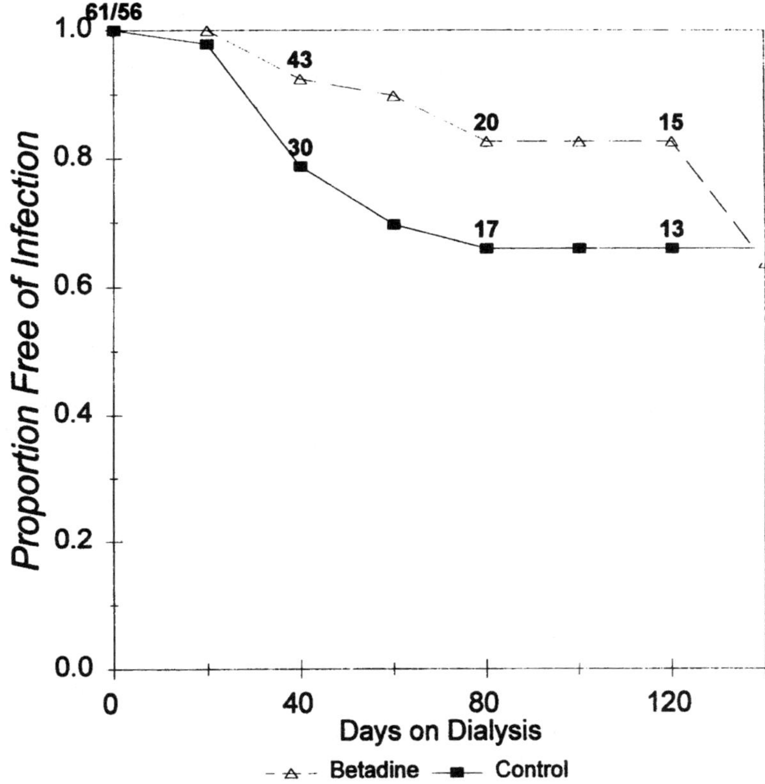

FIGURE 1.—Life table curves for the infectious complications over time for the 2 groups. The povidone-iodine group showed significantly less infections between 40 and 140 days on dialysis compared with the control group ($P = 0.04$, Wilcoxon test). (Courtesy of Waite NM, Webster N, Laurel M, et al: The efficacy of exit site povidone-iodine ointment in the prevention of early peritoneal dialysis-related infections. *Am J Kidney Dis* 29:763–768, 1997.)

Conclusion.—Topical povidone-iodine treatment of patients undergoing peritoneal dialysis resulted in a lower infection rate and a delay in the average time to first infection. The protective effect was lost after 140 days of dialysis. Two povidone-iodine treated patients vs. 10 controls experienced *S. aureus* infection even though the rate of the carrier was 36% in the povidone-iodine group vs. 25% in the control group.

▶ These authors show that the prophylactic use of povidone-iodine ointment diminishes the likelihood of early peritoneal dialysis-related infections. Similar observations have been shown for topically applied mucopuricin. Figure 1 shows a life table analysis of the povidone-iodine treated group compared to the control group, who received standard care that did not involve an antimicrobial or povidone-iodine ointment. Thus, there is increasing evidence that exit-site therapy is important in the prevention of peritonitis.

S.J. Schwab, M.D.

Simultaneous Removal and Replacement of Infected Peritoneal Dialysis Catheters

Majkowski NL, Mendley SR (Children's Mem Hosp, Chicago; Northwestern Univ, Chicago)

Am J Kidney Dis 29:706–711, 1997 1–26

Objective.—Recurrent infection with the same organism for patients undergoing peritoneal dialysis may indicate colonization of the catheter and may require its replacement. Replacement of peritoneal dialysis catheters in infants, children, and young adults and catheter replacements in patients undergoing interval hemodialysis were reviewed and compared.

Methods.—Catheters were replaced in a single step 34 times in 27 patients aged 6 months to 22 years, with recurrent peritonitis, nonresolving peritonitis, and severe exit site or tunnel infection within 30 days after completing antibiotic therapy. Infecting organisms were determined. Peritoneal dialysis was reinstituted within 48 hours after catheter replacement. Stage catheter replacement was generally performed with patients undergoing hemodialysis. Compliance and infecting organisms were determined for patients who discontinued peritoneal dialysis because of recurrent infections. Success was defined as a lack of reinfection within 45 days of catheter replacement.

Results.—Infecting organisms consisted of *Staphylococcus aureus* (37%), *S. epidermidis* (22%), *Pseudomonas* sp(6%), and culture negative (13%). There was no difference in age, ethnic background, or cause of disease between patients who had single-step catheter replacements or those who had staged catheter removal. The procedure was successful in 29 patients. All patients undergoing peritoneal dialysis were maintained on peritoneal dialysis during the catheter replacement period. One infection resulted from intraoperative contamination. There were 5 failures within the 45-day period after replacement. Fifteen of 18 replacements for exit site or tunnel infection were successful. As a result of infection, 18 catheters were removed in a staged procedure with 6 to 65 days off peritoneal dialysis. In half of the staged procedures, the infecting organism was *Pseudomonas* sp, whereas only 6% of single-step procedures were the result of *Pseudomonas* infection. Peritoneal dialysis was discontinued in 22 patients as a result of infection, although the duration of discontinuation was shorter for these patients than for patients with either single-step or staged catheter replacements.

Conclusion.—Simultaneous removal and replacement of infected peritoneal dialysis catheters is effective in treating recurrent infections. The failure rate was low and comparable to results after staged catheter replacement.

► Peritonitis is the single largest barrier to long-term peritoneal dialysis therapy. In general, peritonitis associated with a tunnel tract infection, recurrent peritonitis with the same organism, or peritonitis refractory to antibiotic therapy has required a staged catheter removal and replacement procedure. This staged procedure involves removal of the peritoneal dialysis catheter, a period of antibiotic therapy with hemodialysis and then peritoneal catheter replacement. These authors confirm the previous observation of Swartz and associates[1] that simultaneous removal and replacement of a peritoneal dialysis catheter can have long-term outcome similar to staged removal and replacement. This small study, predominantly in children, shows a significant success rate. The problem with adults not addressed by this paper, is the need to perform very low volume exchanges for the first 3–4 weeks after the new catheter is placed. Perhaps low-volume continuous cyclic peritoneal dialysis is the answer. Nonetheless, the concept of simultaneous removal and replacement is gaining credence.

S.J. Schwab, M.D.

Reference

1. Swartz R, Messana J, Reynolds J, et al: Simultaneous catheter replacement and removal in refractory peritoneal dialysis infections. *Kidney Int* 40:1160–1165, 1991.

Xanthomonas maltophilia Peritonitis in Uremic Patients Receiving Continuous Ambulatory Peritoneal Dialysis

Szeto CC, Li PKT, Leung CB, et al (Chinese Univ of Hong Kong, Shatin)
Am J Kidney Dis 29:91–95, 1997 1–27

Introduction.—Xanthomonas maltophilia, previously known as *Pseudomonas maltophilia*, is an increasingly important nosocomial pathogen. There have been a few reports of *X. maltophilia* peritonitis in patients receiving continuous ambulatory peritoneal dialysis (CAPD). Six cases of *X. maltophilia* peritonitis in patients receiving CAPD are reported.

Patients.—The patients were 45 women and 2 men with a mean age of 52 years. Seen over a 5-year period, the patients represented 1.5% of all cases of peritonitis in the authors' renal unit. In the previous year, 4 of the 6 patients had had another episode of peritonitis. All 4 of these patients had been treated with intraperitoneal imipenem and vancomycin in the 3 previous months.

Outcomes.—The outcomes of medical treatment were poor. All patients required removal of the Tenckhoff catheter, 3 within 3 weeks after the onset of peritonitis. The indication for catheter removal was failure of the effluent to clear up with antibiotics alone in 2 patients and secondary peritonitis in 4. There were no deaths caused by *X. maltophilia* peritonitis per se, but 2 patients died of fungal peritonitis.

Conclusions.—Xanthomonas maltophilia peritonitis is a serious complication in patients receiving CAPD. The prognosis is poor, and the catheter will likely have to be removed. Double antipseudomonal antibiotics should be given as soon as the diagnosis is made. The catheter should be removed promptly if there is no response. There is a risk of opportunistic or secondary infections in patients receiving prolonged multiple antibiotic therapy.

► These authors outline the emergence of *Xanthomonas maltophilia* peritonitis in patients receiving peritoneal dialysis. The treatment outcome for these patients is clearly worse than that for patients with routine gram negative peritonitis. The authors propose that failure to respond rapidly to appropriate antimicrobial therapy should prompt early removal of the catheter to prevent short- and long-term complications when this is the infecting organism.

S.J. Schwab, M.D.

The Anemia of End-stage Renal Disease

Introduction

In one of the most provocative articles of the year, Fishbane et al. suggest that the commonly used iron indices we use to determine when additional iron supplementation is necessary (serum ferritin, serum transferrin saturation) may be woefully inadequate (Abstract 1–28). These authors have an innovative strategy and propose some thoughtful guidelines. In the second study in this section (Abstract 1–29), the authors from Charleston, SC, evaluate screening prior to the initiation of erythropoietin (EPO) therapy and conclude that very limited screening is required for a cost effective initiation of EPO therapy. In the next selection (Abstract 1–30), a French investigator suggests that iron can be administered continuously during the dialysis treatment, preventing the need for recurrent bolus therapy. And, in the following selection (Abstract 1–31), high serum C-reactive proteins are identified as a strong factor in EPO-resistance.

Steve J. Schwab, M.D.

The Evaluation of Iron Status in Hemodialysis Patients
Fishbane S, Kowalski EA, Imbriano LJ, et al (Univ of New York, Stony Brook)
J Am Soc Nephrol 7:2654–2657, 1996 1–28

Introduction.—Iron status in patients with anemia while on hemodialysis has been difficult to determine accurately with the 2 commonly used tests for serum ferritin and transferrin saturation. Using a general hemodialysis population, researchers sought to define the performance of commonly used iron indices in this setting.

Methods.—Patients eligible for the study had a serum ferritin level of less than 600 ng/mL, were on a stable recombinant human erythropoietin (r-HuEPO) dose for at least 2 months, and had no hematologic disease (other than end-stage renal disease) affecting erythropoietin. Forty-seven patients received a course of IV iron dextran, 1,000 mg divided over 10 hemodialysis treatments. Hematocrit values and r-HuEPO doses were recorded at baseline, then every 2 weeks for 3 months. Patients considered to have had iron deficiency at study entry were those who had an increase in hematocrit value of at least 5% or a decrease in the r-HuEPO dose of at least 10% by the end of the study period. All other patients were judged to have adequate iron.

Results.—Thirty-one (66%) patients exhibited the positive erythropoietic response, as defined for the study, after an IV iron course, and 16 (34%) were considered to have adequate iron at baseline. The iron-deficient group did not differ significantly from the group with adequate iron in mean hematocrit values at baseline or at 1 month before baseline (30.3% versus 31.7% and 30.1% versus 31.2%, respectively). The 2 groups also were similar in mean r-HuEPO dose, mean cell volume, mean cell hemoglobin, and red cell distribution width at baseline. Tests for serum ferritin and transferrin saturation were of marginal significance in distinguishing iron-deficient and adequate-iron groups.

Discussion.—The commonly used iron indices examined in this study, whether considered alone or in various combinations, failed to accurately diagnose iron deficiency in hemodialysis patients. Such tests should be interpreted only in the context of the patient's underlying erythropoietin responsiveness. Recommended indicators of inadequate iron stores in r-HuEPO–responsive patients are a serum ferritin level of less than 100 ng/mL or a transferrin saturation value of less than 18%. For r-HuEPO–resistant patients, critical values are a serum ferritin level of less than 300 ng/mL or a transferrin saturation level of less than 27%.

► The determination of adequate iron availability in patients with end-stage renal disease receiving EPO therapy remains controversial. The DOQI panel of the National Kidney Foundation has determined levels of ferritin and transferrin saturation that they believe reflect reasonable iron repletion. The authors of this manuscript question the value of serum levels of iron but argue that iron deficiency is best defined by responsiveness, defined as increasing hemoglobin and hematocrit following the administration of iron. This is an attractive theory. The problem is, no one has defined what level of erythropoietin dose reflects erythropoietin resistance. The authors' approach was to provide a wide range of patients who had serum ferritins less than 600, a test dose of 1,000 mg of intravenous iron divided over 10 treatments. They found a wide range of variability in what patients would be determined to have in inadequate versus adequate iron stores. The authors argue that the commonly used tests for transferrin saturation and serum ferritin are of marginal value if not interpreted in the context of EPO responsiveness. They suggest that in those patients who are responsive to EPO, lower levels of serum ferritin and transferrin saturation are acceptable. In patients who are resistant to EPO, transferrin saturations of 27% or serum ferritin levels of 300 mg/dL should yield more than 90% sensitivity. Because it is difficult to determine what dose of EPO reflects EPO resistance, one could argue that a second reasonable approach is to maintain transferrin and ferritin targets at the levels the authors suggest are appropriate for patients with apparent EPO resistance. Additional investigations of this type are needed to allow us to fully understand the value of iron therapy in our patient population and to lead to rational iron therapy.

S.J. Schwab, M.D.

A Cost-effectiveness Analysis of Anemia Screening Before Erythropoietin in Patients With End-stage Renal Disease

Hutchinson FN, Jones WJ (Med Univ of South Carolina, Charleston)

Am J Kidney Dis 29:651–657, 1997 1–29

Objective.—Although the development of human recombinant erythropoietin (EPO) has resulted in improved quality of life for those with end-stage renal disease (ESRD), the significant cost of treatment requires that EPO be administered in the lowest effective dose. Certain conditions can impair response to EPO. The frequency of aluminum intoxication, hyperparathyroidism, and deficiencies of iron, folate, and vitamin B_{12} in patients beginning dialysis and the cost-effectiveness of screening patients to detect these disorders before starting EPO were studied.

Methods.—Before beginning dialysis, patients with ESRD underwent anemia screening for serum iron, transferrin, aluminum, intact parathyroid hormone, vitamin B_{12}, and folate concentrations. Cost-effectiveness analysis was based on the cost of EPO ($14 for 2,000 U) vs. the cost of the laboratory screening tests.

Results.—During the 36-month study period at Ralph H. Johnson Veterans Affairs Medical Center, 48 patients (3 women) aged 37–78 years with ESRD were screened. Most patients (36) were black and most had ESRD secondary to type II diabetes mellitus or hypertension. Eighteen patients had a low serum iron concentration (7 or less µmol/L), and 25 had a transferrin saturation less than 0.20. One patient was folate deficient. The cost of 1 month of EPO treatment (6,000 U/week) was $172, and the cost of all 5 laboratory screening tests was $152.17. The cost-effectiveness analysis assumed that without screening it would take 1 month before a poor response was seen, and that failure to treat deficient conditions would decrease response to EPO. All screening tests but the transferrin saturation test had a cost-effectiveness ratio greater than 1, meaning that they cost more than they saved.

Conclusion.—Testing transferrin saturation before administering EPO to patients requiring dialysis is cost-effective because this type of iron deficiency is common with anemic patients. Other screening tests add more cost than they save.

► These authors evaluate screening parameters such as folate, vitamin B_{12}, etc., to identify deficiency states that might impair EPO administration. The final analysis shows that, given cost-effective considerations, the only reasonable laboratory screen in patients with progressive chronic renal insufficiency before the initiation of EPO is the determination of iron stores. Thus, sophisticated and extensive testing should be reserved for those patients with chronic renal failure or ESRD who do not respond to routine EPO administration.

S.J. Schwab, M.D.

Continuous Administration of Intravenous Iron During Haemodialysis
Granolleras C, Zein A, Oulès R, et al (Univ Hosp, Nîmes, France)
Nephrol Dial Transplant 12:1007–1008, 1997 1–30

Objective.—Intravenous administration of iron during hemodialysis improves hematocrit levels. Rarely, anaphylactic reactions can result from too rapid an administration of iron in sensitized patients. A safe, simple, and cost-effective technique for continuous administration of IV iron during hemodialysis was developed.

Methods.—Depending on serum ferritin levels and transferrin saturation, the appropriate dose of iron polymaltose is drawn into a 50-mL syringe containing 20 mL N saline and heparin and administered as a continuous infusion at a maximum rate of 7.5 mL/hr. Heparin is given as an IV loading dose (2,500–6,000 U) before the start of the infusion.

Results.—There was a 30% reduction in the average erythropoietin dose required in 18 patients after 4 months of hemodialysis with iron therapy. Mean hematocrit rose significantly from 29 to 31 vol%, serum ferritin increased from 321 to 654 ng/mL, and transferrin saturation grew from 31% to 33%. There were no pharmacologic compatibility problems observed between heparin and iron polymaltose. There were no adverse reactions.

Conclusion.—Slow administration of heparin and iron maltose during hemodialysis increased hematocrit and serum ferritin levels and transferrin saturation and decreased the erythropoietin requirement of patients, with no adverse effects.

► Intravenous iron is becoming a standard of therapy to maintain adequate iron levels to allow effectiveness of erythropoietin (EPO). Indeed, by maintaining iron at higher levels as recommended by the Dialysis Outcome Quality Initiative Practice Guidelines on Anemia Management, it is believed that signficantly less EPO will be required. Because EPO is relatively expensive and iron relatively inexpensive, IV iron infusion will gain further use in future hemodialysis therapy. Currently, iron is administered at the end of the treatment as a bolus injection. These authors described what appears to be a safe and cost-effective method of giving IV iron mixed with saline during the regular dialysis treatment. The iron administered in this study was iron polymaltose, which has not been widely tested in the United States. Nonetheless, they present a potentially important observation with cost-effective complications. The other key issue of the risk of the now rare but always frightening anaphylactic reaction associated with IV iron was not addressed.

S.J. Schwab, M.D.

High C-Reactive Protein Is a Strong Predictor of Resistance to Erythropoietin in Hemodialysis Patients

Bárány P, Divino Filho JC, Bergström J (Karolinska Institutet and Huddinge Univ, Stockholm; Sophiahemmet, Stockholm)

Am J Kidney Dis 29:565–568, 1997 1–31

Background.—Several factors modulate response to recombinant human erythropoietin (EPO) treatment. One of the major causes of resistance to such therapy is inflammation. The relationship between increased serum C-reactive protein (s-CRP) and the EPO dose needed to maintain hemoglobin levels at about 12 g/dL in a group of patients receiving hemodialysis with maintenance EPO was reported.

Methods.—Thirty patients undergoing hemodialysis were included. Twenty-eight received EPO subcutaneously during dialysis, and 2 received EPO in IV injections.

Findings.—The mean weekly EPO dose was 80% greater in patients with s-CRP of 20 mg/L or higher than in patients with s-CRP of less than 20 mg/L. Both EPO dose and s-CRP were correlated inversely with levels of serum albumin and serum iron, which suggests that the main mechanism by which inflammatory cytokines inhibit erythropoiesis is coupled to iron metabolism (functional iron deficiency).

Conclusion.—In patients undergoing hemodialysis, s-CRP is associated with resistance to EPO. This is consistent with the notion that the EPO response may be inhibited by an inflammatory acute phase reaction, mediated by elevated cytokine release. Serum CRP will be a useful predictor of EPO therapy resistance.

▶ The authors of this paper sought to identify factors that may contribute to EPO resistance. Serum C-reactive protein is an acute phase protein generated by the liver, generally in response to inflammation. These authors demonstrate that patients with higher s-CRP levels tend to require higher doses of EPO to achieve a similar hematocrit. In this patient group, this was despite equivalent levels of serum iron, parathyroid hormone, ferritin, etc. The authors also note an inverse relationship of s-CRP with serum iron. Thus, they propose that iron metabolism, i.e., reticuloendothelial blockade or a problem with iron utilization, may be the problem mediated by chronic inflammatory states. Thus, s-CRP identifies patients who likely have an inflammatory state and are less likely to be EPO responsive.

S.J. Schwab, M.D.

Uremic Osteodystrophy

INTRODUCTION

There were 3 selections from this year's literaure for uremic osteodystrophy chosen for the YEAR BOOK (Abstracts 1–32, 1–33, and 1–34). All 3 selections deal with new therapeutic techniques for improving metabolic bone disease in the end-stage renal disease patient—techniques which may ultimately prove superior to 1,25-dihydroxy vitamin D_3 in our patients.

The second article evaluates a new noncalcemic phosphate binder which holds significant promise. In the third study in this section, the histologic prevalence of β-2 microglobulin amyloidosis is evaluated. It provides interesting new observations about where and when this particular molecule is deposited in paients with end-stage renal disease.

Steve J. Schwab, M.D.

Effective Suppression of Parathyroid Hormone by 1α-Hydroxy-Vitamin D_2 in Hemodialysis Patients With Moderate to Severe Secondary Hyperparathyroidism

Tan AU Jr, Levie BS, Mazess RB, et al (West Los Angeles Veterans Affairs Med Ctr; UCLA School of Medicine, Los Angeles; Bone Care Internatl Inc, Madison, Wis)

Kidney Int 51:317–323, 1997 1–32

Background.—Calcitriol deficiency is an important contributing factor to secondary hyperparathyroidism associated with chronic renal failure. Reduced blood calcitriol levels lead to increased secretion of parathyroid hormone (PTH), a result of the loss of the inhibitory action of calcitriol on the parathyroid gland. Although calcitriol has been used extensively to treat patients with secondary hyperparathyroidism, receiving dialysis, its therapeutic index is quite low. A multicenter study was conducted to test the safety and efficacy of an alternative to calcitriol, the vitamin D analog 1α(OH)-vitamin D_2 (1αD_2).

Methods.—Study participants were 24 patients with moderate to severe secondary hyperparathyroidism. All had a duration of hemodialysis of more than 4 months. An 8-week washout period, during which calcitriol was discontinued, was followed by a 12-week treatment period. Blood samples were obtained during both periods for determination of calcium, phosphorus, intact PTH (iPTH), 1α25$(OH)_2D_2$ and 1α25$(OH)_2D_3$ levels. Patients were eligible to enter the treatment phase if a serum iPTH value exceeded 400 pg/ml and the average serum phosphorus level was 6.9 mg/dl or lower during the washout period.

Results.—The starting dose of oral 1αD_2, 4 μg/day or 4 μg 3 times per week, was adjusted to maintain serum iPTH between 130 and 250 pg/ml. The mean baseline serum iPTH level was 672 pg/ml. A significant decrease was observed by the end of the first week of treatment, and a steady decline continued through the 12-week study period (Fig 1). The final dose of 1αD_2 averaged 14.2 μg/week; mean iPTH after treatment was 289 pg/ml. Most (87.5%) patients reached target iPTH levels. There was a small rise in mean serum calcium, from 8.8 mg/dl before treatment to 9.5 mg/dl after treatment. No changes were observed in average serum phosphorus level, the incidence of hyperphosphatemia, or the dose of phosphate binders.

Conclusion.—This is the first study to demonstrate the efficacy of 1αD_2 in lowering serum levels of iPTH in patients with moderate to severe secondary hyperparathyroidism who are receiving hemodialysis. By the

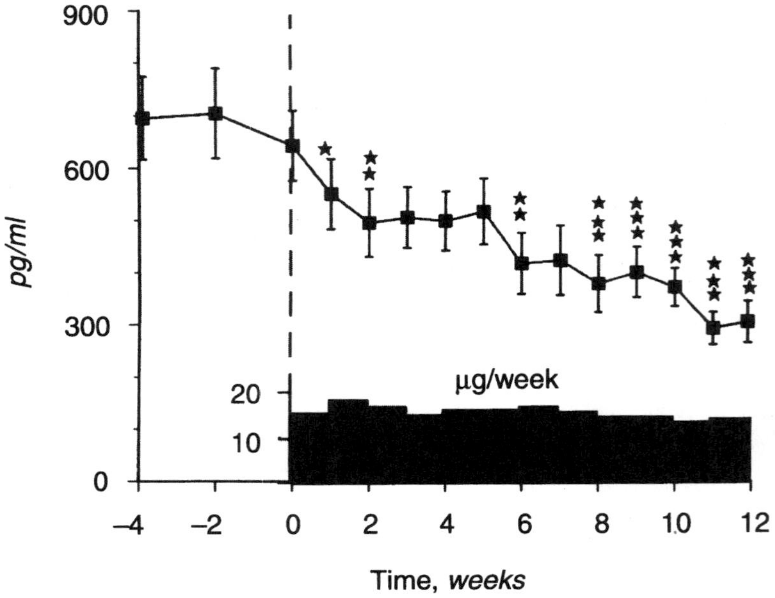

FIGURE 1.—Mean levels of serum intact PTH during the last 4 weeks of washout and treatment with 1 α-hydroxy-vitamin D_2 (1αD_2), with the mean weekly dosage of 1αD_2 shown as solid bars. Data are mean ± SEM. *P* values differ from baseline: $*P < 0.05$; $\dagger P < 0.025$, and $\ddagger P < 0.01$. (Courtesy of Tan AU Jr, Levie BS, Mazess RB, et al: Effective suppression of parathyroid hormone by 1α-hydroxy-vitamin D_2 in hemodialysis patients with moderate to severe secondary hyperparathyroidism. *Kidney Int* 51[1]:317–323, 1997. Reprinted by permission of Blackwell Science, Inc.)

end of the study, serum iPTH in these patients averaged 51% below pretreatment values.

► Calcitriol has been used in both intravenous and oral forms as an effective therapy to lower PTH levels in patients with end-stage renal disease (ESRD). The primary side effect of calcitriol administration has been hypercalcemia. In some cases, this hypercalcemia prevented the effective use of vitamin D to treat secondary hyperparathyroidism. This study is the first trial of another vitamin D analog that promises equal PTH-suppressive ability (see Figure 1) with less tendency toward hypercalcemia. If verified in additional trials, this may well prove to be the medical therapy of choice for secondary hyperparathyroidism in patients with ESRD.

S.J. Schwab, M.D.

Poly[allylamine Hydrochloride] (RenaGel): A Noncalcemic Phosphate Binder for the Treatment of Hyperphosphatemia in Chronic Renal Failure

Chertow GM, Burke SK, Lazarus JM, et al (Harvard Med School, Boston; GelTex Pharmaceuticals Inc, Waltham, Mass; Rogosin Inst, New York; et al)
Am J Kidney Dis 29:66–71, 1997 1–33

Introduction.—Recent strategies to control hyperphosphatemia in patients with end-stage renal disease have included dietary phosphate restriction and the oral administration of calcium and aluminum salts. In a substantial proportion of patients, however, calcium treatment is associated with hypercalcemia and an increased risk of metastatic calcification. A randomized, placebo-controlled trial evaluated the efficacy of cross-linked poly[allylamine hydrochloride] (RenaGel), a cationic polymer that binds phosphate ions through ion exchange and hydrogen bonding.

Methods.—Study participants were 36 patients on maintenance hemodialysis. All had been receiving calcium-based phosphate binders, with or without vitamin D or vitamin D metabolite replacement therapy, at stable doses for at least 1 month before screening. After a 2-week washout phase in which calcium-based phosphate binders were discontinued, patients were randomized to RenaGel or placebo for a 2-week treatment phase, returning to their usual calcium regimen during the last 2 weeks of the study. Laboratory studies and dietary assessments were performed at baseline and after the various study phases.

Results.—The mean maintenance doses of oral calcium were similar at baseline in the placebo-treated (4.4 g/day) and RenaGel-treated (4.1 g/day) groups. The 2 groups also were similar in prevalence of chronic medical conditions, proportion using acetate and carbonate salts, proportion on calcitriol or related vitamin D metabolites, and adherence to the study regimen. At the end of the 2-week treatment phase, serum phosphorus decreased by a mean of 1.2 mg/dL in the RenaGel group and increased by a mean of 0.2 mg/dL in the placebo group. Treatment with RenaGel also led to a significant reduction, compared with placebo, in total serum cholesterol and the low-density lipoprotein cholesterol fraction. RenaGel proved to be as effective as calcium carbonate or acetate as a phosphate binder. A few minor adverse events were reported, 3 in each of the treatment groups.

Conclusion.—In this phase II trial, cross-linked poly[allylamine hydrochloride] (RenaGel) was found to be an effective dietary phosphate binder in patients on hemodialysis. Its potential advantages include lowering of cholesterol, abrogating the need for exposure to aluminum, and allowing intensification of calcitriol or other vitamin D analogue therapy.

► The authors describe a new and apparently effective phosphate binding agent that does not appear to significantly increase serum calcium concentrations. Thus, this agent, if confirmed in additional larger trials, may emerge as an ideal therapy for those patients with low turnover osteomalacia or severe tertiary hyperparathyroidism in whom hypercalcemia limits effective phosphate binding. Its performance in most patients, as compared with generic phosphate binders such as calcium acetate or calcium carbonate, remains to be determined. Nonetheless, a potentially significant new agent may be on the verge of entering our therapeutic armamentarium.

S.J. Schwab, M.D.

Histological Prevalence of β2–Microglobulin Amyloidosis in Hemodialysis: A Prospective Post-Mortem Study

Jadoul M, Garbar C, Noël H, et al (Univ of Louvain, Brussels; Vrije Universiteit Brussel, Bruxelles; Rijksuniversiteit Gent; et al)

Kidney Int 51:1928–1932, 1997 1–34

Introduction.—A prospective study of joint samples obtained at autopsy in patients on hemodialysis (HD) sought to demonstrate the histologic prevalence of β-2 microglobulin amylodiosis (Aβ_2m). Although the prevalence of clinical signs of Aβ_2m has been reported, little is known about the prevalence and localization of histologic Aβ_2m.

Methods.—Participating centers submitted to post mortem those patients who had received HD for at least 1 month and who died while on chronic HD or who died within 1 month after renal transplantation. The 54 patients who provided samples had been on HD for a median of 47 months. Median age at HD onset was 63 years, and median age at time of death was 69 years. A variety of causes of end-stage renal disease (ESRD) were represented in the group. Data gathered included modalities and dates of renal replacement therapy, history of carpal tunnel syndrome, and cause of death. A control group of 34 men (mean age 67 years) without a history of ESRD who died at the coordinating center hospital was randomly selected and submitted to post mortem joint sampling. Diagnosis of amyloidosis was based on a positive Congo red staining with characteristic green–yellow birefringence under polarized light.

Results.—Most of the 153 samples were taken from the sternoclavicular joints, shoulders, and knees. Twenty-six (48%) patients on HD had a diagnosis of Aβ_2m. The size of the Aβ_2m deposits varied considerably among patients, and the prevalence increased with duration of HD (from 21% within 2 years to 100% at more than 13 years). Minute amyloid deposits were detected in 35% of the controls. Multivariate analysis identified both HD duration and older age at HD onset as independent, significant risk factors for the presence of Aβ_2m. Gender and diabetic nephropathy as the cause of ESRD were not significant risk factors.

Conclusion.—β-2 Microglobulin amyloidosis may be seen in the large joints early after HD onset. The overall prevalence in this group (48% after HD for a median of 47 months) was much higher than indicated by clinical or radiologic evidence. Carpal tunnel syndrome was present in only 2%, and radiologic signs of amyloidosis were present in 4%. Because of the frequency of positive findings in the sternoclavicular joint and because of its easy accessibility, this joint appears to be the best site for early detection of Aβ_2m.

► This post mortem study examines the role of β_2-microglobulin deposition in the joints of patients with and without end-stage renal disease. It yields the following interesting observations:

1. Deposition of β_2-microglobulin seems to be most prevalent in the sterno-cleidomastoid joint
2. Deposition is often subclinical without major symptoms
3. The age of the patient, as well as the time of hemodialysis, influence the likelihood of β_2-microglobulin deposition.

This is very interesting but does not shed any light on possible therapies to ameliorate β_2-microglobulin deposition in dialysis patients. The role of various membranes, both biocompatible and nonbiocompatible, high- and low-flux, still await definitive resolution.

S.J. Schwab, M.D.

Continuous Venovenous Hemodialysis

INTRODUCTION

Two articles were selected for inclusion in continuous venovenous hemofiltration and continuous venovenous hemodialysis this year. Both of these observations show that continuous therapy, although promising, is not the complete solution for patients with acute renal failure. In the first study (Abstract 1–35), CVVH, although it clears significant amounts of lactic acid, neither masks nor significantly treats the dramatic acid production that is seen in these conditions. The next article (Abstract 1–36) shows that, despite cytokine removal by CVVH, this procedure has very little effect relative to cytokine production.

Steve J. Schwab, M.D.

Effect of Continuous Venovenous Hemofiltration With Dialysis on Lactate Clearance in Critically Ill Patients

Levraut J, Ciebiera J-P, Jambou P, et al (Centre Hospitalo-Universitaire de Nice, France)

Crit Care Med 25:58–62, 1997 1–35

Introduction.—Continuous venovenous hemofiltration with dialysis would appear to be well suited for management of acute renal failure in the ICU. Previous studies, however, suggest that because a large amount of plasma lactate is filtered with this technique, the blood lactate concentration fails to reflect tissue oxygenation status. A prospective study was designed to determine the effect of continuous venovenous hemofiltration with dialysis on lactate elimination in critically ill patients.

Methods.—The study group included 10 patients with acute renal failure and stable blood lactate concentrations. All were receiving continuous venovenous hemofiltration with dialysis. In a 2-stage investigation, lactate clearance by the hemofilter was calculated by measuring lactate concentrations in samples of serum and ultradiafiltrate. Total plasma lactate clearance was evaluated by infusing sodium L-lactate (1 mmol/kg of body weight) over 15 minutes. Arterial lactate concentration was determined before, during, and after the infusion.

Results.—Patients had a median ultrafiltration rate of 714 ml/hr. The blood lactate concentration did not significantly alter hemofilter clearances of urea and lactate. Median filter clearance of urea was 23.8 ml/min, and median filter clearance of lactate was 24.2 ml/min. The lactate concentration in the ultradiafiltrate did not differ significantly from the lactate concentration in the blood. Thus, the lactate-sieving coefficient was not significantly different from 1. Filter lactate clearance showed a close correlation with the filter urea clearance. The median blood lactate concentration increased from 1.4 to 4.8 mmol/L at the end of the infusion, then returned to 1.6 mmol/L 60 minutes later.

Discussion.—Filter lactate clearance was found to account for <3% of total lactate clearance. Because the lactate removed by continuous venovenous hemofiltration with dialysis is negligible compared with the overall plasma lactate clearance, blood lactate concentration is minimally altered with the technique and remains a reliable marker of tissue oxygenation.

► In this study, continuous venovenous hemofiltration (CVVH) performed with a hemofilter did not clear enough lactate to mask lactic acidosis. It also establishes that CVVH per se is not a treatment for lactic acidosis because it was responsible for only 3% of the lactate removal in the patients studied. Thus, it seems that CVVH, as practiced in this study, although clearing significant amounts of lactic acid, neither masks nor successfully treats lactic acidosis The only treatment for lactic acidosis is reversal of the process that causes the lactic acid.

S.J. Schwab, M.D.

Cytokine Removal and Cardiovascular Hemodynamics in Septic Patients With Continuous Venovenous Hemofiltration

Heering P, Morgera S, Schmitz FJ, et al (Heinrich-Heine-Universität, Düsseldorf, Germany)

Intensive Care Med 23:288–296, 1997 1–36

Introduction.—Acute renal failure (ARF) often develops in critically ill patients with sepsis, and mortality exceeds 60% despite advances in treatment and technical support. Cytokines, which are thought to be important mediators in the pathology of sepsis and septic shock, appear to be removed from the serum of septic, critically ill patients undergoing continuous renal replacement therapies. Patients in an ICU with ARF were studied prospectively to determine the effect of continuous venovenous hemofiltration (CVVH) on plasma levels of cytokines.

Patients and Methods.—The study group included 33 critically ill patients with ARF receiving CVVH. Origin of the ARF was sepsis in 18 patients and cardiovascular disease in 15. All required mechanical ventilation throughout the period of hemofiltration because of acute respiratory failure and all received vasopressive agents to maintain an adequate mean arterial pressure. Hemodynamic monitoring and collection of blood and ultrafiltrate samples were performed before and during the first 72 hours of CVVH.

Results.—Twenty (60%) patients died either in the ICU or before hospital discharge. Septic and nonseptic patients were comparable in main clinical parameters before the initiation of hemofiltration. Septic patients exhibited elevated cardiovascular values for cardiac output (mean 7.2 L/min), cardiac index (mean 4.2 L/min/m^2), and stroke volume (mean 67 mL), and reduced values for systemic vascular resistance (mean 540 dynese cm^{-5}. All hemodynamic values returned to normal within the first 24 hours after the start of CVVH treatment. Tumor necrosis factor-α (TNFα) was significantly elevated in septic patients (mean 1,833 pg/mL) compared with nonseptic patients (mean 42.9 pg/mL) before CVVH. Although TNFα was detected in ultrafiltrate, its levels did not decrease in blood during CVVH treatment. Septic and nonseptic patients did not differ significantly in serum levels of interleukin 1β (IL1β). Detectable levels of other cytokines (TNFα-RII, IL6, IL6R, IL1RA, and IL8) were also measured in the ultrafiltrate, but no significant reduction in plasma level was achieved.

Conclusion.—Hemofiltration treatment seemed to improve cardiovascular hemodynamics in septic patients, although there was no evidence that extracorporeal removal of cytokines achieved a reduction in blood levels. Findings do not support the use of hemofiltration for the primary purpose of eliminating cytokines in multiple organ failure.

► This European study addresses one significant issue: The removal of potentially harmful cytokines by continuous renal replacement therapy does not achieve a reduction in overall cytokine blood levels. It shows that low volume continuous hemofiltration with polysulfone is not able to remove cytokines significantly compared to cytokine production. Thus, the theory that continuous therapy may be superior because of its improved cytokine removal is called forcefully into question.

S.J. Schwab, M.D.

Miscellaneous

INTRODUCTION

The miscellaneous category this year contains 11 selections (Abstracts 1–37 through 1–47). These excellent studies cover the depth and breadth of dialysis therapy. They range from the impact of capitation on free-standing dialysis centers to the effect of dialysis sodium delivery on blood pressure, to the improved preservation of residual renal function in chronic hemodialysis patients with polysulfone dialyzers. We believe each has an important message without lending itself to any one specific category.

Steve J. Schwab, M.D.

Impact of Capitation on Free-Standing Dialysis Facilities: Can You Survive?
McMurray SD, Miller J (Northeast Indiana Kidney Ctrs, Fort Wayne)
Am J Kidney Dis 30:542–548, 1997 1–37

Introduction.—The Medicare program has funded patients with end-stage renal disease since 1973, and in 1994, $11.1 billion was spent caring for these patients. Because the cost is expected to escalate to $20 billion by the year 2000, ways to reduce costs are being sought. One method may be to capitate the care of these patients. The total cost of caring for a group of patients with end-stage renal disease was examined to determine whether capitating the care of these patients is cost-effective.

Methods.—Follow-up evaluation for 1 year was conducted with 6 patients new to dialysis and 29 patients already receiving treatment. The patients had a mean age of 60 years, and 11 of the 35 patients were diabetic. Their cost of care was tracked in the hospital and in the outpatient setting. Of these patients, 22 received dialysis and 13 received continuous ambulatory peritoneal dialysis.

Results.—For all patients, the cost of care was $43,044 per year. Patients already receiving dialysis treatment cost $3,164 less than new patients, primarily because of the hospital expense for new patients. Hemodialysis patients cost $14,570 more to care for than continuous ambulatory peritoneal dialysis patients, primarily because of their increased need for hospitalization. The outpatient and inpatient cost for hemodialysis patients primarily resulted from vascular access expenses. During the study, no patient had a transplantation.

Conclusions.—When comparing the cost of treating these patients in a capitation model, it was discovered that these patients could be successfully treated under a capitation system. A major challenge is reducing the number of hospitalization days to reduce the cost. The goal will be to optimize therapy. There may be opportunities in reducing supply costs and drug costs. As the cost of care continues to escalate, the dialysis market may need to be consolidated.

▶ The authors evaluated the true costs of providing care for patients with end-stage renal disease in a capitated environment. They identified vascular access as their principal cost that was amenable to intervention. Thus, it is clear that as we move toward capitation, aggressive efforts to minimize hospitalization, preferentially by controlling vascular access hospitalizations and outpatient costs, will be mandatory. Thus, the tools we need may be available to allow us to survive in a capitated environment. Clearly, control of hospitalization costs, especially for vascular access, is emerging as a leading problem. Early referral with elective placement of arteriovenous access for hemodialysis patients, specifically arteriovenous fistulas, may be the solution to our capitation woes.

S.J. Schwab, M.D.

Dialysate Sodium Delivery Can Alter Chronic Blood Pressure Management

Flanigan MJ, Khairullah QT, Lim VS (Univ of Iowa, Iowa City)

Am J Kidney Dis 29:383–391, 1997 1–38

Introduction.—Despite improved pharmacotherapy, hypertension is now epidemic in hemodialysis centers. The resurgence of dialysis hypertension has been attributed to a number of factors, but most were not applicable at the study institution. To determine whether the dialysis itself might be a contributing factor, volunteers were assigned to a crossover trial comparing "programmed variable-sodium" with "high-sodium" dialysis.

Methods.—Forty adults agreed to participate in a pretest-posttest crossover study. Patients receiving dialysis on Monday, Wednesday, and Friday received 3.5 months of control followed by 3.5 months of experimental dialysis; the therapy order was reversed for patients treated on Tuesday, Thursday, and Saturday. Control dialysis employed a dialysate sodium of 140 mEq/L; the experimental condition consisted of dialysis with a programmed exponential decrease of dialysate sodium from 155 mEq/L to 135 mEq/L. Dialysate sodium was then held constant at 135 mEq/L for the final half hour of dialysis.

Results.—Eighteen of the 40 patients completed both arms of the 7-month study. The "variable-sodium" program did not substantially alter dialysis efficiency, interdialytic weight gain, or the ability to achieve target weight. Also unaffected were the incidence of dialysis hypotension, saline administration, hypertonic saline use, or quantity of saline administered. Postdialysis blood pressures decreased and antihypertensive drug use was reduced during programmed "variable-sodium" dialysis. Results of ambulatory blood pressure recordings suggested that blood pressure returns to predialysis level by the evening of therapy with "standard dialysis," but this rebound is delayed to the day after treatment with "variable-sodium" dialysis. Patients did have higher postdialysis target weights during the programmed vs. the standard therapy.

Conclusion.—It was proposed that "variable-sodium" dialysis might alter dialysis sodium transfer, thereby improving the blood pressure control of sodium-sensitive patients. Hypertensive and normotensive patients had different blood pressure responses to the programmed therapy. Blood pressure was not reduced in the normotensive group, but 63% of hypertensive patients were able to stop or reduce their medications, and only 1 had to increase medication during "variable-sodium" dialysis.

► The issue of variable sodium vs. fixed sodium has not been resolved. The authors of this study took a different tack in the evaluation of a variable sodium dialysate delivery system. By comparing a fixed sodium dialysate of 140 mEq/L to a variable sodium of 155 to 135 mEq/L, they showed decreases in predialysis blood pressure that persists. The tradeoff for this appears to be an elevated postdialysis weight. However, there were no changes in intradialytic weight gain. In my opinion, the issue still remains unresolved, but one additional piece of the puzzle has now fallen into place.

S.J. Schwab, M.D.

Predictors of the Progression of Renal Insufficiency in Patients With Insulin-Dependent Diabetes and Overt Diabetic Nephropathy

Breyer JA, Bain RP, Evans JK, et al (Vanderbilt Univ, Nashville, TN; George Washington Univ, Washington, DC; Univ of Colorado, Denver; et al)

Kidney Int 50:1651–1658, 1996 1–39

Background.—Nephropathy develops in approximately 35% to 40% of patients with insulin-dependent diabetes mellitus (IDDM). Although microalbuminuria and hypertension are known risk factors for nephropathy in diabetic populations, the factors that predict the progression of renal insufficiency once nephropathy is established have not been examined in large-scale studies. A prospective, double-blind, controlled trial analyzed the impact of numerous baseline characteristics on loss of renal function in patients with established diabetic nephropathy.

Methods.—Thirty clinical centers were involved in the trial, which enrolled 409 patients. Eligibility criteria included age 18 to 49 years, duration of IDDM of 7 years or longer, disease onset before age 30, diabetic retinopathy, urinary protein excretion of 500 mg/day or greater, and a serum creatinine concentration of less than 2.5 mg/dl. Patients were participants in a trial on the effect of captopril on the rate of progression of renal disease. Those randomized to captopril received a dose of 25 mg 3 times daily; those in the control group received placebo. The primary outcome of the study was a doubling of the baseline serum creatinine concentration to at least 2.0 mg/dl. Baseline demographic, clinical, and laboratory parameters were analyzed as risk factors for time to progression of renal disease.

Results.—The study population was primarily Caucasian. More than 70% had serum creatinine levels less than 1.5 at baseline. During a median follow-up period of 3 years, there were 25 serum creatinine doubling events in the captopril group and 43 in the placebo group. Thus, the risk of creatinine doubling was reduced by 48.5% with captopril treatment. Multivariate analysis identified 5 demographic and clinical features that independently predicted nephropathy progression: onset of IDDM later in life, parental diagnosis of IDDM, the presence of edema, increased mean arterial pressure, and an abnormal ECG. Laboratory characteristics predictive of nephropathy progression were a low hematocrit, high blood sugar level, greater protein excretion, and a higher serum creatinine level.

Conclusion.—A number of baseline demographic, clinical, and laboratory variables can help to predict which patients with IDDM and established nephropathy are at increased risk for renal disease progression. Patients so identified can be targeted for early aggressive interventions.

► This study analyzes the database from the angiontensin-converting enzyme inhibitor in an IDDM trial. The trial involved 409 patients with diabetes mellitus and nephropathy. The identification of a series of prestudy factors that were associated with the progression of renal disease in this population is a helpful observation. Expected findings associated with the progression of renal disease include the degree of proteinuria, baseline creatinine level, poor glucose control, and increased blood pressure. Unexpectedly, findings such as insulin-dependent mellitus in a parent and late onset in life also emerged as factors for progression of diabetic nephropathy.

S.J. Schwab, M.D.

Echo Color Doppler Imaging of Carotid Vessels in Hemodialysis Patients: Evidence of High Levels of Atherosclerotic Lesions

Pascazio L, Bianco F, Giorgini A, et al (Univ of Trieste, Italy; Maggiore Hosp, Trieste, Italy)

Am J Kidney Dis 28:713–720, 1996 1–40

Background.—Because cardiovascular disease is an important cause of morbidity and death among patients receiving maintenance hemodialysis, such patients might be thought to have a very high level of atherosclerosis. Risk factors for cardiovascular disease are present more frequently in patients receiving hemodialysis, supporting the hypothesis that atherosclerosis is a cause rather than a result of end-stage renal disease. The relationship between hemodialysis and atherosclerosis was examined in 2 groups of patients, 1 receiving hemodialysis and another matched for age, sex, and pattern of cardiovascular risk factors.

Methods.—The study population included 61 consecutive patients receiving hemodialysis and 61 patients without end-stage renal disease. Each group had 36 men and 25 women with a mean age of 68 years. All patients underwent a clinical examination, routine blood tests, a surface ECG at rest, and echo color Doppler US assessment of the carotid arteries. Each group was divided into 2 subgroups: patients receiving hemodialysis with (59%) and without (41%) cardiovascular events and control subjects with (51%) and without (49%) cardiovascular events.

Results.—The prevalence of arterial hypertension was 86.9% in the hemodialysis group; 67.2% had dyslipidemia, 16.4% had diabetes mellitus, and 45.9% were smokers. Intima media thickening was present in all patients in each group. Patients with uremia had a significantly larger number of vascular plaques (73.8%) than control subjects (44%). In both groups, those with clinical evidence of cardiovascular complications had a high prevalence of carotid lesions. The degree of carotid disease, however, was significantly higher in the dialysis subgroup than in the control subgroup. In all vessels except the common carotid, patients receiving hemodialysis were found to have a greater frequency distribution of atheromatous plaques in carotid vessels than control subjects; this difference was statistically significant.

Discussion.—Patients receiving hemodialysis have a higher degree of atherosclerosis than age- and sex-matched control subjects with similar cardiovascular risk patterns. The level of carotid atherosclerosis among the subgroup of patients receiving hemodialysis without cardiovascular events was very close to that of the control subgroup with cardiovascular events (56% and 58.1%, respectively). It is uncertain whether atherosclerosis is accelerated by uremia and/or hemodialysis; there may be a relationship between progression of atherosclerosis and uremia in the period before dialysis.

▶ In this small study, 61 patients referred for color Doppler analysis of fistula flow in Trieste, Italy, also underwent carotid evaluation. When the patients were compared with age-matched control subjects, carotid disease was found to be present in a much higher percentage of patients receiving hemodialysis. It is possible that the development of atrioventricular access dysfunction may have selected out a group of patients with ESRD with an additional predisposition toward atherosclerosis. However, it supports the contention that even in Italy, where atherosclerosis seems to be much less prevalent than in North American populations, incidence of carotid disease is higher in the patient population with ESRD than in age-matched control subjects.

S.J. Schwab, M.D.

Improved Preservation of Residual Renal Function in Chronic Hemodialysis Patients Using Polysulfone Dialyzers

McCarthy JT, Jenson BM, Squillace DP, et al (Mayo Clinic and Found, Rochester, Minn)

Am J Kidney Dis 29:576–583, 1997 1–41

Background.—Preliminary findings suggest that the use of polysulfone (PS) membranes may help slow the loss of residual renal function in patients with end-stage renal disease with parenchymal renal disease. A retrospective study determined whether rates of loss of residual function in such patients differ between groups receiving hemodialysis exclusively with PS or cellulose acetate (CA) dialyzers.

Methods.—Fifty consecutive patients with residual renal function using PS dialyzers were compared with patients using CA dialyzers. Every 3 months, endogenous urea clearance was assessed in patients with remaining residual function. All patients were observed for 6 or more months using 1 type of dialyzer.

Findings.—The patients using PS dialyzers had a higher delivered Kt/V and mean urea clearance than the patients using CA dialyzers. However, these differences were nonsignificant after 22 to 24 months of dialysis. When patients with identical causes of chronic renal failure were compared, the PS and CA groups with diabetes mellitus, tubulointerstitial disease, and polycystic disease did not differ. Those with parenchymal renal disease had substantially better intrinsic renal function retention when using PS dialyzers. The PS group with parenchymal renal disease had a mean of 23 months before loss of intrinsic renal function, compared with 11 months in the CA group. Patients in the CA group lost renal function at a mean rate of 0.27 mL/min/month compared with 0.14 mL/min/month in the PS group. The rates of renal function loss were 0.29 and 0 mL/min/month in the CA and PS groups, respectively, with parenchymal renal disease. Loss of intrinsic renal function was unaffected by age, sex, or the use of angiotensin-converting enzyme inhibitors or calcium channel blockers.

Conclusion.—The rate of residual renal function loss is slower in patients with nondiabetic parenchymal renal disease receiving chronic hemodialysis with hydrogen peroxide/peroxyacetic acid–reprocessed PS dialyzers and a higher Kt/V than in disease-matched patients using single-use CA dialyzers. The choice of dialyzer membrane may affect intrinsic renal function.

▶ This study suggests that, in certain subclasses of patients, residual renal function is maintained longer with a PS vs. a CA dializer. The principal drawback of this study is that it is not a randomized, prospective trial. Thus, patient populations were not matched for other agents that might also influence loss of renal function e.g., treatment with calcium channel blockers. This difference in loss of renal function was ameliorated by 22 months. Thus, although these results are very interesting, they await confirmation and, even if confirmed, appear to be eliminated by 22 months of therapy.

S.J. Schwab, M.D.

Prognostic Value of Serum Cardiac Troponin I and T in Chronic Dialysis Patients: A 1-Year Outcomes Analysis

Apple FS, Sharkey SW, Hoeft P, et al (Hennepin County Med Ctr, Minneapolis, Minn)

Am J Kidney Dis 29:399–403, 1997 1–42

Background.—In patients with chronic renal failure, false positive increases in creatine kinase MB (CK-MB) often complicate the biochemical diagnosis of acute myocardial infarction. Recently developed monoclonal antibody–based immunoassays specific for cardiac troponin I (cTnI) and cardiac troponin T (cTnT) may help determine whether myocardial injury has occurred without diagnostic electrocardiography.

Methods.—The medical records of 16 patients undergoing chronic renal hemodialysis were reviewed to determine the incidence and prognostic value of increased serum cTnI and cTnT levels during 12 months. The patients were selected randomly without previous knowledge of their cardiac status.

Findings.—Seventy-five percent of the patients initially had elevated serum enzyme-linked immunosorbent assay (ELISA) cTnT levels exceeding 0.2 µg/L. Fifty percent of the patients had serum CK-MB increases of greater than 5 µg/L, and 19% had cTnI increases of greater than 0.8 µg/L. Four patients had fatal myocardial infarctions during the 1-year study. The cardiac event rate was associated with higher elevations of cTnT, CK-MB, and cTnI. Of the 12 survivors, 58% had increased ELISA cTnT levels, and 42% had increased CK-MB levels. None of the survivors had increased cTnI levels.

Conclusion.—Marked increases in cardiac markers tended to indicate a poor prognosis in these patients. However, there was also a high incidence of elevated cTnT and CK-MB levels with no evidence of myocardial injury. The preferred serum marker for detecting myocardial injury in patients with chronic renal disease may be cTnI.

▶ The availability of new serum markers cTnI and cTnT has been suggested as more predictive markers of acute myocardial injury. Levels of MB-CPK in some dialysis patients tend to be chronically elevated. Thus, a more predictive marker in patients with end-stage renal disease would be very helpful. This study suggests that cTnI may be highly specific for myocardial injury in patients with end-stage renal disease. A definitive study surveying a larger dialysis population or a study evaluating acute myocardial infarction will be required to confirm these preliminary observations. This paper, although small, does suggest that relatively few patients will have an elevated level of cTnI in the nonischemic state.

S.J. Schwab, M.D.

Bicarbonate Haemodialysis as a Treatment of Metformin Overdose

Heaney D, Majid A, Junor B (Natl Hosp for Neurology and Neurosurgery, London)

Nephrol Dial Transplant 12:1046–1047, 1997 1–43

Introduction.—The oral hypoglycemic agent metformin is commonly used to treat patients with diabetes mellitus. Excreted largely by the kidneys, metformin can produce severe lactic acidosis in patients with renal insufficiency. In the case reported here, a young man attempted deliberate self-poisoning with metformin.

Case Report.—A man, 29, was seen 2 hours after taking medications prescribed for his father—a large dose of metformin and smaller amounts of glibenclamide and nabumetone. He had a Glasgow Coma Scale (GCS) score of 10/15 at admission and a glucose level of 0.6 mmol/L. Initial treatment included glucose (100 ml 50% administered IV) and oxygen (10 L/min). Gastric lavage was performed when the patient's consciousness level improved. He subsequently had a GCS of 15/15 and a blood glucose level of 18 mmol/L.

The patient complained of nausea and abdominal pain over the next 3 hours and appeared increasingly agitated. Pulse rate was 190 beats/min, systolic blood pressure was 110 mm Hg, and ECG showed multifocal ectopic beats. Serum lactate measurements revealed profound lactic acidosis. The patient's condition improved after he was transferred to the renal unit and hemodialyzed for 10 hours using a sodium bicarbonate buffer. There was a transient deterioration in serum urea and creatinine, but the patient was able to be discharged on the seventh day after admission. He has had no further complications.

Discussion.—Although lactic acidosis associated with metformin toxicity has been reported, deliberate overdoses of the agent are rare. This otherwise healthy patient experienced profound and life-threatening lactic acidosis soon after ingesting the drug. Hemodialysis with bicarbonate as the buffer was an effective treatment, resulting in clearance of metformin and allowing bicarbonate to be given without the risks of IV administration.

► Metformin is a biguanide oral hypoglycemic agent now widely used in the treatment of diabetes mellitus. In chronic renal failure, metformin can induce significant lactic acidosis from the inhibition of pyruvate dehydrogenase. Thus, this agent should not be used in patients with chronic renal insufficiency. Treatment of metformin-induced toxicity and lactic acidosis has been described in one previous case report,[1] which describes the treatment of metformin-induced lactic acidosis with prolonged bicarbonate hemodialysis with complete recovery. The controversy over treatment of lactic acidosis usually is discussed in the setting of tissue hypoxia or liver dysfunction. In the absence of tissue hypoxia, as shown in this case report, hemodialysis can correct the lactic acidosis by allowing aggressive bicarbonate infusion. Whether this will be the standard of care is unclear. What is clear is that in heroic instances there are at least case reports of hemodialysis treatment of the lactic acidosis associated with metformin. As newer agents enter the market, it is possible that metformin lactic acidosis will be relegated to historical interest.

S.J. Schwab, M.D.

Reference

1. Gan SC, Barr J, Arieff AI, et al: Biguanide-associated lactic acidosis case report and review of the literature. *Arch Intern Med*, 152:2333–2336, 1992.

Uremic Pruritus: Roles of Parathyroid Hormone and Substance P

Cho Y-L, Liu H-N, Huang T-P, et al (Veterans Gen Hosp, Taipei, Tawian; Natl Yang-Ming Univ, Taiwan)

J Am Acad Dermatol 36:538–543, 1997 1–44

Introduction.—Pruritus is a problem experienced by many patients receiving hemodialysis. Because some studies report the disappearance of intractable itching after parathyroidectomy, secondary hyperparathyroidism has been proposed as a possible cause. In other reports, hemodialysis-related pruritus was reduced by topical capsaicin, an agent that deletes substance P from peripheral neurons. A 2-phase study examined the role of parathyroid hormone (PTH) and substance P in uremic pruritus.

Methods.—Study participants were 30 men and 15 women who had been receiving maintenance hemodialysis for at least 3 months. In phase 1, patients were divided into 3 groups according to degree of pruritus: none, mild, and moderate to severe. No other cause for itching was identified,

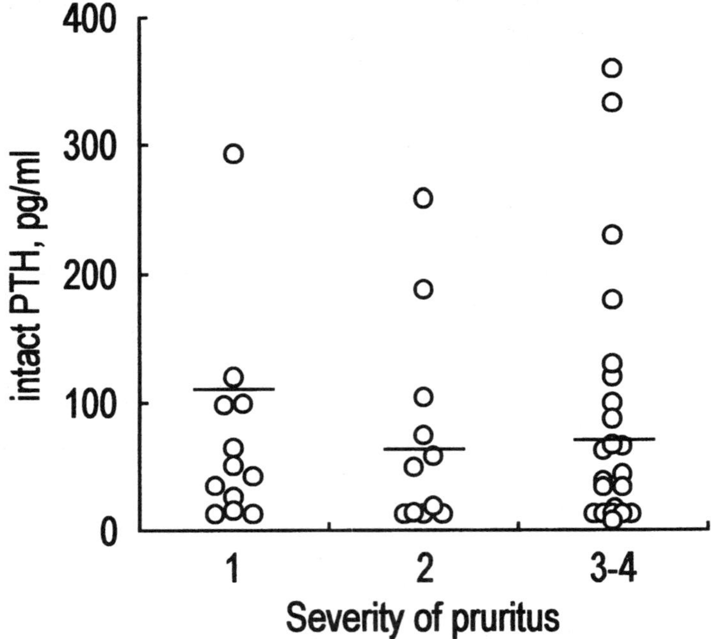

FIGURE 1.—Scatterplot of serum intact PTH values in hemodialysis patients with none (*1*), mild (*2*), and moderate to severe (*3–4*) pruritus. (Courtesy of Cho Y-L, Liu H-N, Huang T-P, et al: Uremic pruritus: Roles of parathyroid hormone and substance P. *J Am Acad Dermatol* 36:538–543, 1997.)

and no relief had been gained from antipruritic agents. Serum calcium, phosphate, and intact PTH levels were measured in all patients. In the second phase of the study, patients with moderate or severe pruritus were classified into subgroups on the basis of intact PTH levels (low, ≤35 pg/ml versus high, >35 pg/mL). A double-blind, placebo-controlled, crossover trial evaluated the benefits of topical capsaicin (0.025% cream). Pruritus was assessed at weekly intervals.

Results.—Serum concentrations of calcium, phosphate, and intact PTH (Fig 1) did not differ among the 12 patients without pruritus, the 11 with mild pruritus, and the 22 with moderate to severe pruritus. The 3 groups also were similar in mean age, sex, cause of uremia, and average duration of hemodialysis. Phase 2 of the study showed capsaicin cream to be significantly more effective than placebo in improving the itching score. Of 22 patients, 19 had complete resolution of pruritus or significant relief after active treatment.

Conclusion.—Severity of uremic pruritus showed no relationship to the patient's serum intact PTH level, and levels of serum intact PTH did not significantly change during treatment. Topical capsaicin is an effective treatment for uremic pruritus, possibly through its effect on substance P, which may act as a neurotransmitter.

► In this interesting trial, the authors subdivide patients by degree of pruritus and attempt to correlate this degree of uremic pruritus with PTH levels. When this subdivision was performed (Fig 1), there was no correlation between the severity of pruritus and the measurement of the intact parathyroid hormone level. Thus, a relationship between elevated intact PTH and symptoms of uremic pruritus could not be associated. Although this observation will conflict with some prior observations, this is the first randomized prospective trial to evaluate degree of pruritus in a substantial group of patients. The good news is that capsaicin seems to alleviate pruritus in most of the patients tested. Given the extreme discomfort this causes many of our patients, further research in this vital area is required.

S.J. Schwab, M.D.

Gynecologic and Reproductive Issues in Women on Dialysis

Holley JL, Schmidt RJ, Bender FH, et al (Univ of Rochester, NY; West Virginia Univ, Morgantown; William Beaumont Hosp, Royal Oak, Mich)

Am J Kidney Dis 29:685–690, 1997 1–45

Introduction.—Few studies have examined menstrual patterns in women on hemodialysis, and little is known about the interactions of erythropoietin, prolactin, and ovulation. Issues related to women's health were examined in a group of 76 patients, age 55 years or younger at the start of dialysis, who completed a questionnaire. Also studied were 115 women, older than 55 years at the start of dialysis, whose records were reviewed for estrogen replacement therapy.

Methods.—The questionnaire covered topics such as the menstrual periods (regularity, duration, flow, menopause), pregnancies, recombinant human erythropoietin (r-HuEPO) treatment, sexual activity, use of counseling about contraception, and woman-focused health care questions.

Results.—Of the 76 women who completed the entire questionnaire, 59% were white, and 29% were African-American. The median age of this group was 36.9 years at the start of hemodialysis and 41.7 years at the time of the study. Most (90%) were receiving r-HuEPO, and 70% had been pregnant at least once; 4 of the 179 pregnancies had occurred while the patient was on hemodialysis. Thirty-two women were currently menstruating; 19 of these reported irregular periods, and flow was often heavier after the start of dialysis. Regularity of periods was not influenced by r-HuEPO treatment. The median age at menopause was 47 years. Although 50% were sexually active, only 36% used birth control, and few (13%) had discussed such issues with their nephrologist. Yearly Pap smears were reported by 63% and mammograms by 73%, but only 5% of women who were older than 55 years at the start of dialysis were receiving estrogen replacement therapy.

Discussion.—Compared with previous reports suggesting that only 10% of premenopausal women on dialysis menstruate regularly, 42% of the women in this study were menstruating. This difference may be attributed to the use of r-HuEPO treatment and its possible effects on hypothalamic function. Further studies are needed that focus on the gynecologic concerns of women on dialysis, including the potential for pregnancy and the effects of estrogen replacement therapy.

▶ This questionnaire-based study evaluates women's health issues in an end-stage renal disease patient population. As such, it provides a starting point for further evaluation in this area. Currently, the role of birth control methods, oral contraceptives, and estrogen replacement therapy in postmenopausal women remains to be defined. The effect of estrogen replacement therapy on bone loss, bone density, and other bone-related complications remain unstudied.

S.J. Schwab, M.D.

Uremia Therapy in Patients With End-Stage Renal Disease and Human Immunodeficiency Virus Infection: Has the Outcome Changed in the 1990s?

Ifudu O, Mayers JD, Matthew JJ, et al (State Univ of New York, Brooklyn; Nephrology Found of Brooklyn, NY)

Am J Kidney Dis 29:549–552, 1997 1–46

Background.—Previous studies have reported limited survival in patients with HIV infection receiving hemodialysis. Thus, the decision to begin uremia treatment in HIV-infected patients with advanced renal failure has become an ethical dilemma. Outcomes in patients with end-stage renal disease (ESRD) and HIV infection receiving hemodialysis were reviewed.

Patients and Findings.—All 34 HIV-infected patients with ESRD undergoing hemodialysis in 1 hospital-based and 3 community-based outpatient hemodialysis facilities in Brooklyn, New York, were included in the cross-sectional survey study. The patients were 26 men and 8 women, aged a mean of 42 years. Ninety-one percent were black, and 9% were Hispanic. Eighty-five percent had AIDS. Fifty-nine percent had a history of IV drug abuse. Only 18% were being treated with an antiretroviral drug. Acquired immune deficiency syndrome was presumed to be the cause of renal failure in 68% of the patients. The mean HIV infection duration was 50.5 months, and the mean ESRD duration was 57 months. The mean total CD4 count was 140 cells/µL, the mean hematocrit was 28%, and the mean serum albumin concentration was 3.5 g/dL. All patients were being treated with erythropoietin to correct anemia. The hemodialysis sessions lasted a mean of 3.5 hours 3 times a week.

Conclusion.—The survival of patients with HIV-associated ESRD treated with hemodialysis is apparently better than the dismal rates reported in the 1980s. Because ESRD in HIV-infected patients does not necessarily signal near-term death, the decision regarding initiating renal replacement therapy in such patients should be individualized.

▶ This study is a cross-sectional survey of patients with HIV infection in Brooklyn, New York. Despite the inherent limitations of a cross-sectional "snapshot," it is clear that survival of patients with HIV has improved. The early papers showing uniform progression to death within 6 months are no longer the norm. The reason for these increased survivals is less clear. The authors acknowledge that the change in the clinical definition of AIDS, now based primarily on CD4 counts, may merely allow earlier identification of this patient population. Nonetheless, they point out the need for survival studies in HIV-positive patients to determine the appropriate role of renal replacement therapy.

S.J. Schwab, M.D.

Prealbumin Is the Best Nutritional Predictor of Survival in Hemodialysis and Peritoneal Dialysis

Sreedhara R, Avram MM, Blanco M, et al (Long Island College Hosp, Brooklyn, NY)

Am J Kidney Dis 28:937–942, 1996 1–47

Background.—The survival rate is poor for patients in the United States who undergo dialytic therapy for end-stage renal disease (ESRD). Malnutrition appears to be a major contributor to this high mortality rate compared with that of patients in Europe and Japan. Risk factors for early death during treatment for ESRD include age; diabetes; hypertension; and serum levels of albumin, cholesterol, and creatinine. In a previous study, the authors identified an association between a serum prealbumin level less than 30 mg/dl and lower survival at 36 to 48 months after the start of hemodialysis (HD) or peritoneal dialysis (PD). A group of patients receiving HD and PD was followed up to compare the relative risks of mortality of prealbumin with that of other markers.

Methods.—The study group included 111 patients receiving HD and 78 patients receiving PD who were undergoing dialytic therapy between June 1991 and March 1992. Monitoring continued through May 1996. Variables examined for their effect on survival included age; race; gender; diabetic status; and serum concentrations of albumin, creatinine, cholesterol, and prealbumin.

Results.—The HD and PD groups were both predominantly black (55% and 53%, respectively); slightly more than one third in each group had diabetes. Mean patient age was 59.9 in the HD group and 54.0 in the PD group. The majority of patients receiving PD had a base line serum albumin level of at least 3.5 g/dl (62%), a creatinine level of at least 9 mg/dl (74%), a cholesterol level of at least 200 mg/dl (62%), and a prealbumin level of at least 30 mg/dl (68%); corresponding percentages in the HD group were 86%, 80%, 24%, and 33%. A higher relative risk (RR) of death in patients receiving HD correlated with older age, diabetes, and a serum prealbumin level less than 30 mg/dl. For patients receiving PD, older age and the presence of diabetes correlated with a higher RR of death than in the general population. A prealbumin level less than 30 mg/dl was the strongest nutritional variable predictive of death in patients receiving HD (RR = 2.64); in patients receiving PD, the RR was 1.8.

Conclusion.—Prealbumin level appears to be the best single nutritional predictor of survival in patients with ESRD. In both HD and PD groups, observed and expected survival was significantly higher in those with enrollment prealbumin greater than 30 mg/dl.

▶ This relatively small study seeks to find additional predictors of death caused by ESRD. Serum albumin and serum creatinine have been reported as predictors of survival in several large retrospective studies. These authors argue that prealbumin may have even more predictive value. More definitive clinical trials in large patient populations are required before it can be determined that prealbumin is more predictive than other nutritional parameters.

S.J. Schwab, M.D.

2 Transplantation

Introduction

The past year in transplantation has been one of consolidation of knowledge without major diagnostic or treatment advances. Despite some outstanding contributions to the understanding of mechanisms involved in rejection and progressive renal failure, no significant advances have been made in ameliorating chronic allograft failure, a major problem following transplantation.

New immunosuppressive agents have been introduced, such as the humanized anti-CD2 antibody. Clinicians are gradually learning how to use other recently introduced drugs such as tacrolimus and the microemulsion formulation of cyclosporine. The mechanisms of renal damage from cyclosporine in either the original or microemulsion formulation and their contributions to chronic allograft failure remain unsolved issues.

In terms of patient management, there have been some recent insights gained, but no real blockbuster changes which impact standard patient management. From outcomes data, it is still clear that the major problem for renal transplantation in this country is a shortage of donors. The recent move toward more living unrelated transplants has been embraced by most transplant centers; however, at the same time, national sharing of organs has become somewhat controversial in that cold ischemia time has emerged as a very important factor in long-term kidney allograft survival. Kidney/pancreas transplantation also continues to be a procedure that is of great benefit to individual patients when successful, but it is frequently complicated by perioperative complications and carries an uncertain impact on chronic diabetic-induced micro- and macrovascular changes.

William Bennett, M.D.

Mechanisms of Damage to Transplanted Kidneys

Molecular Executors of Cell Death–Differential Intrarenal Expression of Fas Ligand, Fas, Granzyme B, and Perforin During Acute and/or Chronic Rejection of Human Renal Allografts

Sharma VK, Bologa RM, Li B, et al (New York Hosp/Cornell Med Ctr; Hennepin County Med Ctr, Minneapolis)

Transplantation 62:1860–1866, 1996 2–1

Background.—Two distinct cytolytic pathways have been described. In 1, the interaction between the Fas antigen and its ligand results in apoptosis. In the other, the pore forming protein perforin and the serine protease granzyme N contribute to DNA fragmentation and cell death. The intrarenal expression of these molecular executors of cell death was studied in light of the potential participation of cytolytically active cellular elements in the antiallograft repertory.

Methods.—Eighty human renal allograft biopsy specimens were studied. Intrarenal expression of Fas antigen, Fas ligand, granzyme B, and perforin was identified using reverse transcriptase-polymerase chain reaction. Display of messenger RNA (mRNA) was correlated with the Banff histologic diagnosis of renal allografts.

Findings.—Intrarenal expression of Fas ligand mRNA and of granzyme B mRNA was found to be a correlate of acute, but not chronic, rejection. In the absence of rejection, Fas ligand mRNA was not detectable. The intrarenal coexpression of members of each lytic pathway and that of both pathways were associated with acute rejection. In addition, there was a direct correlation between the histologic severity of acute rejection and intrarenal coexpression of mRNA encoding Fas ligand, Fas, granzyme B, and perforin (Fig 3).

Conclusion.—These data demonstrate the differential expression of the 2 major lytic pathways in acute and chronic allograft rejection. Specific treatment aimed at the cytotoxic attack molecules may be effective in preventing and/or treating acute rejection.

► The treatment of renal allograft rejection remains imperfect, both in its prevention and in management once it is clinically obvious. What is clear, however, is that allograft rejection shortens patients' 1-year graft survival rates compared with patients who are acute rejection free, and, perhaps more importantly, has long-term consequences on the observed half-life of cadaver transplants. Thus, understanding the mechanisms of cell death becomes extremely important in designing treatments that will prevent or manage the renal damage caused by rejection.

Dr. Sharma et al. examined the renal expression of molecular species that cause cell death in human allograft biopsy specimens. They characterized the 2 distinct cytolytic pathways. There is an interaction between Fas antigen and its ligand that usually results in accelerated programmed cell death and an additional pathway in which the protein perforin and the protease

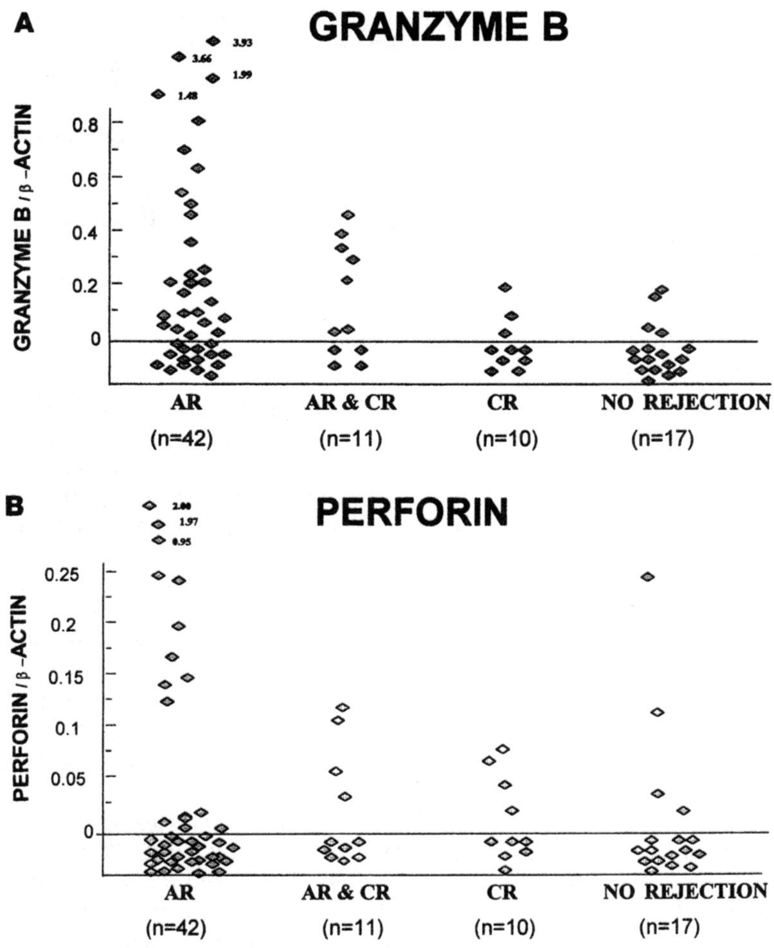

FIGURE 3.—Quantification of intrarenal expression of messenger RNA (mRNA) encoding granzyme B or perforin. The steady state levels of granzyme B mRNA (**A**) and of perforin mRNA (**B**) were measured by semiquantitative reverse transcriptase–polymerase chain reaction and normalized against the β-actin mRNA control. *Abbreviations*: *AR*, acute rejection; *CR*, chronic rejection. (Courtesy of Sharma VK, Bologa RM, Li B, et al: Molecular executors of cell death–differential intrarenal expression of fas ligand, fas, granzyme B, and perforin during acute and/or chronic rejection of human renal allografts. *Transplantation* 62[12]:1860–1866, 1996.)

granzyme B contribute to cell death. These studies demonstrate that the expression of messenger RNA for these 2 proteins correlated with acute rejection but did not correlate with chronic rejection, and, most importantly, that evidence of these pathways was absent in the absence of acute rejection.

The implications of this study are that processes that lead to acute and chronic rejection may be different and it may take separate strategies to manage them. The authors are to be congratulated for taking the molecular techniques and applying them to human tissues. The fact that major cytolytic pathways are expressed in biopsy specimens during acute rejection of human renal transplants may lead to more precise diagnosis and more effective treatments for acute rejection, which, unfortunately, still involves 30% to 50% of patients at most transplant centers, even under maximum immunosuppression.

W. Bennett, M.D.

Quantitative Detection of Immune Activation Transcripts as a Diagnostic Tool in Kidney Transplantation

Strehlau J, Pavlakis M, Lipman M, et al (Harvard Med School, Boston; McGill Univ, Montreal)

Proc Natl Acad Sci U S A 94:695–700, 1997 2–2

Background.—Current procedures for the diagnosis of renal allograft rejection rely upon detection of graft dysfunction and the presence of a mononuclear leukocytic infiltrate. The typical finding of azotemia and mild cellular infiltration is often inconclusive, and the diagnosis must await the response to antirejection therapy. A molecular approach, utilizing reverse transcription polymerase chain reaction (RT-PCR) of multiple immune activation genes was used to diagnose renal allograft rejection episodes.

Methods.—Sixty renal allograft core biopsies obtained for surveillance or to diagnose graft dysfunction were used to quantify intragraft gene expression of 15 immune activation genes by competitive RT-PCR. The results of these assays were compared to results of clinicopathologic analysis based upon the Banff criteria and the response to antirejection treatment.

Results.—During acute renal allograft rejection episodes, intragraft expression of interleukin (IL)-7, IL-10, IL-15, Fas ligand, perforin, and granzyme B but not IL-2, interferon-γ, or IL-4, was significantly increased. Amplified RANTES and IL-8 gene transcripts were sensitive, but nonspecific, markers of rejection. The simultaneous RT-PCR assay of perforin, granzyme B, and Fas ligands identified acute rejection with 100% sensitivity and 100% specificity. Effective treatment with antirejection therapy resulted in rapid downregulation of the expression of these genes.

Conclusions.—Clinical renal allograft rejection episodes are associated with the expression of a specific subset of immune activation genes. Simultaneous RT-PCR assay of perforin, granzyme B, and Fas ligand gene expression is an effective and reliable method for the diagnosis and follow-up of acute renal allograft rejection. The accuracy and potential for rapid analysis of this technique suggests it may be useful in the clinical management of patients receiving renal transplants.

► The diagnosis of renal allograft rejection is of primary importance for management of patients receiving renal transplants. Because most of the allografts that survive over the first 1–2 years, and that are later lost, succumb to chronic allograft rejection, and because chronic rejection has as its most important risk factor, acute rejection, the accurate diagnosis of acute rejection is paramount. Using competitive RT-PCR in allograft core biopsies, Strehlau et al. used sophisticated techniques to look for immune activation transcripts for diagnostic purposes. The finding that specific intragraft expression of IL-7, IL-10, IL-15, Fas ligand, perforin, and granzyme B were associated strikingly with the histologic diagnosis of rejection and changed in response to antirejection treatment may allow more effective and more specific diagnosis of rejection than the currently used clinical means. For all practical purposes, with modern immunosuppressive therapy, the suspicion of rejection rests on a decrease in a glomerular filtration marker, namely, the serum creatinine, and other indirect clues. A rapid diagnostic test for rejection would be welcomed and probably would be dissociable from the serum creatinine. If these techniques work out, they may represent a substantial advance in the clinical management of renal transplantation.

W. Bennett, M.D.

Blockade of T-Cell Costimulation Prevents Development of Experimental Chronic Renal Allograft Rejection

Azuma H, Chandraker A, Nadeau K, et al (Harvard Med School, Boston)
Proc Natl Acad Sci U S A 93:12439–12444, 1996 2–3

Background.—Chronic rejection, the most common cause of human allograft failure after the first year posttransplant, appears to be mediated by alloantigen-dependent and alloantigen-independent mechanisms. T-cell recognition of alloantigens is the key initial event leading to allograft rejection. One of the 2 signals required by T cells for full activation is a "costimulatory" signal, which is mediated in part by the T-cell accessory module CD28 interacting with the B7 family of molecules on antigen-presenting cells. The role of T-cell costimulatory blockade was investigated in a model of chronic renal allograft rejection.

Methods.—In experimental acute allograft rejection models, blocking CD28–B7 T-cell costimulation by systemic administration of CTLA4Ig, a fusion protein that binds B7 molecules on the surface of antigen-presenting cells, prevents rejection. An established transplantation model using male rats as graft recipients and donors was used to test the effect of CTLA4Ig therapy on the process of chronic renal allograft rejection. Five experimental groups of F344 into LEW renal allograft recipients were examined and compared: no treatment (4 animals, group 1), a single injection of CTLA4Ig (0.5 mg intraperitoneally) on day 2 posttransplant (14 animals, group 2), L6 control Ig (0.5 mg intraperitoneally) on day 2 posttransplant (6 animals, group 3), a short-term low-dose regimen of cyclosporine (CsA) (5 mg/kg/day for 10 days, subcutaneously) (19 animals, group 4), and the low-dose CsA protocol and day 2 CTLA4Ig therapy in combination (13 animals, group 5).

Results.—Most of the controls in groups 1 and 3 died by 8 weeks after transplant, and only 1 of the 10 animals survived more than 100 days. Group 4 animals given the low-dose CsA protocol had a 70% survival rate at greater than 8 weeks, but progressive proteinuria started to develop in these animals between 8 and 12 weeks after transplant and signs of chronic rejection appeared by 16–24 weeks. Early graft loss was prevented in groups 2 and 5 by treatment with CTLA4Ig alone or with low-dose CsA, and 90% of animals survived more than 8 weeks. Compared with CsA-alone treated controls, allografts of CTLA4Ig-treated animals showed attenuation of lymphocyte and macrophage infiltration and activation at 8, 16, and 24 weeks.

Conclusions.—In this experimental model, early blockade of the CD28–B7 T-cell costimulatory pathway prevented the development and evolution of chronic renal allograft rejection. Findings provide support for the hypothesis that T-cell recognition of alloantigen and activation are critical early events in the processes leading to chronic rejection.

▶ Chronic allograft failure continues to be an unsolved problem in renal transplantation. Despite the use of potent immunosuppressive drugs such as CsA and tacrolimus with their increased short-term (1- and 2-year) allograft survival rates, the half-life for cadaveric renal transplants in the United States has not increased significantly in the CsA era. Most physicians agree that chronic rejection is the most common cause of this phenomenon, although a role for nonimmunologic progression factors and CsA itself cannot be excluded. Azuma and colleagues, using a well-characterized model of chronic rejection in the rat, showed that blocking T-cell costimulation by the administration of a fusion protein that binds to the B7 molecule on antigen-presenting cells, prevents rejection and induces tolerance. The use of strategies in the development of compounds that block T-cell costimulation may have widespread application in clinical transplantation. Further evolution of this exciting work is awaited with great interest.

W. Bennett, M.D.

Modulation of Eicosanoid Metabolism in Endothelial Cells in a Xenograft Model: Role of Cyclooxygenase-2

Bustos M, Coffman TM, Saadi S, et al (Duke Univ, Durham, NC)

J Clin Invest 100:1150–1158, 1997 2–4

Background.—Organs transplanted between species undergo rejection mediated by the reaction of the recipient's xenoreactive antibodies and complement with the donor organ's blood vessel endothelial cells. This reaction leads to a loss of vascular integrity and the development of microthrombi, which is termed hyperacute rejection. If hyperacute rejection is averted, acute vascular xenograft rejection can develop, which is characterized by diffuse intravascular coagulation, inflammation, and ischemia. Acute vascular xenograft rejection may occur as a result of acti-

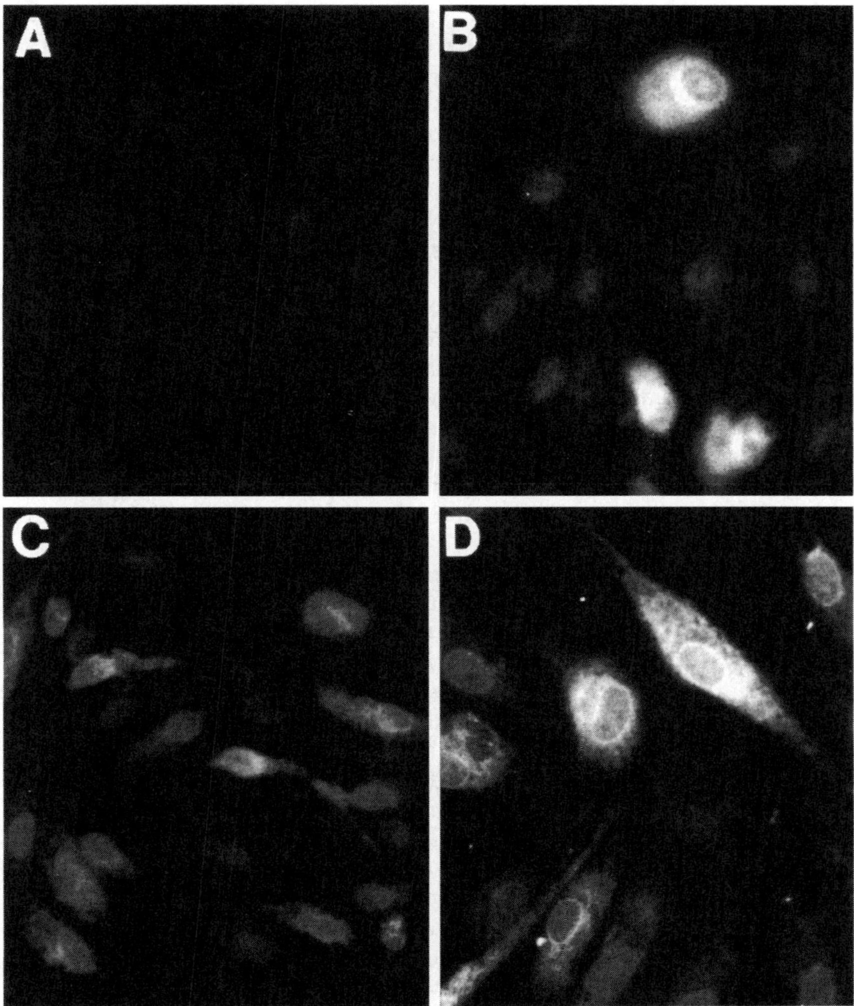

FIGURE 4.—Immunofluorescence localization of cyclooxygenase-2 in resting endothelial cells and endothelial cells stimulated by xenoreactive antibodies and complement. Binding of anti–cyclooxygenase-2 antibodies to porcine endothelial cells was investigated by direct immunofluorescence. **A**, resting endothelial cells. Cyclooxygenase-2 was not detectable. **B**, endothelial cells incubated with xenoreactive antibodies and complement for 6 hours. Cyclooxygenase-2 is detected close to the nucleus; (original magnification, ×400). **C**, endothelial cells stimulated with xenoreactive antibodies plus complement for 14 hours. The level of cyclooxygenase-2 protein was increased as is the number of positive endothelial cells; (original magnification, ×200). **D**, endothelial cells stimulated with xenoreactive antibodies plus complement for 24 hours, Cyclooxygenase-2 protein remained positive and is located in the cytoplasm; (original magnification ×400). (Reproduced from Bustos M, Coffman TM, Saadi S, et al: Modulation of eicosanoid metabolism in endothelial cells in a xenograft model: Role of cyclooxygenase-2 *J Clin Invest* 100:1150–1158, 1997, by copyright permission of The Rockefeller University Press.)

vation of graft endothelial cells, also mediated by xenoreactive antibodies and complement. Complement stimulates the synthesis of lipid inflammatory mediators or eicosanoids. Cyclooxygenase (Cox) is a rate-limiting enzyme in the synthesis of eicosanoids. A model of xenograft/host interaction was utilized to examine the effect of the reaction of xenoreactive antibodies and complement with endothelial cells on the expression of eicosanoids and Cox.

Methods.—Porcine aortic endothelial cells were isolated, characterized, and cultured in vitro. These cells were incubated with dilute human serum as a source of xenoreactive antibodies and complement. The supernatants were tested for eicosanoid levels by radioimmunoassay. Eicosanoid expression was also detected by Northern blot analysis. Immunofluorescence was used to detect proteins within the cells.

Results.—Resting cultured porcine aortic endothelial cells released prostaglandin I_2 into the culture medium, but after stimulation with human serum containing xenoreactive antibodies and complement, these cells released prostaglandin I_2 and thromboxane A_2. Serum from which either antibodies or complement had been removed was not effective. Altered eicosanoid metabolism was associated with induction of Cox-2 and thromboxane synthase, but not Cox-1(Fig 4). The induction of Cox-2 was not induced by complement directly, but required the synthesis of interleukin (IL)-1α, as an autocrine factor. Incubation with an Il-1α receptor antagonist inhibited induction of Cox-2 by endothelial cells.

Conclusions.—Porcine aortic endothelial cells stimulated with xenoreactive antibodies and complement from human serum were studied as a model of acute vascular xenograft rejection. Endothelial cells stimulated by xenoreactive antibodies and complement induced Cox-2 and produced greater amounts of prostaglandins and thromboxane. However, complement did not induce eicosanoid production directly, but induced the synthesis of IL-1α, which acted as an autocrine factor to induce the change in eicosanoid metabolism in the endothelial cells. This change in eicosanoid metabolism may explain the vascular injury, focal ischemia, and thrombosis observed in acute vascular rejection.

► Xenografting of organs between species is looked upon as the future of transplantation considering the limited donor organ supply. The primary barrier for this to happen clinically on a large scale is antibodies in the recipient that are reactive to the xenograft donor endothelial cells. These antibodies also interact with recipient complement. This process leads to hyperacute rejection with occlusion of small vessels. A separate process may take place over the next few days in which diffuse intravascular coagulation and ischemia resulting from acute vascular xenograft rejection occurs even when hyperacute rejection is avoided. The experiments using aortic endothelial cells stimulated with xenoreactive antibodies and complement showed that lipid inflammatory mediators are released with induction of Cox-2 and thromboxane synthase but not Cox-1. This mediator's release was not induced by complement, but required production of IL-1 acting locally as an autocrine factor. These findings have implications for local regulation of blood flow in xenografts and also give the potential of interrupting therapeutically at least 1 of the important pathways in xenograft rejection.

W. Bennett, M.D.

Immunosuppression

A Phase I Trial of Humanized Anti-interleukin 2 Receptor Antibody in Renal Transplantation

Vincenti F, Lantz M, Birnbaum J, et al (Univ of California, San Francisco; Hoffmann-LaRoche Inc, Nutley, NJ)

Transplantation 63:33–38, 1997 2–5

Introduction.—Interleukin (IL) 2 and its high-affinity IL-2 receptor (IL-2R) are involved in the clonal proliferation of T cells that mediate rejection of organ allografts. Murine monoclonal anti-interleukin 2 α chain receptor (Tac) antibodies are limited in efficacy by a short half-life and the development of antibodies to the heterologous protein. The safety, pharmacokinetics-dynamics, and immunosuppressive effect of a humanized anti-Tac antibody (HAT) were studied in 12 renal transplant patients.

Methods.—Ten patients had a living-related donor and 2 underwent cadaver organ transplantation. All received the same immunosuppressive drug regimen: prednisone, azathioprine, and cyclosporine. Randomization was to 1 of 4 treatment arms: HAT at 2 dosage levels (0.5 mg/kg or 1.0 mg/kg) and according to 2 dosing schedules (weekly or every other week) for a total of 5 doses given IV over 30 minutes. The first dose was given within 12 hours before transplant surgery and the remaining 4 doses after surgery according to the schedule of each treatment arm. Recipients of living-related donor organs were compared with 17 historical controls treated with an identical immunosuppressive regimen except for HAT.

Results.—The patient group had a mean age of 45 years; etiology of end-stage renal disease was glomerulonephritis in 5 patients, diabetes mellitus in 3, polycystic kidney disease in 1, and unknown in 3. No serious side effects were attributed to the HAT infusions, and no patient had systemic or local side effects or delayed adverse events from HAT therapy. A rejection episode occurred at day 7 but was successfully treated with OKT3. This patient, a woman who had received a cadaver organ, was in the lowest HAT dose treatment arm. None of the HAT-treated patients with living-related donors had a rejection episode during their first post-transplant year. During a similar follow-up period, 6 (41%) of the historical controls had a rejection episode. None of the transplant patients had malignancies or opportunistic infections. A patient in whom low-titer anti-HAT antibodies developed maintained high serum HAT concentrations throughout the study period. No changes in the percentage of absolute counts of CD3 cells or T-cell subsets were reported after HAT therapy, but there were significant decreases in the number of circulating lymphocytes that expressed free Tac.

Conclusions.—This is the first reported clinical trial to use a humanized anti–IL-2R antibody in renal transplant recipients. Therapy with HAT appeared to be effective in preventing episodes of rejection and was not associated with local or systemic side effects. The long half-life of HAT allows the dose interval to be extended, prolonging effective immunosuppressive therapy.

► The early results of clinical trials of humanized anti–IL-2R antibody are very encouraging. Conventional induction immunosuppression with OKT3 or polyclonal antibody preparations is not completely satisfactory because of high cost, the necessity for daily injections, and in the case of OKT3, cytokine release causing side effects. The murine antibodies that were developed against the IL-2R were limited in clinical trials by short half-lives and the development of anti-mouse antibodies. Thus, early studies with a humanized antibody to the IL-2Rα are encouraging. Little rejection was noted, and most importantly, there were no first-dose reactions or other side effects. The number of lymphocytes that expressed the IL-2R was decreased, and most importantly, the half-life was markedly prolonged, allowing dosing regimens that provide for excellent induction with a limited number of doses. Further clinical trials are ongoing and look promising.

W. Bennett, M.D.

Tacrolimus Therapy for Refractory Acute Renal Allograft Rejection: Definition of the Histologic Response by Protocol Biopsies

Woodle ES, Cronin D, Newell KA, et al (Univ of Chicago)

Transplantation 62:906–910, 1996 2–6

Introduction.—A tacrolimus-based regimen has been used at the study institution for more than 2 years as treatment for acute refractory renal allograft rejection. Essential elements of the therapy include its initiation early in the rejection process, aggressive dosing, and the use of protocol biopsies for histologic monitoring. The therapeutic regimen was described and the outcome was reported for 23 patients.

Patients and Methods.—Patients were 12 women and 11 men with a mean age of 38.3 years. Twelve were black, 10 were white, and 1 was Asian. The etiology of renal disease was insulin-dependent diabetes mellitus in 9 patients, hypertension in 5, chronic glomerulonephritis in 5, polycystic kidney disease in 2, and obstructive uropathy in 2. None had chronic rejection. Both cyclosporine and azathioprine were discontinued 24 hours before the start of tacrolimus therapy, which was initiated at a dosage of 0.3 mg/kg/day divided in 2 daily doses. The dose was increased to achieve levels between 25 and 40 ng/mL if necessary to achieve reversal of rejection. After documented histologic reversal and at least 6 weeks without recurrent rejection, the tacrolimus dose was decreased to provide levels between 8 and 15 ng/mL. Protocol biopsies were performed at defined intervals to determine the histologic response to tacrolimus therapy.

Results.—A total of 92 biopsies (average 4 per patient) were performed, 23 before the start of tacrolimus therapy and 69 during treatment. Initial biopsy specimens showed mild acute rejection in 64% of patients and moderate acute rejection in 36%. Biopsy specimens obtained 1 week after the start of tacrolimus therapy revealed no rejection in 60%, improvement in 13%, no change in 20%, and worsening rejection in 7%. Histologic changes at 1 week were not correlated with improvement in serum creatinine. Increases in tacrolimus dosing brought about rejection reversal or improvement in the 27% of patients who showed no histologic improvement (or worsening) after 1 week of treatment. There were 8 episodes of recurrent rejection, including 6 diagnosed by protocol biopsies alone. Tacrolimus nephrotoxicity was not apparent during the first 2 weeks, but this finding was common (39% of patients) later in the course (median time 60 days) of therapy.

Discussion.—A lack of correlation between renal function and histology during tacrolimus therapy indicates that serum creatinine levels may be a poor indicator of early response. Protocol biopsy specimens obtained at 1- to 2-week intervals early during treatment and at longer intervals thereafter, define the histologic response, help guide clinical decisions, and can detect clinically silent recurrent rejection or tacrolimus nephrotoxicity.

▶ The approval of tacrolimus therapy for renal transplantation has been eagerly awaited. Both the United States and international trials have shown small differences in favor of tacrolimus for 1-year graft and patient survival. The major attractiveness of tacrolimus is that it can be used for rescue of refractory acute rejection. The study of Woodle et al. documents a large protocol biopsy experience when tacrolimus is used in this way for refractory acute rejection. The protocol biopsies were useful in that some episodes of rejection were diagnosed histologically without a clinical counterpart. Consistent with clinical experience, the tacrolimus dose and blood level were not helpful in determining which patients had either silent or clinically evident rejection. This study also documented that tacrolimus can produce pathologic changes similar to those seen with cyclosporine immunosuppression, including arteriolar hyaline changes and interstitial fibrosis. The impressive improvement of more than 60% using strict pathologic criteria after 2 weeks of tacrolimus therapy in patients with refractory acute rejection is very encouraging. At our own center, we are becoming more comfortable with tacrolimus for prophylaxis and rescue therapy in renal transplantation.

W. Bennett, M.D.

Methylprednisolone Exposure, Rather Than Dose, Predicts Adrenal Suppression and Growth Inhibition in Children With Liver and Renal Transplants

Sarna S, Hoppu K, Neuvonen PJ, et al (Univ of Helsinki)
J Clin Endocrinol Metab 82:75–77, 1997 2–7

Background.—Adverse effects can develop in some patients receiving even very low doses of glucocorticoids. In other patients, the usual therapeutic doses cannot achieve the desired effects. Glucocorticoid exposure rather than the dose may predict the development of adverse effects in children given long-term glucocorticoid therapy.

Methods.—Sixteen liver and 10 renal transplant recipients, aged 2.6 to 15.8 years, were studied. All were receiving triple immunosuppression. Serum total methylprednisolone (MP) and cortisol were assessed before and up to 10 hours after peroral administration of MP. The children's heights were measured 6 months before and after the study day.

Findings.—The MP dose was unassociated with serum cortisol levels and change in height standard deviation score. The area under the serum MP time vs. concentration curve was related inversely to serum cortisol level and to height standard deviation score. This was the best predictor of adrenal function and growth.

Conclusion.—The area under the curve of MP predicted adrenal suppression and growth inhibition better than dose in this group of glucocorticoid-treated children with liver transplants. Dosing according to the area under the curve in children receiving long-term glucocorticoid therapy may greatly decrease the incidence of adverse effects without affecting treatment efficacy.

► The spectrum of glucocorticoid toxicity is familiar to all physicians managing transplant patients. The ratio of the dose-to-adverse effect profile, however, is far from clear. Many patients receiving low doses of steroids have major complications whereas those receiving large doses often have rejection episodes. In a pediatric population, adverse effects of steroids on growth and development are extremely important. In teenagers, the adverse cosmetic effects of steroids can be devastating, leading to noncompliance.

Sarna et al. found that the MP dose in milligrams per kilogram was not associated with serum cortisone values. As in many situations in which drug metabolism is genetically determined, serum MP levels vs. time curves are the best predictor of growth and adrenal function. Obviously, this is not practical in all patients undergoing transplantation. However, in children where growth inhibition is such a disastrous side effect of steroids, it might be prudent to further explore better pharmacologic ways to monitor the amount of therapy that a patient is actually receiving.

W. Bennett, M.D.

Safety and Tolerability of Cyclosporine Microemulsion Versus Cyclosporine: Two-Year Data in Primary Renal Allograft Recipients

Pescovitz MD, for the Neoral Study Group (Indiana Univ, Indianapolis; Univ of Arkansas, Little Rock; Univ Hosps of Cleveland, Ohio; et al)

Transplantation 63:778–780, 1997 2–8

Introduction.—The benefits of cyclosporine (CsA) therapy in solid-organ transplant recipients can be affected by wide variations in its absorption, which lead to marked interindividual and intraindividual variability in the agent's pharmacokinetic behavior. The new microemulsion formulation of CsA (CsA-ME) has improved bioavailability in de novo renal transplant patients. The safety and tolerability of CsA and CsA-ME were compared in 101 renal transplant recipients.

Methods.—In this double-blind, parallel-group multicenter study, 50 patients were randomly assigned to receive CsA and 51 to receive CsA-ME. Patients were given soft gelatin capsules to be taken every 12 hours during the 2-year observation period. Dosages were adjusted according to the standard practice of each center, using whole-blood CsA trough levels. The initial dosage at the time of transplantation was 5 mg/kg administered twice a day.

Results.—The first year of treatment was completed by 29 patients in the CsA-ME group and 26 in the CsA group; all but 1 of these 55 patients continued with the second year of the study. During the second-year extension period, the 2 treatment groups had similar CsA trough blood levels. Mean dosages at the end of 2 years were 4.6 mg/kg per day for CsA-treated patients and 3.8 mg/kg per day for CsA-ME–treated patients. The mean CsA trough levels at study conclusion were 187 and 210 ng/mL for CsA-treated and CsA-ME–treated patients, respectively. There were no deaths during the second year of the study, and although adverse events were common (96% of each group), none required the patient to discontinue treatment. Renal function, as measured by serum creatinine levels, and blood pressure were comparable over time in the CsA and CsA-ME groups.

Conclusions.—After 2 years of treatment, this multicenter study of de novo renal transplant recipients failed to show any significant differences between CsA and CsA-ME groups in laboratory measurements of hepatic, metabolic, or hematologic function. The 2 groups also had similar blood pressure values, renal function, and CsA blood trough levels.

► The new CsA-ME formulation (CsA Neoral) has been widely adopted by transplant centers around the world. This new formulation has more rapid and complete absorption from the gastrointestinal tract than the conventional formulation (Sandimmune). Aside from difference in price favoring the new preparation, it has been difficult to show benefit in terms of number of acute rejection episodes, 1-year graft survival, or patient survival. This multicenter double-blind study of 101 recipients randomly assigned to receive one or the other preparation is probably the best designed of these studies and indeed shows no significant difference in any parameters measured. Without clear-cut benefit of a clinical advantage, many groups have elected not to switch stable patients to the new preparation. Indeed, switching between formulations is difficult unless careful pharmacokinetic analyses are made because CsA Neoral trough levels before the next dose are unreliable in determining the shape of the area under the drug concentration curve. Many examples of CsA nephrotoxicity and some examples of acute rejection caused by rapid metabolism are available in the literature. Furthermore, the use of data from the nontransplant indications of Sandimmune to

Neoral is not warranted unless clinical trials establish the safety of the new preparation.

W. Bennett, M.D.

Prediction of Cyclosporine Area Under the Curve Using a Three-Point Sampling Strategy After Neoral Administration

Gaspari F, Anedda MF, Signorini O, et al (Instituto di Ricerche Farmacologiche Mario Negri, Bergamo, Italy; Ospedali Riuniti, Bergamo, Italy)

J Am Soc Nephrol 8:647–652, 1997 2–9

Introduction.—Cyclosporine A (CsA) is an effective treatment for many disorders and has significantly improved outcome in organ transplantation. The immunosuppressive agent also causes toxic side effects, however, and accurate monitoring of dosage is important. Currently, measurement of the area under the curve (AUC) requires a number of blood samples to be taken during a 12-hour span. A study of kidney transplant recipients sought to determine whether a limited sampling strategy reflected the actual AUC better in patients treated with Neoral than in those given Sandimmune.

Methods.—Eligible patients received kidney transplants 6 months or more before starting the study, had stable CsA dosages for more than 1 month, and stable renal function. During a 2-week stabilization period, the 20 patients received Sandimmune as the trial drug at the same previous maintenance dose. Blood CsA trough levels were measured to determine individual therapeutic windows. After 2 weeks, each patient's 12-hour CsA pharmacokinetic profile was measured after the morning dose of Sandimmune. Patients were then shifted to Neoral at a 1:1 dose ratio, with the daily dose adjusted to maintain the CsA trough level in the established individual therapeutic window. The CsA pharmacokinetics were again evaluated after 2 weeks.

Results.—Pharmacokinetic profiles were more consistent and reproducible after Neoral than after Sandimmune administration. For Neoral, stepwise multiple regression analysis of CsA blood levels showed the best results in AUC prediction with 3 sampling points: 1.5, 8, and 11 hours after dosing. Because blood sampling at 8 and 11 hours is not feasible in routine clinical practice, sample points from 1 to 3 hours after Neoral dosing were considered. A 3-point strategy of 0, 1, and 3 hours after Neoral dosing yielded the best results, providing an excellent correlation between measured and predicted AUC ($r = 0.989$). When a similar analysis was employed after Sandimmune, AUC prediction was poor.

Conclusion.—For patients treated with Neoral, an adequate and accurate prediction of the daily exposure to CsA can be obtained by a simplified sampling strategy that requires blood collection at 0, 1, and 3 hours after Neoral administration. This strategy requires less blood, is less uncomfortable for the patient, and reduces staff time and costs.

► The monitoring of trough cyclosporine blood levels has become routine in clinical practice to estimate the patient's exposure to the drug. It had been hoped that monitoring and adjusting trough blood levels would lead to safe and effective therapy. This hope has not been fully realized since it is now apparent that therapeutic whole blood concentrations can be associated with nephrotoxicity or rejection. With the introduction of cyclosporine Neoral, the problem is further compounded because of the early concentration peak achieved with Neoral followed by more rapid metabolism. Whereas, the 12-hour level is more reliable in the same patient day to day, it is a poor predictor of the area under the concentration curve and thus the total exposure of the patient to the drug. Gaspari et al. have shown that 3 sampling points, 1.5, 8, and 11 hours after Neoral dosing gives a very good prediction of the actual area under the concentration curve. They further document that using levels at 0, 1, and 3 (predose) hours after dosing gives an excellent correlation between measured and predicted area under the curve and should be more suitable for use in clinical practice. These same timepoints after Sandimmune ingestion were associated with unacceptable error. Whether this abbreviated pharmacokinetic approach will find acceptance in the clinical practice will depend on further analysis of its utility in predicting clinical endpoints such as allograft rejection and acute cyclosporine nephrotoxicity. What is clear, however, is that 12-hour trough level monitoring of cyclosporine Neoral can be misleading in terms of the actual drug exposure.

W. Bennett, M.D.

Conversion From Cyclosporine A to Azathioprine Treatment Improves LDL Oxidation in Kidney Transplant Recipients

van den Dorpel MA, Ghanem H, Rischen-Vos J, et al (Univ Hosp Rotterdam, The Netherlands; Erasmus Univ, The Netherlands)

Kidney Int 51:1608–1612, 1997 2–10

Introduction.—Graft survival is significantly improved with the use of cyclosporine A (CsA) after organ transplantation. Hypertension and hyperlipidemia frequently develop in patients treated with CsA, which may contribute to the high incidence of cardiovascular morbidity and mortality in organ recipients. It has been suggested that oxidative modification of low-density lipoproteins (LDL) is important in the initiation and progression of atherosclerosis. Lipid peroxidation may be facilitated in vitro and in vivo by CsA. Several parameters of LDL oxidizability were assessed in renal transplant recipients who were switched from CsA to azathioprine (AZA)-based immunosuppressive treatment.

Methods.—At 6 months or longer after renal transplantation, 19 patients were randomized to either continue CsA treatment or convert from CsA- to AZA-based immunosuppression. During CsA treatment and 16 weeks after randomization, patients were evaluated for susceptibility of LDL to in vitro oxidation, LDL particle size, plasma titers of IgG and IgM antibodies against oxidized LDL, and plasma LDL subclass patterns. Patients also underwent measurements of arterial pressure, glomerular filtration rate, and renal blood flow (estimated from clearance of radiolabeled thalamate and hippurate).

Results.—There was a decrease in plasma concentrations of total cholesterol, LDL, cholesterol, and triglyceride. There was no change in plasma HDL cholesterol. During the CsA phase, plasma LDL was significantly more susceptible to in vitro oxidation. With conversion to AZA, the LDL size increased and titers of IgM- and IgG-autoantibodies against oxidized LDL decreased significantly. Five of 13 patients with an atherogenic LDL subclass pattern B changed to pattern A after conversion. Patients converted to AZA had a decrease in mean arterial pressure and a significant increase in renal function.

Conclusion.—Compared to AZA therapy, CsA administration seems to increase the susceptibility of LDL to in vivo and in vitro oxidation. Combined with lower arterial pressure and improved renal function, conversion to AZA from CsA may decrease the risk of atherosclerosis in renal transplant recipients.

► Hyperlipidemia following renal transplant is a potent risk factor for cardiovascular disease. Since the most common cause of death in kidney transplant patients is cardiovascular disease, and since this may occur despite good function of the transplant, attention must be directed toward management of those risk factors that can minimize this problem. While cyclosporine is a superior immunosuppressant and has improved short-term survival rates in renal transplantation, the drug has been associated with unfavorable plasma lipid profiles. Oxidative modification of LDL cholesterol is an important factor in progression of atherosclerosis. This shows that during cyclosporine therapy, plasma LDL is more susceptible to in vitro oxidation than during the time when the same patient is treated with azathioprine. The most atherogenic LDL subclass was present in the majority of patients receiving cyclosporine, and in 5 of these patients, the pattern changed following conversion to azathioprine. In addition to these effects on lipids, mean arterial pressure and renal function improved significantly after conversion. It would be of interest to know if these same patterns of improvement in LDL oxidation might be achieved with medical therapy in patients continuing on cyclosporine. This obviously is an important point for long-term immunosuppressive drug strategy.

W. Bennett, M.D.

Cyclosporine Protects Glomeruli From FSGS Factor via an Increase in Glomerular cAMP

Sharma R, Sharma M, Ge X, et al (Med College of Wisconsin, Milwaukee)
Transplantation 62:1916–1920, 1996 2–11

Background.—In patients with recurrent focal segmental glomerulosclerosis (FSGS) after transplantation, cyclosporine results in proteinuria remission. Sera from patients with recurrent FSGS can increase the glomerular albumin permeability. Increased glomerular cAMP concentrations can change the permeability characteristics of glomeruli in vitro. Whether the increased glomerular levels of cAMP were associated with the protective effects of cyclosporine (CsA) on an increase in glomerular albumin permeability by FSGS sera was determined.

Methods.—Glomeruli from rats given intraperitoneal CsA, cremophore, or saline for 5 days were incubated with a 1:50 dilution of serum from 3 patients with FSGS or pooled normal human serum before calculation of glomerular albumin permeability. Glomerular cAMP was assessed by radioimmunoassay and glomerular ultrastructural changes by transmission electron microscopy.

Findings.—Serum from the patients with FSGS markedly increased albumin permeability of glomeruli from rats given saline or cremophore. However, albumin permeability of glomeruli from CsA-treated rats was not increased by any FSGS sample. Glomerular cAMP increased fivefold in rats given CsA compared with the cremophore- and saline-treated rats. After CsA treatment, glomerular basement membrane appeared to be thickened, and the lamina densa had an irregular appearance. There were no ultrastructural changes in glomerular epithelial or endothelial cells.

Conclusion.—Cyclosporine may have a direct protective effect on the glomerular filtration barrier in FSGS. Increased levels of glomerular cAMP by CsA may play an important role in protecting the glomerular albumin permeability effect of the FSGS factor. It may also contribute to proteinuria remission in patients with FSGS.

► Focal and segmental glomerulosclerosis is a relatively common cause of renal failure in children and in many adults. A circulating humoral factor is present in many cases of this disease, resulting in prompt recurrence of the disease after kidney transplantation. Savin and associates have previously reported the presence of a circulating factor in the plasma of patients with recurrent focal and segmental glomerulosclerosis which is associated with increased glomerular permeability to albumin.[1] The study abstracted here extends these observations and strikingly demonstrates the protection of isolated rat glomeruli by cyclosporine treatment. Furthermore, the protection was associated with increases in glomerular cyclic AMP. These data are best demonstrated in Figure 3 from the original article.These intriguing observations form a rational basis for pharmacotherapy of focal and segmental glomerulosclerosis in primary renal disease caused by this process in children and adults.

W. Bennett, M.D.

Reference

1. Savin VJ, Sharma R, Sharma M, et al: Circulating factor associated with increased glomerular permeability to albumin in recurrent focal segmental glomerulosclerosis. *N Engl J Med* 334:878, 1996.

Patient Management

Diagnostic Contribution of Renal Allograft Biopsies at Various Intervals After Transplantation

Kon SP, Templar J, Dodd SM, et al (Royal London Hosp)
Transplantation 63:547–550, 1997 2–12

Background.—The gold standard for assessing episodes of graft dysfunction in the early posttransplant period is renal allograft biopsy. However, later renal biopsies done for graft dysfunction or as part of routine care have not been critically evaluated.

Methods.—Two hundred sixty-three consecutive renal allograft biopsy specimens at 1 center were analyzed. One hundred seventeen were performed in the first 3 months (group 1); 60, between 4 and 12 months (group 2); and 86, more than 12 months after transplantation (group 3).

Findings.—A significant reduction in the frequency of acute rejection was noted in group 3 compared with groups 1 and 2. The frequency of chronic rejection was significantly greater in group 3 than in groups 1 and 2. Acute tubular necrosis occurred almost exclusively in group 1. Cyclosporin A nephrotoxicity was an important cause of graft dysfunction in all 3 groups, with no significant differences. The biopsy report prompted management changes for 72% of group 1 patients, 75% of group 2 patients, and 19% of group 3 patients.

Conclusion.—Late renal allograft biopsies are usually not helpful in patient management. Thus, such biopsies should only be performed as a last resort.

▶ Renal allograft biopsy has proven to be the standard for diagnosing renal allograft dysfunction, particularly in the early posttransplant period. It is obvious that no nonbiopsy technique is well enough accepted or validated to avoid the need for histologic examination of the allograft. Clearly, in the early postoperative period when rejection, ischemic renal injury, and drug toxicity are the major differential diagnosis, biopsies are useful.

The report by Kon et al. shows that almost three quarters of patients undergoing biopsy during this interval had major changes in management based on the biopsy findings. These authors, however, performed biopsies on patients at later intervals after transplant and at 6 months, the biopsy resulted in major changes in therapy, based on the findings. A much smaller percentage of patients had management changes based on biopsy findings performed 1 to 2 years after transplantation. In the patients who did have abnormal biopsy specimens at late times post transplant, cyclosporin A nephrotoxicity was the overwhelming diagnosis, and this diagnosis probably would have been possible without the need for biopsy. Thus, it is clear that the major utility of a transplant biopsy occurs in the first months after transplantation when the differential diagnosis between acute allograft rejection and drug toxicity is difficult. Late renal biopsies very seldom add to information needed for proper patient management.

W. Bennett, M.D.

Treatment of Postrenal Transplant Erythrocytosis: Long-Term Efficacy and Safety of Angiotensin-converting Enzyme Inhibitors

MacGregor MS, Rowe PA, Watson, MA, et al (Western Infirmary, Glasgow, Scotland; Derriford Hosp, Plymouth, England)

Nephron 74:517–521, 1996 2–13

Introduction.—Postrenal transplant erythrocytosis (PRTE) is diagnosed in up to 22% of all renal transplants, occurs despite good graft function, and can lead to serious thrombotic complications. Several short-term studies with small numbers of patients have shown angiotensin-converting enzyme inhibitors (ACE-I) to lower hemoglobin (Hb) in PRTE, but the longer-term safety and efficacy of this treatment is not known. Therefore, patients who received an ACE-I for a median of 13 months to control PRTE were studied.

Methods.—Patients were selected for treatment on the basis of erythrocytosis, defined as a Hb level of 17 $g \cdot dL^{-1}$ or greater in men and 16 $g \cdot dL^{-1}$ or greater in women, or an ongoing requirement for venesection to maintain Hb below these levels. Forty-three of the 52 patients were men; the mean age at start of ACE-I treatment was 46.5 years. Glomerulonephritis was the primary renal disease in 46% of cases; 62% of patients had been receiving hemodialysis and 37%, continuous ambulatory peritoneal dialysis. Thirty patients were treated with lisinopril and 22 with enalapril, reaching a maximum daily dose of 5 mg.

Results.—Mean Hb levels decreased in both men (from 16.7 to 14.9 $g \cdot dL^{-1}$) and women (from 15.8 to 14.2 $g \cdot dL^{-1}$) after 3 months of ACE-I treatment (Fig 1). Because most patients were being managed with venesection, Hb was lower than the intervention threshold. The maximum effect of ACE-I was seen by 3 months, and lisinopril and enalapril yielded similar results. Mean systemic arterial blood pressure showed significant decreases at both 6 months and 12 months. Serum creatinine and serum potassium levels were unchanged throughout the treatment period. Sixteen patients had the ACE-I withdrawn, primarily because of deterioration in renal function and/or anemia. These and other complications were all reversible. The agents were ineffective in 3 patients.

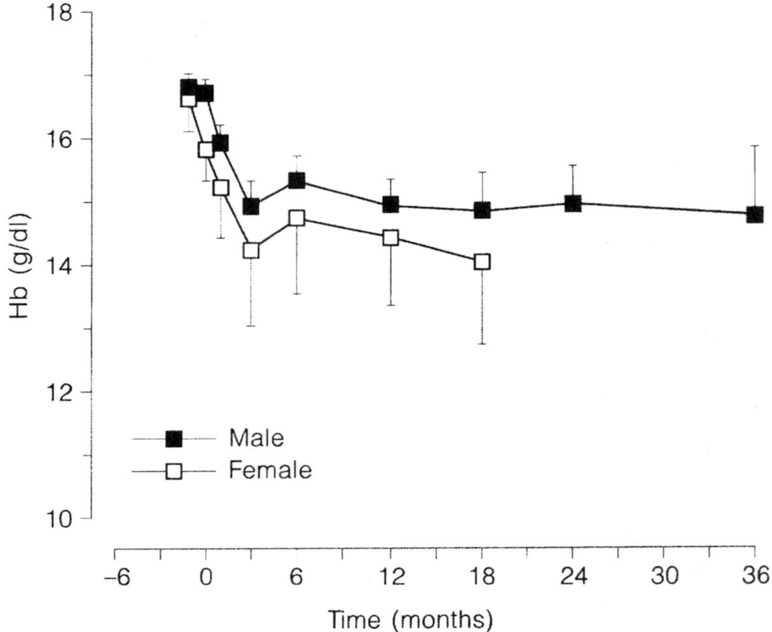

FIGURE 1.—Change in hemoglobin Hb with time, divided according to gender. Angiotensin-converting enzyme inhibitor ACE-I was commenced at time 0. *Points* are means with 95% confidence intervals. After withdrawal of ACE-I, patients are excluded from the analysis. (Courtesy of MacGregor MS, Rowe PA, Watson MA, et al: Treatment of postrenal transplant erythrocytosis: Long-term efficacy and safety of angiotensin-converting enzyme inhibitors. *Nephron* 74:517–521, copyright 1996, S. Karger AG, Basel, publisher.)

Conclusions.—Lisinopril and enalapril are safe and effective when used in the long-term treatment of PRTE. Low doses of the drugs were adequate, and complications were neither serious nor irreversible. Compared with venesection treatment, ACE-I is more convenient and more effective.

▶ Erythrocytosis after renal transplantation can be a potent risk factor for thrombotic complications, including stroke and other cardiovascular events. Erythrocytosis affects approximately 20% of all transplant recipients, and while its pathogenesis is still not completely understood, the efficacy of ACE inhibitors has provided a simple, safe treatment of this disorder. Most groups start such treatment when the hematocrit is in the high 40s or low 50s based on the realization that the blood viscosity rises abruptly with hematocrits greater than 53%. The experience of MacGregor et al. is instructive, with stable hematocrits during follow-up of up to 3 years (Fig 1). This therapy is, of course, not free of complications such as hyperkalemia and overshoot anemia, as well as drug-related declines in renal function. It is prudent to start with very low doses of ACE inhibitor and gradually increase the doses. Early evidence suggests that the angiotensin II receptor antagonist will be equally effective for this purpose.

W. Bennett, M.D.

No Trend Toward a Spontaneous Improvement of Hyperparathyroidism and High Bone Turnover in Normocalcemic Long-term Renal Transplant Recipients

Dumoulin G, Hory B, Nguyen NU, et al (Centre Hospitalier Universitaire, Besançon, France)

Am J Kidney Dis 29:746–753, 1997 2–14

Introduction.—It is not known how the parathyroid gland adapts to graft restoration of renal function. Excessive parathyroid hormone (PTH) secretion remains common in renal transplant recipients, even those with normal renal function. Calcium-regulating hormones, calcium-phosphate metabolism, and serum osteocalcin were evaluated as a marker of bone remodeling in 82 normocalcemic renal transplant recipients (6–73 months previously) with good renal function.

Methods.—Recipients and 82 well-matched healthy control subjects underwent fasting serum samples for: PTH, 1,25-$(OH)_2$, 25(OH)D, osteocalcin, total and ionized calcium, phosphate, creatinine, and albumin and 24-hour urinary phosphate and creatinine. Subgroups consisting of 25 members of each group underwent matching of serum creatinine and creatinine clearance.

Results.—Excessive PTH secretion was observed in transplant recipients, compared to control subjects (6.9 pmol/L vs 3.0 pmol/L). The recipient group had significantly higher bone turnover than control subjects (osteocalcin 16.6 µg/L vs 8.0 µg/L). An inappropriate PTH secretion was observed in recipients, as demonstrated by a slightly higher ionized calcium level than in control subjects. Creatinine clearance and serum creatinine were similar in the subgroups of 25 control subjects and recipients matched for creatinine clearance. In the subgroup of recipients, serum PTH, osteocalcin, ionized calcium, and serum 1,25-$(OH)_2D$ were significantly higher, compared to control subjects. Serum phosphate, TRP, and Tmp/GFR were significantly lower in recipients than in control subjects.

Conclusion.—Compared to control subjects, renal transplant recipients had excessive secretion of PTH, renal phosphate wasting, and high bone turnover. Recipients had an adequate 1,25-$(OH)_2D$ synthesis. There was no biologic evidence of a spontaneous improvement of these bone mineral disturbances after renal transplantation. The positive association between PTH levels and serum osteocalcin emphasizes the contribution of PTH to high bone turnover in long-term renal transplant recipients.

► Metabolic bone disease is present in some form in nearly every patient who will undergo kidney transplantation. Following transplantation with normalization of renal function, metabolic bone disease is thought to improve. However, some of the medications used in transplantation, such as corticosteroids and calcineurin-inhibiting immunosuppressive drugs (cyclosporine, tacrolimus) may increase bone turnover. It had been thought that patients with persistent hyperparathyroidism would spontaneously improve with a prolonged period of normal renal function. This was thought to be the rule in patients who had relatively normal serum calcium levels posttransplant. The data of Dumoulin et al. put this idea to rest. They observed 82 normocalcemic renal transplant recipients with excellent renal function and matched them to healthy control subjects for age and sex. The important results of their study are that even following successful renal transplant, there is excessive parathyroid hormone secretion and high bone turnover. The long-term effects of this on bone health is, of course, unknown, but much more study is indicated to assess the consequences of prolonged hyperparathyroidism. This could even have a role in progressive renal dysfunction over time (chronic allograft failure), which is so common in transplant recipients.

W. Bennett, M.D.

Monoclonal Gammopathy After Intense Induction Immunosuppression in Renal Transplant Patients

Passweg J, Thiel G, Bock HA (Kantonsspital Basel, Switzerland)

Nephrol Dial Transplant 11:2461–2465, 1996 2–15

Background.—Monoclonal gammopathy, a potential premalignant state, is not uncommon after transplantation. A large renal transplant recipient population was evaluated to determine the incidence, clinical course, and risk factors of monoclonal gammopathy.

Methods.—The 1982–1991 charts of all renal transplant recipients were reviewed in Basel. During the period of this study, 490 transplants were performed in 451 patients. Patients were examined annually and underwent standard renal and hematologic parameter determinations, complete history and physical examinations, and protein- and immunoelectrophoresis. The study group included all patients who had at least 1 year of follow-up by January 1994. All patients with pre-existing gammopathy were excluded. The final study group consisted of 390 kidney transplants. Initial immunosuppression consisted of cyclosporine A (CsA) with or without prednisone (Pred) from 1982 to 1984, CsA + Pred +ATG-Fresenius (antithyroglobulin) (ATG-F) from 1985 to 1986, CsA + Pred + azathioprine (Aza) from 1987 to 1988, and CsA + Aza+ Pred + either ATG-F or OKT3 (quadruple immunosuppression) from 1989 until the end of the study. Immunosuppression was reduced to CsA alone whenever possible.

Findings.—Among the 390 transplants included in this study, 46 cases of clonal gammopathy were detected. Thirty of those were detected within the first 2 years of follow-up. Of the 46 gammopathies, 35 were monoclonal and 11 were bi- or triclonal. There was a predominance of IgG and κ light-chain subtypes. Gammopathy was transient in 17 patients. The 5-year cumulative gammopathy incidence was 10.7%, significantly higher than the rate in the general population. Gammopathy was never observed to progress to multiple myeloma over the 1- to 10-year follow-up in this patient group. One patient did have Kaposi's sarcoma. The incidence of gammopathy was significantly higher in patients receiving transplants after 1989, than in those receiving transplants before 1989. This date coincides with the introduction of quadruple induction immunosuppression therapy. The risk of acquiring gammopathy within 2 years of transplantation was 14.7% after quadruple induction therapy, but only 3.0% without this type of therapy. The risk for patients receiving quadruple therapy with OKT3 was 24.5%, significantly higher than 11.8% for those who received quadruple therapy with ATG-F. Discriminant analysis indicated that the type of immunosuppression, but not age or year of transplant, was an independent risk factor for the development of gammopathy.

Conclusions.—Monoclonal gammopathy appears to be common after renal transplantation. The risk of gammopathy is higher among patients receiving quadruple induction immunosuppression regimens, particularly if those regimens include OKT3. These patients require monitoring for the potential early detection of malignant transformation.

► The increased incidence of malignancy after renal transplant with immunosuppressive therapy is of concern to all clinicians making the decision on the modality of treatment for an individual patient with end-stage renal disease. Careful screening for cancer is done preoperatively and then surveillance is maintained in the postoperative state, particularly in patients who have heavy treatment for acute rejection. Monoclonal gammopathy, both of solid organs and bone marrow, has been observed after transplantation, but its course is not well characterized. In the general population, monoclonal gammopathy may be a prelude to multiple myoloma and other lymphoproliferative diseases. Passweg et al. report a rather large experience of monoclonal gammopathy occurring after renal transplantation. The risk of development of this condition is higher for patients receiving induction immunosuppression, particularly if it contains OKT3. Although the exact significance of this is unclear, the authors' admonition that patients be observed carefully for development of malignant transformation is prudent, because the follow-up in this series was very short. It is also worthwhile to note that the 5-year cumulative incidence of this condition was 10.7%. Only longer term follow-up studies will ascertain the significance of this finding and its relationship to induction immunosuppression.

W. Bennett, M.D.

Technetium-99m-MAG3 Scintigraphy in Acute Renal Failure After Transplantation: Marker of Viability and Prognosis

Tulchinsky M, Dietrich TJ, Eggli DF, et al (Pennsylvania State Univ, Hershey)

J Nucl Med 38:475–478, 1997 2–16

Introduction.—A retrospective review of patients who had renal nuclear medicine scans for suspected early posttransplantation kidney dysfunction was conducted to assess the prognostic value of technetium-99m-mercaptoacetyltriglycine (MAG3), a recently introduced renal tubular radiopharmaceutical agent. The hypothesis was that cortical uptake of MAG3

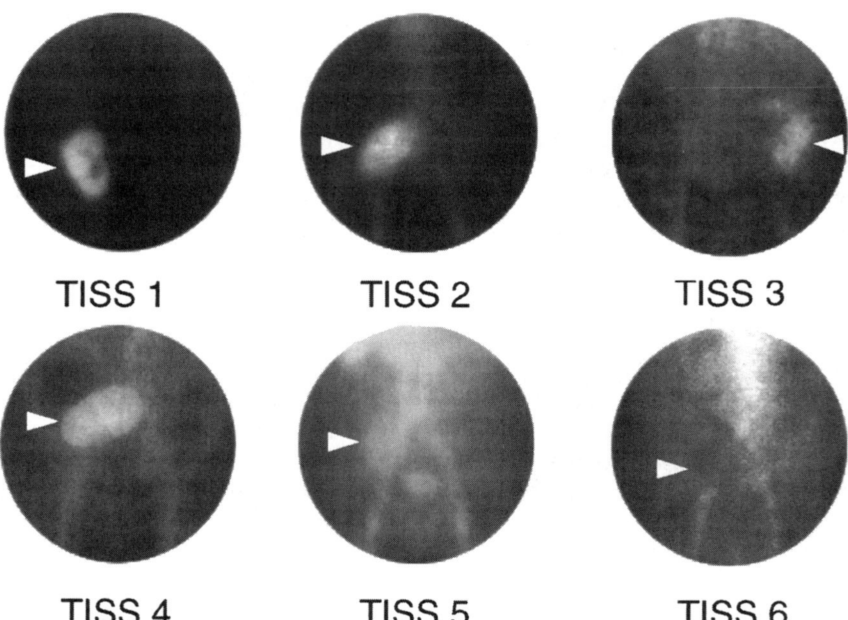

FIGURE 1.—Representative images illustrate corresponding tubular injury severity scores (TISS). These images are summations of frames acquired for 75 seconds, starting from the end of the first minute after injection. (Reprinted by permission of the Society of Nuclear Medicine, from Tulchinsky M, Dietrich TJ, Eggli DF, et al: Technetium-99m-MAG3 scintigraphy in acute renal failure after transplantation: Marker of viability and prognosis. *J Nucl Med* 38:475–478, 1997.)

would parallel the amount of residual viable tubular mass—poor uptake implying irreversible damage and good uptake predicting improvement in renal function.

Methods.—Sixty-four patients underwent renal scintigraphy at the study institution from October 1990 through September 1994; scans were requested for suspected early postransplantation kidney dysfunction. In 52 cases, there was early postoperative failure to make urine and rising serum creatinine or both. Renal scintigraphy was performed on an urgent basis. A cortical uptake phase image, consisting of a 2-minute image acquired 1 minute after MAG 3 administration, was visually analyzed for the amount of MAG 3 extraction by the transplant. A qualitative 6-level grading system was used, yielding a tubular injury severity score (TISS): the higher the score, the lower the residual tubular viability (Fig 1).

Results.—Six patients sustained irreversible renal failure and had to undergo removal of the transplant within 1 month after surgery. In the remaining 58 patients, renal function improved sufficiently to sustain dialysis-free living for 1 year after transplantation. All 5 patients with a TISS of 5 or 6 lost the transplant, whereas only 1 of 10 patients with a TISS of 4 required transplant removal. Renal transplant function was recovered in all patients with a TISS less than 4.

Conclusion.—If patients with early postoperative renal transplant dysfunction could be accurately assessed for the likelihood of functional recovery, those certain to lose the transplants could benefit from early termination of immunosuppression and transplant removal. The findings in this series of patients suggest that MAG3 scans with the cortical uptake phase image offer an accurate prognosis of transplant outcome.

▶ Delayed graft function is an important prognostic factor for chronic renal allograft failure. In addition, knowing the prognosis of a patient with delayed graft function is important in planning hospital discharge, intensity of follow-up, and, indeed, the frequency of surveillance for acute rejection, superimposed on the delayed allograft function. Tulchinsky et al., using the radioisotope MAG3, have shown a relatively simple imaging technique, which uses the isotope count in the kidney cortex 1 minute after administration of the isotope. This index was correlated with recovery from delayed graft function. The authors used a scoring system for ranking the nuclear medicine studies, and in 64 patients, tests proved to be useful in ascertaining prognosis. A prospective study of this relatively simple technique is needed. The images obtained and their scoring system are shown in Figure 1.

W. Bennett, M.D.

The High Prevalence of Severe Early Posttransplant Renal Allograft Pathology in Hepatitis C Positive Recipients

Cosio FG, Sedmak DD, Henry ML, et al (Ohio State Univ, Columbus)

Transplantation 62:1054–1059, 1996 2–17

Background.—Approximately 10% to 15% of American recipients of renal allografts have serum antibodies to hepatitis C virus (HCV). There are reasons to believe that HCV may have a negative impact on graft survival. To evaluate the impact of HCV infection on the early posttransplant period, allograft complications during the first 6 months after renal transplantation were examined at a single institution.

Study Design.—The study group consisted of 32 adult recipients of renal allografts who were HCV+ (R-HCV), 48 recipients who were HCV− and received cadaveric renal allografts from HCV+ donors (D-HCV), and 204 HCV− recipients who received HCV− cadaveric kidneys control. Hepatitis C virus serology was available for all recipients. All patients in the study group received transplants at the Ohio State University from 1993 to 1994 and were treated with an immunosuppressive protocol. Renal allograft biopsies performed during the first 6 months posttransplant were analyzed by physicians blinded to the HCV status of the patients.

Findings.—The prevalence of acute tubulointerstitial rejection was not significantly different among these 3 groups of patients. Both R-HCV and D-HCV patients had a significantly greater prevalence of acute transplant glomerulopathy than control patients. Acute vascular rejection and chronic vascular rejection were significantly more prevalent in R-HCV patients than in control patients. Chronic vascular rejection was diagnosed sooner in R-HCV than in control patients.

Conclusions.—These results reveal that HCV+ recipients of renal transplants have a higher prevalence of severe acute pathologic changes in their allografts shortly after transplantation than HCV− allograft recipients. Chronic vascular rejection is also more prevalent and develops earlier in HCV+ recipients. The previously reported association between HCV and acute transplant glomerulopathy was also confirmed. The effect of HCV infection on long-term renal allograft survival is an issue of concern and requires further study.

▶ The problem of HCV in renal transplantation is controversial. Ten percent of eventual candidates from dialysis units have antibodies to this virus. The pathologic changes in renal allografts in recipients who were already HCV-positive or who have HCV from an HCV donor are striking. Also, the presence of vascular rejection of both acute and chronic types is alarming. These data seem to be confirmed by the recent study of Stehman-Breen et al.,[1] showing an increased risk of kidney failure and death in recipients of 137 kidney pancreas transplants at the University of Washington. The relative risk of death was almost 4 times as great as in patients without HCV infection, and these deaths were the result of liver failure as opposed to the deaths in uninfected control patients, which were primarily cardiovascular. Interestingly, pancreatic allograft failure was not impacted by HCV. Thus, the current policy of using HCV donors for HCV-positive recipients or using HCV-positive donors at all will have to be closely followed in the next few years.

W. Bennett, M.D.

Reference

1. Stehman-Breen CO, Psaty B, Emerson S, et al: Association of hepatitis C virus infection with mortality and graft survival in kidney-pancreas transplant recipients. *Transplantation* 64:281–286, 1997.

Results

Preemptive Cadaveric Renal Transplantation: Clinical Outcome
Roake JA, Cahill AP, Gray CM, et al (Univ of Oxford, England)
Transplantation 62:1411–1416, 1996 2–18

Introduction.—Current practice regarding renal transplantation for patients with end-stage renal disease and no available living donor is to establish such patients on chronic dialysis, then consider them for a cadaveric transplant program. With preemptive cadaveric renal transplantation (PCRT), the procedure is performed before the predicted time at which renal replacement therapy would be required. Because there are both benefits and disadvantages to each strategy, the results of conventional cadaveric renal transplantation were compared with those of PCRT.

Methods.—Between 1975 and 1995, 116 transplants performed at the Oxford Transplant Center fulfilled criteria for PCRT. A cohort of 116 patients who were dialysis dependent before transplantation was matched to the preemptively transplanted patients by recipient age and sex, year transplanted, initial immunosuppression, and, if possible, ABO group.

Results.—On the whole, patient survival was significantly better after PCRT, and this advantage continued to increase with time. The long-term survival advantage of PCRT suggests that the difference was not an effect of transplanting patients earlier in the course of their disease. Graft survival was also significantly better in the PCRT group; actuarial graft survival was 84.3% at 1 year and 72.8% at 5 years for PCRT. Corresponding graft survival rates for the control group were 72.8% and 56.9%, respectively. Much of the difference in graft survival could be attributed to the excess deaths among controls (24 vs.10), but there was a trend toward better graft survival after excluding death with a functioning graft as a cause of failure. Findings were similar when analysis was limited to the 100 patients managed on cyclosporin A–based protocols. Among surviving grafts, the 2 groups did not differ in graft function as assessed by plasma creatinine levels.

Conclusions.—Both patient and graft survival were better when patients with end-stage renal disease were preemptively transplanted than when they were transplanted after being established on chronic dialysis. There was a trend toward more late deaths among controls, probably because fewer patients selected for PCRT had diabetes or renal vascular disease. Whereas PCRT appears to be safe and clinical outcome is good, this management practice may deny organs to patients who are already dialysis dependent.

▶ Most patients who consult with transplant physicians seeking information regarding renal transplantation during the course of chronic renal failure desire to be transplanted before dialysis. The implications both for cadaver organ supply and financial matters are a matter of some concern and interest. The data of Roake et al. are the first to compare outcomes of preemptive transplantation with cadaveric transplantation done at the more usual levels of renal dysfunction. Not surprisingly, patient and graft survival were significantly better in the preemptive group. This was not explainable by better patient survival because when death with the functioning graft was excluded as a variable, differences still persisted. However, renal function was no different at 1, 2, and 3 years after transplant. Thus, while preemptive renal transplantation is safe, the issue as to the effect of widespread implication of this policy on utilization of a precious resource, namely cadaver kidneys, and financial costs must be factored in. A comprehensive analysis including time loss from work, economic aspects of instituting dialysis, and many other factors should be considered. The issue remains controversial, particularly for patients with diabetes in whom transplantation earlier in the course of chronic renal failure has been strongly advocated by some.

W. Bennett, M.D.

Donor Age and Graft Function

Gellert S, Devaux S, Schönberger B, et al (Humboldt Univ, Berlin; Friedrichshain Hosp, Berlin)

Pediatr Nephrol 10:716–719, 1996 2–19

Background.—Previous research has raised the question as to how kidney function adapts when donors and recipients are of different ages and body sizes. Survival and renal function of cadaveric donor grafts according to donor age were investigated.

Methods.—One hundred five children with 114 kidney grafts were studied. Forty-six children, with a median age of 11.8 years, received their first graft from child donors whose median age was 7 years. The remaining 59 children, aged a median 12.1 years, received a first graft from adult donors aged a median of 34.4 years. Thirty recipients were treated with azathioprine and prednisolone, and 75 were given cyclosporin A and prednisolone. Glomerular filtration rate (GFR) and the effective renal plasma flow (ERPF) were assessed 1 to 48 months after transplantation.

Findings.—Graft survival did not differ significantly between the groups. In addition, GFR did not differ between groups. Two to three months after transplantation, the mean GFR in pediatric graft recipients was 62 mL/min/1.73 m^2, compared with 61 mL/min/1.73m^2 in adult graft recipients. In the first month after transplantation, ERPF in adult graft recipients was significantly greater than in pediatric graft recipients, a difference that disappeared at the fourth to the sixth month. The ERPF of grafts from pediatric donors was a mean 279 mL/min/1.73m^2, compared with 273 mL/min/1.73 m^2 in adult donor grafts. Compared with the single-kidney GFR and ERPF in an age-matched group of probands with minor diseases, mean GFRs of pediatric and adult donor grafts increase to 118% and decreased to 60%, respectively, 2–3 months after transplantation. After 4–6 months, ERPFs in pediatric and adult grafts were 96% and 50%, respectively.

Conclusion.—Mean GFRs and ERPFs were comparable in child recipients of pediatric and adult kidney grafts in relation to the body surface area of the recipient 2–3 months after transplantation. Graft function appears to adapt to the requirement of the recipient.

► There has always been a question about the fate of donor kidneys from children. This recent study by Gellert et al. observed a large number of patients with kidney transplants coming from pediatric donors with a mean age of 7 years, as well as pediatric recipients who received a first transplant from adult donors. There was no difference in allograft survival between those receiving pediatric and adult transplants. There was also no difference observable in GFR between pediatric and adult donors 2 to 3 months after the transplantation was performed. Although renal blood flow estimated by the iodine-125 hippurate clearance was increased shortly after transplantation in recipients of adult donors, this difference disappeared by the fourth to sixth month after transplantation. This rather large experience would seem to emphasize the difficulty in extrapolating from experimental animal models in which progression factors can be viewed in isolation from the clinical situation. Although theoretical concerns still exist, this paper gives reassurance to those who use adult kidney donors for pediatric recipients.

W. Bennett, M.D.

Impact of Acute Rejection and Early Allograft Function on Renal Allograft Survival

Cosio FG, Pelletier RP, Falkenhain ME, et al (Ohio State Univ, Columbus)
Transplantation 63:1611–1615, 1997 2–20

Introduction.—Understanding the relationship between acute rejection (AR), graft function, and graft survival can enhance understanding of chronic transplant nephropathy and its prevention. The relationship between AR and graft function was assessed in 843 adult recipients of first cadaveric renal grafts to determine the impact of these factors alone or in combination.

Findings.—Follow-up was a minimum of 3.5 years. During follow-up, 23% of patients died and 15% lost their allograft. Patients were placed in 1 of 4 groups, depending on history of AR and concentration of serum creatinine during the first 6 months after transplantation. There were no significant between-group differences in death censored allografts in: group 1 (376 patients) no AR and low SCr_{6mo}, group 2 (117 patients) no AR and elevated SCr_{6mo}, or group 3 (185 patients) AR and low SCr_{6mo}. Compared to these 3 groups, the 165 patients in group 4 with AR and elevated SCr_{6mo} had a significantly worse graft survival. In group 4, 32% of patients had an elevated SCr at 10 days after transplantation (SCr_{10d}, before onset of AR, that was higher than or equal to SCr_{6mo}). Using these observations, the implications of SCr_{10d} concentration on graft prognosis were evaluated. There was a weak correlation between SCr_{10d} and graft survival. An elevated SCr_{10d} was significantly correlated with other potential risk factors for graft survival: male recipient, older donors, heavier recipients, and the posttransplant factors of increasing numbers of AR, high posttransplant blood pressure, and lower doses of cyclosporine.

Conclusion.—When correlated with AR, graft dysfunction predicts poor graft survival. Acute rejection predicts poor allograft survival only when correlated with graft dysfunction. The SCr_{10d} may be considered an indicator of risk factors from the donor and recipient and predicts a higher risk of acquiring additional risk factors in the early transplantation period.

▶ There is considerable debate about prognostic factors for chronic allograft failure. It is clear from retrospective data that acute rejection is a major risk factor for chronic rejection, and that delayed graft function, presumably due to ischemia reperfusion injury, predisposes the kidney to immunologic events independently shortening the half-life of a kidney transplant. The retrospective analysis of a single center experience in 843 recipients of first-cadaver transplants observed for a minimum of 3.5 years attempts to put these risk factors into perspective. The elevation of serum creatinine level at 10 days (a surrogate for delayed graft function) correlated inversely with graft survival; however, in combination with other risk factors such as older donors, male recipients, and obese patients, and, most importantly, acute rejection episodes and high posttransplant blood pressure, predicted poor graft survival. If there was no early graft dysfunction, acute rejection was not associated with a bad long-term prognosis. Thus, further attempts to minimize cold ischemia time and thus, delayed graft function, as well as potent immunosuppression to delay or prevent acute rejection, should improve long-term allograft survival.

W. Bennett, M.D.

Absence of Deleterious Effect on Long-term Kidney Graft Survival of Rejection Episodes With Complete Functional Recovery

Vereerstraeten P, Abramowicz D, De Pauw L, et al (Université Libre De Bruxelles, Brussels, Belgium)

Transplantation 63:1739–1743, 1997 2–21

Introduction.—Long-term graft outcome is known to be adversely affected by rejection episodes (RE) that occur early in the course of kidney transplantation, but little is known about the impact of the severity of early RE or of factors predictive of severity. These questions were examined in a retrospective study of 487 adult recipients of cadaver kidney transplants.

Methods.—The patients received 582 kidney transplants during the period from August 1983 to December 1995. Biopsy-proven RE occurring during the first year after transplantation were graded as benign (without loss of graft function), severe (partial loss of graft function), or irreversible (return to dialysis). Grafts were then divided into 4 groups: group 1 included 267 grafts free of RE; group 2, 101 grafts with benign RE; group 3, 65 grafts with severe RE; and group 4, 58 grafts with irreversible RE. At the end point of all statistical analyses of graft survival (May 31, 1996), 25 patients had not completed the first posttransplant years and were excluded from survival analyses.

Results.—In multivariate analyses, variables significantly associated with the occurrence of RE during the first posttransplant year were primary immunosuppression with cyclosporine rather than with OKT3 monoclonal antibody, the number of HLA-B + DR mismatches, and younger age of recipient. Among patients with rejection, OKT3 monoclonal antibody prophylaxis was used less often in group 4 (irreversible RE) patients than in patients with reversible RE (groups 2 and 3). No single factor differentiated patients with benign RE from those with severe RE. Graft survival at 1 year was significantly lower in patients with severe RE than in those with no RE or benign RE. Eight-year survival rates were 89% for the no RE or benign RE groups and 60% for the severe RE group. There was a significant correlation between graft survival after 1 year and serum creatinine value.

Discussion.—The severity of RE occurring during the first posttransplant year appears to have an important impact on graft function. Rejection episodes classified as benign, with no loss of graft function during the first year, do not have a negative impact on long-term kidney graft outcome.

▶ The greatest risk factor for chronic allograft rejection is the occurrence of acute rejection. Acute rejection increases the relative risk of chronic rejection up to eightfold. The retrospective analysis of 582 cadaver kidney transplants showed that acute rejection, if there was return to baseline serum creatinine, was associated with graft survival the same as in patients without acute rejection episodes. This was in distinction to rejections not returning to baseline creatinine or requiring dialysis which were associated with a much inferior prognosis for long-term graft function. The mystery of chronic allograft failure and the significance of a single rejection episode continues to be controversial. It is important to note that pathologic evidence of rejection in routine allograft biopsies with no renal dysfunction can have the same Banff pathologic score as clinically diagnosed rejection episodes. Studies like this cast some doubt on the use of acute rejection per se as a surrogate marker for long-term benefits of new antirejection therapies. Although long-term studies of renal structure and function are expensive to define the utility of new immunosuppressive therapy, they are required if replacement of older regimens that have proved effective are to be abandoned.

W. Bennett, M.D.

Kidney Transplant Recipients Who Die With Functioning Grafts: Serum Creatinine Level and Cause of Death

West M, Sutherland DER, Matas AJ (Univ of Minnesota, Minneapolis)
Transplantation 62:1029–1030, 1996 2–22

Background.—In analyzing transplant survival statistics, standard practice is to include "death with function" (DWF) as a graft loss. The University of Minnesota renal transplant group has suggested that the data be analyzed with and without DWF as a graft loss to increase the evaluable information available from these data. To determine whether patients with DWF had kidney impairment that hastened their death, the serum creatinine level and cause of death were determined in a series of renal transplant recipients who died with functional grafts.

Study Design.—Between 1985 and 1994, 1,932 kidney transplants were performed for 1,806 recipients at the University of Minnesota. Of this patient group, 220 recipients died with functional grafts. The charts of these patients were reviewed to evaluate time from transplant to death, serum creatinine level, and cause of death.

Findings.—The most common cause of death was infection in 22%. Other causes were myocardial infarction in 17%, sudden death in 15%, cerebrovascular accident in 11%, and carcinoma in 10% of cases. Recipients who died with functional grafts had normal kidney function throughout the posttransplant period. The average serum creatinine level was 2 mg/100 mL at all time points assessed, including just before death.

Conclusions.—These findings lend support to the contention that kidney transplant recipients who die with functional grafts should be analyzed separately when transplant outcome is evaluated. In this large group of kidney transplant recipients, there was no evidence that impaired renal function contributed to any DWF death.

► It is well known that patients who die of cardiovascular disease with a functioning kidney transplant represent an increasing percentage of those patients who have late allograft loss. In diabetic patients, this is even more striking. West and colleagues at the University of Minnesota looked at the records of 1,932 kidney transplant patients in 1,806 recipients in the decade between 1985 and 1995. Of the 220 patients who died with functioning grafts, largely of cardiovascular or infectious reasons, serum creatinine values were no different than in the general population of transplant patients done during this time period. These data support the idea that renal dysfunction does not hasten or is not related directly to death with a functioning graft, but instead, cardiovascular and infectious disease risk factors are paramount. This puts the burden of altering these risk factors, both by anticipating them before the transplant and managing them posttransplant, on the transplant physician.

W. Bennett, M.D.

Delayed Graft Function: Risk Factors and Implications for Renal Allograft Survival

Ojo AO, Wolfe RA, Held PJ, et al (Univ of Mich; Dept of Veteran Affairs Med Ctr, Ann Arbor, Mich)

Transplantation 63:968–974, 1997 2–23

Background.—Delayed graft function (DGF) of a cadaverous kidney transplant is the most common allograft complication of the immediate posttransplant period. A large cohort analysis was performed to determine

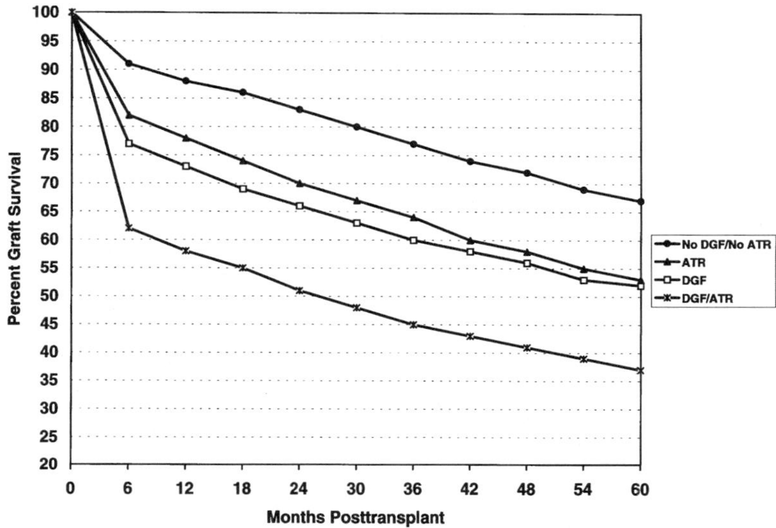

FIGURE 1.—Cox-adjusted cumulative 5-year graft survival stratified by the occurrence of delayed graft function and/or acute rejection (*circle*, no delayed graft function/no acute rejection; *triangle*, acute rejection; *square*, delayed graft function; *, delayed graft function/acute rejection). (Courtesy of Ojo AO, Wolfe RA, Held PJ, et al: Delayed graft function: Risk factors and implications for renal allograft survival. *Transplantation* 63[7]:968–974, 1997.)

whether DGF was an independent prognostic factor of short- or long-term graft survival.

Study Design.—Data from the U.S. Renal Data System prospectively compiled on 37,216 primary cadaveric renal transplants between 1985 and 1992 for which complete information was available were used for this study. Allograft status was studied until death, dialysis, transplant loss, or December 1993. Delayed graft function was defined as at least 1 dialysis treatment during the first postoperative week.

Findings.—Cold ischemia time was significantly associated with DGF. There was a 23% increase in DGF risk for each 6 hours of cold ischemia. Acute transplant rejection occurred significantly more frequently in DGF grafts. Delayed graft function was an independent predictor of 5-year graft loss (Fig 1). In those recipients with both DGF and acute rejection, the 5-year graft survival rate was only 35%. Zero-HLA mismatch improved graft survival by 10% to 15%. However, the 5-year graft survival rate in HLA-mismatched kidney grafts without DGF was significantly higher than in zero-mismatched kidney grafts with DGF.

Conclusions.—Delayed graft function is an independent prognostic factor for both short- and long-term kidney graft survival. The deleterious effect of DGF is more severe than the deleterious effect of HLA-mismatching. The best predictor of DGF is cold ischemia time. Further effort must be made to reduce cold ischemia time for donor organs to decrease the incidence of DGF and associated graft failure.

▶ The authors, using the large U.S. Renal Data System database, analyze the relationship between cold ischemia time, DGF, acute rejection, and graft survival. These data are extremely important in terms of national policies for organ sharing. With the recent information about living unrelated donor transplants doing as well as living related donor transplants, the issue of whether or not cadaveric donor grafts with long ischemia times and, thus, inferior outcomes at 1 and 5 years, should continue to be used if a living donor graft is available needs to be reanalyzed. The complex issue of fairness, as well as the ethics of using living donors who do not have a close biological relationship with the recipient, will need to be re-examined. Most transplant experts favor expanding the donor pool by using living unrelated donor transplants. This article gives them a good scientific basis for doing that, because the long cold ischemia times necessary for widespread national sharing clearly compromise the outcome regardless of the degree of HLA match. The 5-year graft survival in HLA mismatched kidneys *without* DGF was higher than 0-mismatched kidneys *with* DGF. This was highly statistically significant, and has implications for public policy. The authors' conclusion that the deleterious impact of DGF is more severe than that of poor HLA matching has now been stated publicly by a strong proponent of tissue matching.[1]

W. Bennett, M.D.

Reference

1. Terasaki P: Living unrelated kidney donation: The U.S. experience. Presented at Plenary Symposium: Living unrelated donor transplantation—progress and potential. San Antonio, Tex, November, 1997.

Pre-Transplant and Donor Issues

Laparoscopic Bilateral Nephrectomy: Results in 11 Renal Transplant Patients

Fornara P, Doehn C, Fricke L, et al (Univ of Lübeck, Germany)
J Urol 157:445–449, 1997 2–24

Introduction.—Some patients who have undergone renal transplantation have hypertension that does not respond to treatment. In such cases, removal of native kidneys is an effective means of normalizing blood pressure. Eleven renal transplant patients underwent bilateral laparoscopic nephrectomy for treatment of hypertension. Results were compared with those achieved after bilateral open nephrectomy.

Methods.—The 11 patients underwent laparoscopic bilateral nephrectomy between August 1994 and October 1995. Renal transplantations, 9 cadaveric and 2 from living-related donors, were all successful, but 3 patients were considered to have poor renal function with a serum creatinine concentration of 400–600 μmol/L. The indication for nephrectomy in each case was poorly controlled hypertension, assumed to be induced by the native kidney. Controls were a historical group of 10 patients who underwent bilateral open nephrectomy with the transperitoneal approach between November 1989 and January 1996.

Results.—Mean operative time was 195 minutes for the laparoscopy group vs. 145 minutes for the open surgery group. Mean estimated blood loss was 345 mL overall in the laparoscopic group and 280 mL in the open surgery group. One patient required conversion from laparoscopy to an open operation because of bleeding from the left renal artery. Postoperative morphine requirements were significantly higher in the open surgery than in the laparoscopy group (mean 44 mg vs. 14 mg). Patients in the laparoscopic group started oral intake and mobilization 1 day postoperatively, had a mean hospital stay of 4.2 days, and returned to normal activities at a mean of 14 days. All of these events were prolonged in the open surgery group (mean 3.5 days, 10.7 days, and 36 days, respectively). At a mean follow-up of 10.4 months, blood pressure had improved significantly in 8 patients (73%) who underwent laparoscopy. Six patients (60%) in the open surgery group had significantly decreased arterial blood pressure at 42 months of follow-up.

Conclusions.—Laparoscopic nephrectomy, first reported in 1990, is now performed at many centers. Although requiring more operative time than open procedures, laparoscopic techniques often result in less postoperative pain and shorter periods of hospitalization and convalescence. Results in this series of patients suggest that bilateral laparoscopic nephrectomy is a safe, feasible procedure, that may benefit select patients with drug-resistant hypertension after renal transplantation.

► Fornara et al. have demonstrated the feasibility of laparoscopic bilateral nephrectomy after renal transplantation. The indications for this procedure would be poorly controlled hypertension, infection, or neoplasm. The availability of minimally invasive techniques is very appealing in an immunosuppressed patient. Reductions in hospital stay, postoperative analgesia, and blood loss are indeed impressive. Clayman's group have even removed polycystic kidneys laparoscopically.[1] Sometimes in polycystic kidney disease, cystic kidneys continue to grow after transplantation and are a source of discomfort and other problems for the patients. As urologists become experienced with laparoscopic techniques, bilateral nephrectomy for a variety of indications will probably become more widely used.

W. Bennett, M.D.

Reference

1. Elashry OM, Nakada SY, Wolf JS Jr, et al: Laparoscopy for adult polycystic kidney disease: A promising alternative. *Am J Kidney Dis* 27:224–233, 1996.

Evaluation of Voiding Cystourethrography Prior to Renal Transplantation

Glazier DB, Whang MIS, Geffner SR, et al (St Barnabas Med Ctr, Livingston, NJ)

Transplantation 62:1762–1765, 1996 2–25

Background.—Routine pretransplantation assessment of the lower urinary tract includes voiding cystourethrography in many centers. The necessity for this evaluation was investigated.

Methods and Findings.—Five hundred seventeen fully evaluable transplant candidates were included in the review. Thirteen voiding cystourethrograms (VCUGs) (2.5%) were abnormal. Three patients with reflux alone did not need intervention before transplantation. Four with diminished bladder capacity had hydrodistention. Two patients increased their capacity to more than 150 mL. Two failed distention; 1 of them needed an ileal conduit, the other needed an augmentation cystoplasty. Three patients had increased postvoid residual (PVR), and 2 began clean intermittent catheterization. One needed prostate resection for benign prostatic hypertrophy. A patient with reflux and reduced bladder capacity declined therapy. Another patient, with reflux and increased PVR, began clean intermittent catheterization and was cleared for transplant surgery. Stroke occurred in 1 patient with diminished bladder capacity and increased PVR; the patient was then excluded from the transplantation program. All 13 patients with abnormal VCUGs had a urologic history. Overall, only 56 patients assessed had a urologic history.

Conclusion.—Voiding cystourethrography is a distressing and costly examination. These data show that this evaluation can be limited to transplant candidates with a previous urologic history.

► Transplantation is a very expensive medical procedure which involves a lengthy pretransplant evaluation and has many potential transplant complications. One of the routine tests obtained by most centers as part of the pretransplant assessment of the lower urinary tract is a VCUG.

Glazier et al. evaluated the clinical utility of the routine use of this procedure. They studied 517 patients and found only 13 with abnormal VCUGs (2.5%). Of these 13, 3 patients did not require intervention because they had only low-level reflux. The remaining patients required either hydrodistention of the bladder or interventions for PVR. Most importantly, all of the 13 patients with abnormal study results had prior urologic histories and of the 517 patients studied, only 56 patients fell into this category. With the cost of each VCUG approaching $600, it would seem prudent to limit these studies to patients with prior urologic histories. Studies such as this that question routine practices which are costly and, thus, focus them on subgroups at particular risk would seem to be prudent for many of the clinical strategies now used that, although logical, have never been shown to be cost effective.

W. Bennett, M.D.

Pregnancy After Donor Nephrectomy

Wrenshall LE, McHugh L, Felton P, et al (Univ of Minnesota, Minneapolis)
Transplantation 62:1934–1945, 1996 2–26

Background.—Women considering donating a kidney often ask whether unilateral nephrectomy will impair their future ability to have children. One group of kidney donors were surveyed to investigate this question.

Methods and Findings.—Two hundred twenty women who had donated a kidney between 1985 and 1992 were surveyed. The response rate was 65%. Thirty-three of the 144 responders became pregnant after donation. The total number of pregnancies was 45. Three fourths of the pregnancies went to term with no difficulties. Miscarriage occurred in 13.3%, preeclampsia in 4.4%, gestational hypertension in 4.4%, proteinuria in 4.4%, and tubal pregnancy in 2.2%. Difficulties occurring in another 4 pregnancies necessitated preterm hospitalization. Overall, morbidity was 8.8%. There were no pregnancy-related deaths and no fetal abnormalities. There were no cases of persistent hypertension, proteinuria, or changes in renal function. None of these findings differed significantly from outcomes in the general population. Infertility was a problem in 8.3% of the survey respondents, compared with 16.7% worldwide.

Conclusion.—Donor nephrectomy does not appear to be detrimental to the prenatal course or outcome of pregnancies after donation. The incidence of perinatal complications in this series was comparable to that in the general population.

► The use of living-related donors for renal transplantation is associated with superior short- and long-term graft survival. The benefits of minimizing cold ischemia time have led to the use of living-unrelated donors, with results that are also extremely successful. Questions continue to arise regarding the safety of this procedure for the donor.

Wrenshall et al. have surveyed a large number of women who underwent donor nephrectomy between 1985 and 1992. The striking results indicate that pregnancy in a woman with a single kidney after organ donation is extremely safe. There were no fetal abnormalities reported, and, importantly, no problems with proteinuria or persistent hypertension. None of the pregnancy complications observed exceeded their prevalence in the general population. The authors investigated whether organ donation resulted in infertility and, indeed, the incidence of this occurrence was less than the reported worldwide incidence. Thus, the nephrologist counseling families for living-related or living-unrelated transplantation can be relatively optimistic regarding subsequent pregnancy and its outcome.

W. Bennett, M.D.

National Kidney Allograft Sharing: A Decision Analysis

Feldman HI, Roth DA, Fazio I, et al (Univ of Pennsylvania, Philadelphia; Temple Univ, Philadelphia; St Joseph's Hosp, Paterson, NJ)
Transplantation 64:80–88, 1997 2–27

Introduction.—Some investigators proposed a more extensive national sharing of kidney allografts when 1-year allograft survival was found to be better in recipients of nationally shared allografts with 0 histocompatibility (HLA) mismatches than in recipients of locally distributed allografts. Because logistic barriers to expanding organ sharing are large, a decision analysis was undertaken to estimate the improvement in allograft survival that would result from expanding organ sharing.

Methods.—Four allograft-sharing strategies were compared: no national sharing, national sharing of allografts matched at 6 HLA alleles, national sharing of allografts matched at 4 or more alleles, and national sharing of allografts matched at 2 or more alleles. The probability of delayed allograft function, which has a negative impact on long-term allograft survival and may occur more often with national allograft sharing, was incorporated into the decision model. Data sources included the United States Renal Data System and the United Network for Organ Sharing.

Results.—The third strategy, which shares allografts matched at 4 or more alleles, was found to be the optimal strategy with the longest mean allograft survival. Differences among the 4 sharing strategies were small, however, and the optimal strategy would increase mean allograft survival approximately 0.04 years per allograft (compared with the current approach of matching at 6 HLA alleles). Compared with the use of allografts locally, the net gain for the entire United States would be 50 allograft-years annually. The decision model comparing outcomes before and after the use of cyclosporine yielded a mean allograft survival of 6.07 years after and 3.79 years before the drug's introduction. Thus, the impact of cyclosporine was much greater than that anticipated with national sharing of kidney allografts.

Discussion.—The efforts required to implement greater national sharing of cadaveric kidney allografts would yield only slight improvement in overall mean allograft survival. Costs of the proposed national organ sharing would be considerable, and racial inequities in kidney transplantation might be magnified.

► This interesting paper attempted to answer the question of whether massive sharing of cadaver organs would increase the kidney allograft survival in the United States. A model was developed in which end-stage renal disease patients were analyzed using 4 possible allocation strategies ranging from no sharing to sharing of kidneys matched at 6 HLA alleles, matched at 4 or more alleles, and sharing kidneys only matched at 2 or more alleles. The authors incorporated delayed allograft function as defined by need for dialysis into their decision model. Since more widespread sharing would increase cold ischemia time and thus the incidence delayed graft function, kidney survivals at each level of HLA match were obtained from the United Network for Organ Sharing database. While sharing organs that were more highly matched gave better mean survival, it was marginally better than lesser degrees of match presumably because of the greater cold ischemia time that is required with sharing. The model, when applied to data before and after the cyclosporine era, showed the anticipated effect of cyclosporine in doubling the average allograft's survival time. However, this study questions the wisdom of an expensive national organ sharing program if that program is achieved at the expense of longer cold ischemia time. This suggests that prompt transplantation of locally acquired organs gives the best results regardless of the match attained.

W. Bennett, M.D.

Procurement and Allocation of Solid Organs for Transplantation

Hauptman PJ, O'Connor KJ (Harvard Med School; Boston; New England Organ Bank, Newton, Mass)

N Engl J Med 336:422–428, 1997 2–28

Sources of Organs.—Although most organs for transplantation are obtained from brain-dead donors, the number of organs (mostly kidneys) from living related donors is increasing, with 35% of transplanted kidneys coming from relatives. Patients receiving organs from a relative may have better long-term outcomes, except for organs from brain-dead donors with no HLA mismatches. A small number of organs (mostly kidneys) are from unrelated donors, usually spouses. The rate of graft survival of spousal-donated kidneys is higher than for cadaveric kidneys, even with a greater degree of HLA mismatching (Table 1). Results of organ donations from asystolic cadavers are poor for uncontrolled (dead on arrival or failed resuscitation) but better for controlled (patients requesting no resuscitation) donations.

TABLE 1.—Number of Organ Donors in the United States, 1988–1994

Donor	1988	1989	1990	1991	1992	1993	1994
				no. of donors			
Cadaveric*	4,083	4,017	4,512	4,528	4,521	4,862	5,104
Living							
Related	1,754	1,824	2,027	2,308	2,412	2,713	2,814
Unrelated	71	90	98	111	160	185	196

Note: Data are from the 1995 annual report of the U.S. Scientific Registry for Transplant Recipients and the Organ Procurements and Transplantation Network.

*This category includes all brain-dead donors with intact circulation and asystolic donors reported to the United Network for Organ Sharing.

(Reprinted by permission of the *New England Journal of Medicine*, from Hauptman PJ, O'Connor KJ: Procurement and allocation of solid organs for transplantation. *N Engl J Med* 336:422–428, Copyright 1997, Massachusetts Medical Society.)

TABLE 2.—Criteria for Allocating Cadaveric Kidneys

Criterion	Points
Waiting time*	
Longest wait	1.0
>365 days	0.5(additional)
HLA-B or DR mismatches	
0	7.0
1	5.0
2	2.0
Presensitization of recipient (≥80%)†	4.0
Child	
<11 yr	3.0
11–18 yr	2.0

*The time on the waiting list is calculated according to the recipient's ABO blood type. A maximum of 1.0 point is given to the recipient with the longest waiting time, and shorter waits are assigned proportionally smaller values. For example, if there are 75 patients of blood type A waiting for kidneys, the patient with the longest wait is assigned 1.0 point (73/75), the patient whose rank order of waiting is 60th is assigned 0.8 point (60/75), and so forth.

†The presentation criterion applies only in local lists.

(Reprinted by permission of the *New England Journal of Medicine*, from Hauptman PJ, O'Connor KJ: Procurement and allocation of solid organs for transplantation. *N Engl J Med* 336:422–428,

Allocation of Cadaveric Organs.—The 1984 National Organ Transplant Act created the Organ Procurement and Transplantation Network for developing national policies for transplantation, and along with the Omnibus Reconciliation Act of 1986 and the Transplants Amendment Act of 1990, controls allocation of organs for transplantation. The Health Care Financing Administration (HCFA) certifies organ procurement organizations, which act as intermediaries between donor hospitals and histocompatibility testing facilities in the allocation process. These procurement organizations include professional education, hospital development, and donor-awareness campaigns.

Organ-specific allocation is based on algorithmic matching of organs with potential recipients (Table 2). Other allocation factors considered include HLA matching, pretransplantation cross-match, waiting time, medical urgency, and donor size. How well the allocation system works is unknown. There need to be standardized criteria for accepting donors. The influence of geographic differences in death rates and demographic aspects needs to be factored in. Patient access to transplantation centers and results for patients and transplantation centers need to be evaluated. Insuring an increasing supply of organs for transplantation and the equitable allocation of those organs will require the continued vigilance of all involved in the process.

► Hauptman and O'Connor have provided an extensive review of the current situation in procurement and allocation of solid organs for transplantation. This article provides the reader with an up-to-date summary of the current state-of-the-art. It is clear from Table 1 that the number of cadaveric donors in the United States has remained relatively flat. This is despite massive education attempts and data that the public, when queried, is willing to serve as organ donors. The growing trend toward living unrelated donors should become increasingly more evident with inclusion of recent data. However, the overall picture remains substantially below the level that is required for effective transplantation of all patients who could benefit by the procedures. The authors summarize the controversial use of brain-dead cadaver donors, and because of the need for more donors, the effort to pursue this source of organs again. Although the ultimate hope for the future lies in such things as xenotransplantation, most experts think that this is still 5–10 years away, with barriers such as prevention of rejection, zoonoses, and other substantial ethical and logistical problems. A summary of the current United Network for Organ Sharing database and the system of allocation is crisply reviewed for the reader, and the criteria for allocation of cadaver kidneys are summarized as well in Table 2. This article is a must for all who need to counsel patients about transplantation options.

W. Bennett, M.D.

Kidney–Pancreas Transplantation

Analysis of Early Readmissions After Combined Pancreas-Kidney Transplantation

Stratta RJ, Taylor RJ, Sindhi R, et al (Univ of Nebraska, Omaha; Clarkson Hosp, Omaha, Neb)
Am J Kidney Dis 28:867–877, 1996 2–29

Background.—Combined pancreas-kidney transplantation (PKT) is slowly becoming an accepted therapeutic alternative to continued insulin therapy in patients with insulin-dependent diabetes mellitus (IDDM) and progressive renal failure. Most pancreas transplantations (87%) performed in the United States have involved a simultaneous kidney transplantation (KTX) in the setting of imminent or projected renal failure. The combined procedure, however, has had a higher morbidity rate than KTX alone. The early morbidity associated with combined pancreas-kidney transplant (PKT) was retrospectively analyzed in 98 patients.

Methods.—The 98 consecutive PKTs were performed at a single center during a 5-year period. Forty-seven patients were already dialysis dependent and 51 would soon require dialysis. A preoperative workup sought to determine the patient's operative risk, establish the absence of exclusion criteria, and document end-organ complications. Patients eligible for combined PKT had secondary diabetic complications and nephropathy; for those not already receiving dialysis, a creatinine clearance of less than 40 mL/min was required. A cardiovascular evaluation was used to assess operative risk. Organs were procured from heart-beating cadaveric donors.

Results.—After a mean follow-up of 2.6 years, PKTs had a patient survival rate of 96%, a kidney survival rate of 90%, and a pancreas graft survival rate of 88%. Two deaths, 2 kidney graft losses, and 4 pancreas graft losses occurred in the first 3 months after PKT. Readmissions were common in the first 3 months, with 73 patients returning to the hospital on

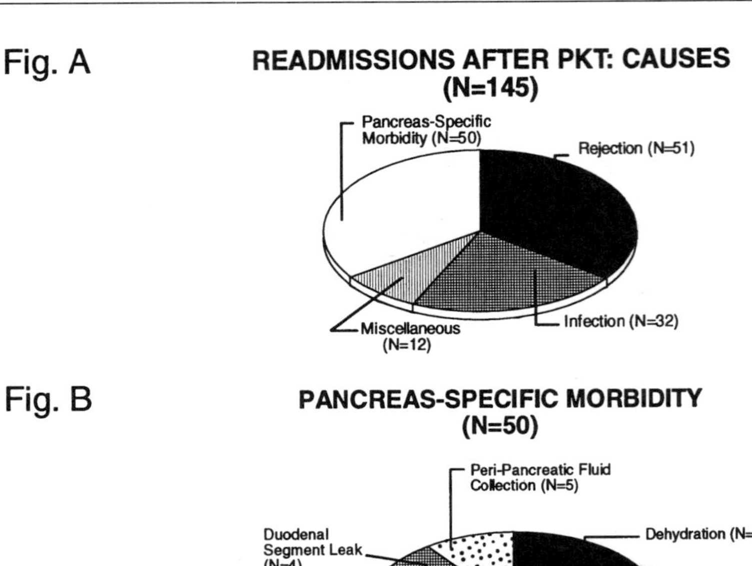

FIGURE 5.—**A**, causes of readmission in the first 3 months after pancreas-kidney transplant (PKT) in 98 consecutive recipients. **B**, etiology of pancreas-specific morbidity as a cause for readmission in the first 3 months after PKT. (Courtesy of Stratta RJ, Taylor RJ, Sindhi R, et al: *Am J Kidney Dis* 28:867–877, 1996.)

145 occasions during this period. Forty-seven readmissions occurred in the first week. Common causes of readmission were rejection, pancreas-specific morbidity, and infection (Fig 5). Thirteen patients underwent reoperation during a readmission. The mean total length of hospitalization in the first 3 months after PKT was 31 days, and the mean time required for return to work or normal activity was 4 months.

Conclusions.—During the course of the study period, the incidence, timing, causes, and duration of readmissions after PKT has remained unchanged. Thus, PKT is associated with a fixed morbidity, with early readmission in nearly 50% of patients. One third of readmissions are necessitated by pancreas-specific morbidity. Candidates for combined PKT should be carefully selected and fully informed about the unique morbidity of the procedure.

► Simultaneous PKT is now being advocated by some transplant groups as the option of choice when a type I diabetic reaches end-stage renal disease. The major issue now is the morbidity surrounding the addition of the bladder-drained pancreas operation to a standard kidney transplant. Stratta et al. have reviewed their large experience retrospectively. The initial hospital stay was 3 times as long as a standard kidney transplant, and only one quarter of patients in their 98-patients series had no readmissions to the hospital. The morbidity rate, most importantly early readmissions after initial discharge, occurred in nearly half of the patients, and morbidity related to the pancreas accounted for the vast preponderance of cases (Fig 5). Because the evidence of beneficial effects on complications of diabetes is slim, it is most important to have proper patient selection such that individuals who undergo simultaneous PKT are prepared for the added morbidity that generally follows the procedure. Clearly, the push for pancreas transplantation is largely patient driven. Physicians should not underestimate the attractiveness of not requiring insulin to a diabetic recipient. A well-motivated and informed patient ready to undergo the rigors of this procedure will obviously do the best.

W. Bennett, M.D.

Peripheral Vascular Disease After Kidney–Pancreas Transplantation in Diabetic Patients With End-stage Renal Disease

Morrissey PE, Shaffer D, Monaco AP, et al (Beth Israel-Deaconess Med Ctr, Boston; Harvard Med School, Boston)

Arch Surg 132:358–362, 1997 2–30

Background.—Peripheral vascular complications (PVCs) are greatly increased in diabetic patients. Theoretically, replacement of the malfunctioning pancreas with a functioning one should reduce these complications by achieving euglycemia. This study evaluated the rate of PVCs after either kidney transplantation alone or kidney-plus-pancreas transplantation in patients with diabetes.

Methods.—The study group included 39 diabetic patients with a kidney-plus-pancreas transplant. The control group included 65 diabetic patients with a kidney transplant only. Both groups received long-term immunosuppressive therapy. Peripheral vascular complications were defined as any midfoot or limb amputation caused by arterial occlusive disease (amputations resulting from an ulcer were not included), an ischemic ulceration that required treatment, lower-extremity bypass surgery, or angioplasty.

Findings.—Allograft function after 6 months was slightly better in the group that received a kidney transplant alone. Of patients undergoing kidney-plus-pancreas transplantation, 35 of 39 patients (90%) were no longer taking insulin at the end of the study, indicating euglycemia. The group that received a kidney transplant alone had more atherosclerotic risk factors, yet the pretransplantation incidence of PVCs was similar in both groups. After transplantation, however, the patients receiving a dual transplant experienced significantly more PVCs than the patients receiving a kidney-only transplant (46% vs. 31%).

Conclusion.—Diabetic patients receiving a kidney-plus-pancreas transplant enjoyed drastic improvements in their dependence on insulin. However, this group actually had more PVCs after transplantation than the group that received a kidney transplant alone. These contradictory findings indicate that, whereas pancreas transplantation can improve some measures of diabetic function, it has no effects—or perhaps even detrimental ones—on other complications of diabetes, such as peripheral vascular disease.

▶ One of the difficult decisions for the nephrologist when recommending a transplant for patients with type 1 diabetes with end-stage renal disease is whether to perform a simultaneous kidney-pancreas transplant or to pursue a kidney transplant alone. The combined procedure has more morbidity and a high rehospitalization rate. One of the prime theoretical benefits for the patient in achieving an insulin-free, nondiabetic state is stabilization or improvement of macrovascular disease.

Although theoretically appealing, the data of Morrissey et al. are disappointing. Patients who received kidney transplants alone—despite a higher pretransplant profile of atherosclerotic risk factors including coronary artery disease and serum lipids—did worse than the simultaneous kidney-pancreas transplant patients. Although the peripheral vascular disease before transplant was comparable, there were actually PVCs in the patients with successful kidney pancreas transplants.

The authors conclude—and nephrologists should note, for discussions with their patients—that there was little improvement in peripheral vascular disease and, in fact, a tendency toward worse disease in the patients with a functioning pancreas allograft. A role for increased endogenous insulin liberated systemically, not into the portal system, might provide an explanation for these results, which seem, at first look, somewhat counterintuitive.

W. Bennett, M.D.

3 Hypertension

A Clinical Trial of the Effects of Dietary Patterns on Blood Pressure

Appel LJ, for the DASH Collaborative Research Group (Johns Hopkins Univ, Baltimore, Md; Brigham and Women's Hosp, Boston; Merck, Westwood, Mass; et al)

N Engl J Med 336:1117–1124, 1997 3–1

Introduction.—Numerous dietary changes have been recommended for the prevention and treatment of hypertension, including weight control, reduced salt intake, reduced alcohol consumption, and increased potassium consumption. Trials of vegetarian diets have resulted in reduced blood pressure for normotensive and hypertensive subjects. However, trials testing individual nutrients, often in the form of dietary supplements, have shown little effect. The effects of diet on blood pressure were assessed in a multicenter, randomized dietary study.

Methods.—A total of 459 adults with a systolic blood pressure of less than 160 mm Hg and a diastolic blood pressure of 80–95 mm Hg were studied. For the first 3 weeks of the study, all patients received a control diet with a fat content typical of the average U.S. diet; the control diet contained few fruits, vegetables, and dairy products. Then, the patients were randomly assigned to receive the control diet, a diet high in fruits and vegetables, or a combination diet that was high in fruits, vegetables, and low-fat dairy products and had reduced levels of saturated and total fat. The patients' sodium levels and body weight were held steady at all times.

Results.—Mean blood pressure at baseline was 131/85 mm Hg. Compared with patients assigned to the control diet, those assigned to the combination diet had a 5.5 mm Hg reduction in systolic blood pressure and a 3.0 mm Hg reduction in diastolic blood pressure. Patients receiving the diet high in fruits and vegetables had a 2.8 mm Hg reduction in systolic blood pressure and a 1.1 mm Hg reduction in diastolic blood pressure. One hundred thirty-three patients had hypertension, defined as a blood pressure of 140/90 mm Hg or greater. In this group, the combination diet yielded a 11.4/5.5 mm Hg reduction in blood pressure. For individuals without high blood pressure, the reduction was 3.5/2.1 mm Hg.

Conclusions.—Blood pressure can be lowered by following a diet high in fruits, vegetables, and low-fat dairy foods, and low in saturated and total fat. This combination diet provides an additional nutritional approach to the prevention and treatment of hypertension. It achieves significant reductions in blood pressure with no change in body weight, a sodium intake of about 3 g/day, and an alcohol intake of no more than 2 drinks per day.

▶ The Dietary Approaches to Stop Hypertension (DASH) study is an important study in which a clear and significant lowering of both systolic and diastolic blood pressure was observed by dietary intervention in both normal and hypertensive individuals. The most important finding was in the hypertensive subgroups in which the systolic and diastolic blood pressure reductions were similar in magnitude (SBP 11 mm Hg and DBP 5 mmHg) to those typically seen in monotherapy pharmacologic interventions. Thus diet was as good for mild hypertension as many drug interventions. The mechanism of blood pressure lowering was not elucidated, and a number of factors could be responsible for the reductions in blood pressure observed in the fruit and vegetable and combination diet groups. One important factor could be dietary calcium, which is increased by low-fat dietary product intake. High dietary calcium intake has been shown to lower blood pressure in both animal and human studies, including in patients with salt-sensitive hypertension. A shortcoming of the study was its short duration, and longer follow-up is needed to show that such dietary intervention has an important impact on cardiovascular disease or mortality. But, if lifestyle changes including such diets could be achieved, then this hypothesis could be tested.

R.D. Toto, M.D.

Endogenous Erythropoietin Correlates With Blood Pressure in Essential Hypertension

Schmieder RE, Langenfeld MRW, Hilgers KF (Univ of Erlangen-Nürnberg, Germany)

Am J Kidney Dis 29:376–382, 1997 3–2

Introduction.—To stimulate erythropoiesis, human recombinant erythropoietin (EPO) is administered to anemic patients with renal insufficiency. An increase of arterial blood pressure is observed in about 30% of these patients with end-stage renal disease that requires new or additional antihypertensive treatment. When administered intravenously to healthy humans, erythropoietin has been shown to have proliferative effects on endothelial cells and has been shown to increase vascular resistance. Therapy with human recombinant EPO has been linked to a higher risk of blood pressure elevation for patients with a family history of hypertension. In patients with essential hypertension who are characterized by an elevation of total peripheral resistance in the early stage, endogenous erythropoietin might play a pathogenic role.

Methods.—There were 42 untreated patients with a mean age of 51 ± 9 years who had essential hypertension classified as stage 1 or 2 according to the World Health Organization. Measurements were taken of erythrocyte count, hemoglobin, hematocrit, renal hemodynamics with paraaminohip-

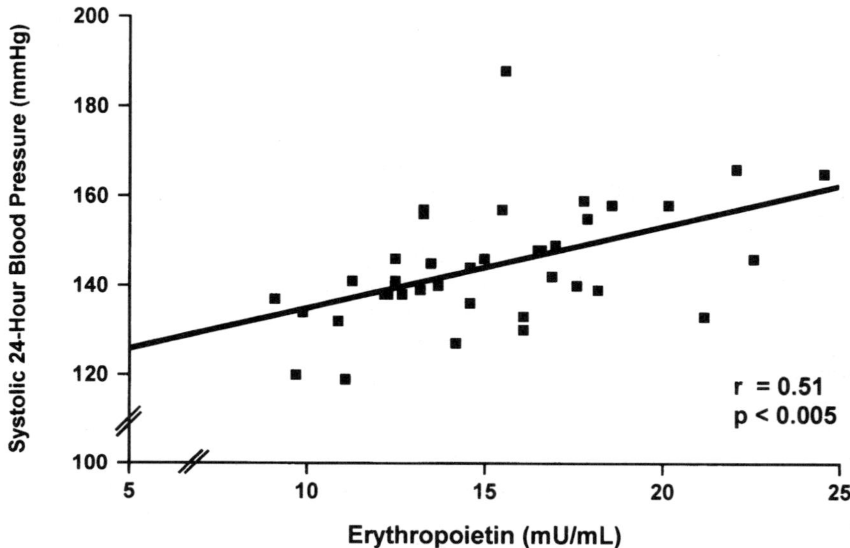

FIGURE 2.—Relation of endogenous erythropoietin concentrations and 24-hour systolic ambulatory blood pressure. (Courtesy of Schmeider RE, Langenfeld MRW, Hilgers KF: Endogenous erythropoietin correlates with blood pressure in essential hypertension. *Am J Kidney Dis* 29:376–382, 1997.)

purate and insulin clearance, cardiac output with echocardiography and Doppler sonography, and 24-hour blood pressure. The mean diastolic blood pressure was 93 ± 8 mm Hg and the mean systolic blood pressure was 145 ± 13 mm Hg. There was an average EPO concentration of 15.3 ± 3.7 mU/mL, which was within the normal range.

Results.—The ambulatory systolic and diastolic blood pressure was more elevated with the higher erythropoietin concentrations (Fig 2). There was a correlation between total peripheral resistance as determined by echocardiography and sonography and the concentration of endogenous erythropoietin. Renal plasma flow and renal blood flow were found to be progressively reduced, and renal vascular resistance progressively increased with increasing erythropoietin concentrations. Endogenous EPO concentrations were not related to hematocrit, hemoglobin, or erythrocyte count.

Conclusion.—The level of arterial blood pressure is related to endogenous EPO, which is mediated by an increase in total peripheral resistance in human essential hypertension. Endogenous EPO may be an aggravating or even promoting factor in the pathogenesis of essential hypertension, as is evidenced by erythropoietin's showing proliferative and vasoconstrictive effects on the endothelium in experimental studies.

► Administration of EPO to patients with end-stage renal disease on dialysis is known to significantly increase blood pressure in about 20% of patients. Numerous investigators have searched for the causal relationship between EPO dosing and its pressure response in dialysis patients; to date the precise mechanism of hypertension in EPO-treated patients is unknown. In this study, Schmieder and associates measured endogenous EPO levels in patients with stage I and II essential hypertension (World Health Organization criteria). The subjects underwent ambulatory blood pressure monitoring as well as measurements of renal plasma flow (RPF) and glomerular filtration rate (GFR). In these 42 untreated hypertensives, the researchers found that the plasma EPO level correlated directly with the blood pressure. Moreover, there was an inverse correlation between EPO level and RPF and a direct correlation with renal vascular resistance. The finding of the positive correlation between systolic blood pressure and EPO levels was independent of the hematocrit. In fact, it appeared to be slightly inversely correlated with the EPO level, although this was not statistically significant. The interesting finding in this study is that the EPO is correlated with the level of blood pressure, suggesting that the EPO may have either a direct or an indirect effect on vascular resistance, which in turn is associated with higher blood pressure and reductions in RPF and GFR. Experimental data support the vasoconstrictor effect of EPO as well as an effect on increasing endothelial proliferation. Furthermore, EPO receptors have been identified in endothelial cells in some studies. However, injecting EPO directly does not generally result in high blood pressure. If the present findings are confirmed by additional studies, it may turn out that EPO plays a role in either the pathogenesis or promotion of essential hypertension.

R.D. Toto, M.D.

Sodium Restriction Shifts Circadian Rhythm of Blood Pressure From Nondipper to Dipper in Essential Hypertension

Uzu T, Ishikawa K, Fujii T, et al (Natl Cardiovascular Ctr, Osaka, Japan)
Circulation 96:1859–1862, 1997 3–3

Introduction.—More serious end-organ damage, such as left ventricular hypertrophy, microalbuminuria, and cerebrovascular disease, has been seen in essential hypertensive patients who do not have a nocturnal fall in blood pressure (considered the nondipper type) than in patients whose blood pressure falls during the night (considered to be dippers). A previous study found that in patients with the sodium-sensitive type of essential hypertension, blood pressure failed to fall during the night, especially while on a high-sodium diet. The nocturnal fall in blood pressure may be restored by sodium restriction in these patients. It was clarified whether the amount of sodium intact affected the nocturnal fall and circadian blood pressure rhythm.

Methods.—There were 42 patients with essential hypertension who were given a high-sodium diet of 12–15 g of NaCl per day for 1 week and a low-sodium diet of 1–3 g/day for 1 week. An automatic oscillometric device was used to measure blood pressures every hour for 24 hours on the last day of each diet.

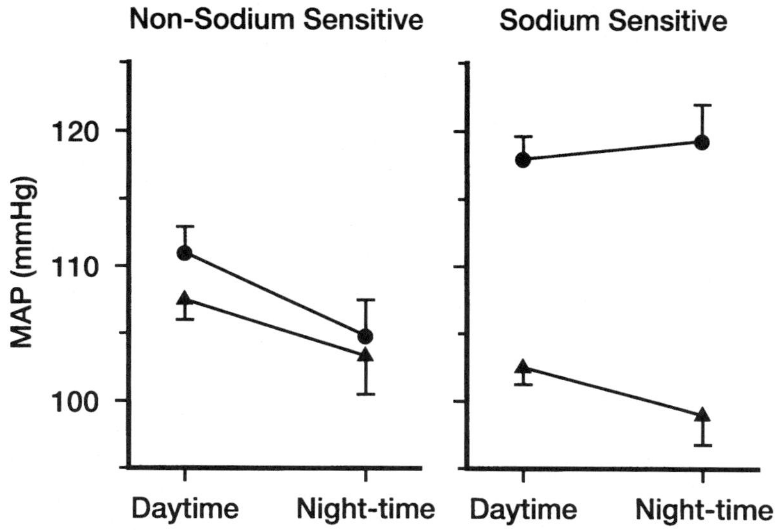

FIGURE 1.—Effects of mean arterial pressure of sodium restriction and nocturnal fall as well as their interaction in non-sodium sensitive (*left*) and sodium-sensitive (*right*) types of essential hypertension. Two-way anaylsis of variance and analysis of covariance with repeated measures clearly demonstrated the presence of an interaction (alternating action; $P < 0.05$) in the sodium-sensitive type only, indicating that diminished nocturnal blood pressure decline was restored by sodium restriction, and circadian rhythm of blood pressure was shifted from nondipper to dipper in this type of essential hypertension. *Black circle* and *black triangle*, mean arterial pressure values during high- and low-sodium diets, respectively. Error bars indicate either the upper or the lower half of the 95% confidence interval. (Courtesy of Uzu T, Ishikawa K, Fuji T, et al: Sodium restriction shifts circadian rhythm of blood pressure from nondipper to dipper in essential hypertension. *Circulation* 96[6]:1859–1862, 1997.)

Results.—On the basis of 10% or more change in 24-hour mean arterial pressure caused by sodium restriction, 21 patients were classified as non–sodium sensitive and 21 were classified as sodium sensitive. In the non–sodium-sensitive patients, nocturnal blood pressure fall was significant but not in the sodium-sensitive patients. Only in the sodium-sensitive patients was there a significant interaction between sodium restriction and nocturnal fall in blood pressure. The degree of the nocturnal fall was affected by sodium restriction in these patients. A positive relationship with sodium sensitivity was seen in changes in the nocturnal fall induced by sodium restriction. There was a negative relationship seen with the nocturnal fall before sodium restriction.

Conclusion.—The sodium-sensitive type has a diminished nocturnal fall, which is restored by sodium restriction, indicating that the circadian rhythm of blood pressure shifted from a nondipper to a dipper pattern (Fig 1). In the non–sodium-sensitive type, the nocturnal fall is not affected by sodium restriction, and the circadian rhythm remains of the dipper variety.

▶ It has been postulated that the lack of nocturnal fall in blood pressure (nondipper) is associated with more serious end-organ damage, including left ventricular hypertrophy, microalbuminuria, and cerebrovascular disease as compared with nocturnal fall in blood pressure (dipper).

The normal circadian rhythm in which blood pressure decreases at night (non-dipper) has been attributed to numerous factors. In this particular study, the authors sought to determine whether lowering salt intake in salt-sensitive non-dippers could restore the normal circadian rhythm. Indeed, they found that during salt restriction the normal pattern of nocturnal decline in blood pressure was restored in salt-sensitive hypertensives as illustrated in the right panel of Figure 1. Salt restriction reduces baseline mean arterial pressure during the daytime in salt-sensitive individuals (*closed triangle*). Remarkably, nocturnal mean arterial pressure increased during salt excess and decreased during salt restriction in the salt-sensitive patients.

The implication of this study is that the reduced ability to excrete a sodium load in salt-sensitive patients may determine circadian rhythm of blood pressure. The authors hypothesize that when sodium intake is high, defect in sodium excretion capability in salt-sensitive hypertensives becomes evident, thus elevating mean arterial pressure during the night to compensate for diminished daytime diureses (pressure naturises). This is an interesting hypothesis that should be tested in this salt-sensitive population. It may provide further insights into the relationship between non-dippers' rhythm and target organ damage risk. In this regard, a number of studies indicate that non-dippers are at greater risk for renal disease, presumably in part as a result of glomerular capillary hypertension, which is associated with proteinuria glomerular sclerosis in progressive renal failure.

R.D. Toto, M.D.

The Angiotensinogen T235 Variant and the Use of Antihypertensive Drugs in a Population-based Cohort

Schunkert H, Hense H-W, Gimenez-Roqueplo AP, et al (Univ of Regensburg, Germany; Univ of Münster, Germany; Institut für Epidemiologie, Munich-Neuherberg, Germany, et al)

Hypertension 29:628–633, 1997 3–4

Introduction.—The angiotensinogen T235 allele has been associated with high blood pressure in white, black, and selected Japanese populations. The common change of methionine to threonine at residue 235 of mature angiotensinogen (M235T) has been linked to hypertension. This study assesses the potential of the M235T change to represent a genetic marker related to blood pressure levels and subsequent use of antihypertensive medication in the general population.

Methods.—The T174M and M235T allele status and angiotensinogen plasma levels were determined in a cross-sectional sample of 634 middle-aged research subjects (48.4% males and 51.6% females).

Results.—There was no correlation between T174M allele status and angiotensinogen levels, blood pressure, or use of antihypertensive drugs. There were 418 research subjects with at least 1 copy of the T235M allele. They had significantly higher systolic and diastolic blood pressures and were 1.6-fold more likely to use antihypertensive drugs than the 216

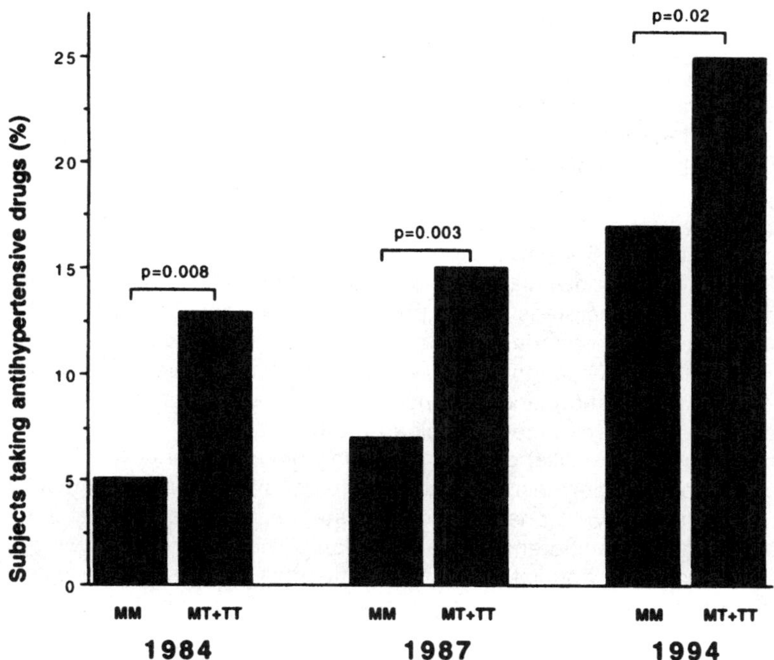

FIGURE 1.—Association between M235T allele status and number of research subjects (percentage) taking at least 1 antihypertensive agent to control blood pressure. Research subjects homozygous for the M235 allele (MM, n = 216 consumed antihypertensive drugs significantly less often than research subjects heterozygous or homozygous for the T235 allele (MT plus TT, n = 418). This association was consistently observed in all surveys carried out on these individuals in 1984, 1987, and 1994. (Courtesy of Schunkert J, Hense H-W, Gimenez-Roqueplo AP: The angiotensinogen T235 variant and the use of antihypertensive drugs in a population-based cohort. *Hypertension* 29:628–633, 1997.)

research subjects who were homozygotes for the M235 allele. Research subjects who were carriers of the T235 allele were 2.1-fold more likely to take 2 or more antihypertensive drugs. The excess risk associated with this allele seems to be responsible for 22.5% of all antihypertensive drugs taken. These findings had already been demonstrated in 2 previous surveys conducted on the same individuals over 10 years (Fig 1). The T235 allele was associated with higher angiotensinogen plasma levels, systolic pressure, and more intensive antihypertensive medication than that in homozygotes for the M235 and T235 alleles.

Conclusion.—The angiotensinogen T235 allele was responsible for a substantial proportion of antihypertensive drug use in this cohort of middle-aged, population-based white research subjects.

► The role of genetic predisposition and regulation of hypertension in the population with essential hypertension remains an area of intense investigation. In recent years, mutations in the angiotensinogen gene have been shown to be associated with a predisposition to elevated blood pressure. In particular, the mutation of methionine to threonine at the amino acid 235 of angiotensinogen has been associated with an increase in systolic and diastolic blood pressure.

The study by Schunkert et al. takes these observations a step further by showing that, in a selected population cohort mutations at this same locus are associated with not only higher blood pressures but also at requirement for greater hypertensive therapy (see Fig 1). As Figure 1 indicates, research subjects homozygous for the M235 allele consumed antihypertensive drugs significantly less often than research subjects either heterozygous or homozygous for the T235 allele. Importantly, this observation was found repeatedly in the same individuals during a 10-year period. Furthermore, it was found that the angiotensinogen phenotype was associated with higher plasma angiotensinogen levels, that is, those patients homozygous for the defining wild type had significantly lower levels than those homozygous for the threonine mutation, and intermediate levels were seen for those heterozygote for the methonine–threonine mutation.

This study has implications for predicting blood pressure levels and the response to antihypertensive therapy in the population with essential hypertension. There may be pharmacologic strategies that are more effective in patients with the angiotensinogen mutations. These strategies will require careful studies in populations, and multicenter studies will probably be required because of the relatively low number of individuals, homozygous for the threonine mutation.

R.D. Toto, M.D.

Polymorphisms of α-Adducin and Salt Sensitivity in Patients With Essential Hypertension

Cusi D, Barlassina C, Azzani T, et al (Univ of Milan, Italy; S Raffaele Hosp, Milan, Italy; Prassis-Sigma Tau Research Inst, Settimo Milanese, Milan, Italy et al)

Lancet 349:1353–1357, 1997 3–5

Introduction.—Genetic alterations in tubular reabsorption may be a cause of hypertension according to studies of hypertensive and normotensive strains of rats and in human beings with essential hypertension. This effect seems to be affected by cytoskeleton proteins. Through changes in the actin cytoskeleton, adducin, an α/β heterodimeric protein, is thought to regulate cell-signal transduction. There has been an association between some allelic markers close to the α-adducin locus and hypertension. The effect of the α-adducin polymorphism on linkage of the α-adducin locus to hypertension, on a functional mutation in the α-adducin gene associated with hypertension in at least 2 independent populations, and on the influence of α-adducin on the relation between renal sodium handling and blood pressure was analyzed.

Methods.—In 137 hypertensive sibling-pairs, linkage analysis of 3 DNA markers at different distances from the α-adducin locus (20–2500 Kb) was conducted. Genotyping for the α-adducin polymorphism was performed

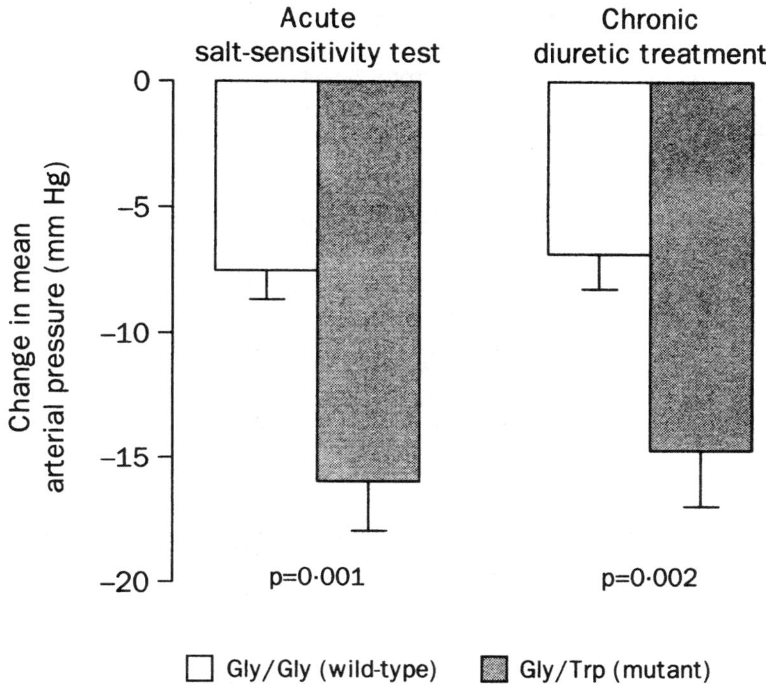

FIGURE.—Mean Standard error decrease in arterial pressure after acute salt-sensitivity test or chronic diuretic treatment. (Courtesy of Cusi D, Barlassina C, Azzani T, et al: Polymorphisms of α-adducin and salt sensitivity in patients with essential hypertension. *Lancet* 349:1353–1357.)

on 477 hypertensive and 322 normotensive individuals. In hypertensive individuals with and without the 460 Trp α-adducin allele, the blood-pressure response to acute and chronic changes in sodium balance was studied.

Results.—In the sibling-pair study, significant linkage was found for all 3 markers. With increasing distance from the α-adducin locus, the extra shared alleles and the significance level for linkage decreased. Hypertension and the 460 Tp mutation were significantly associated. The decrease in mean arterial pressure was greater in 65 patients who were heterozygous for the mutant allele (gly/Tp) than in 21 wild-type homozygotes in the salt-sensitivity tests that was conducted to assess the acute blood-pressure response to changes in body sodium in 86 hypertensive patients (Figure). The mean decrease for heterozygous patients was 15·9 mm Hg, and for the wild-type homozygotes, it was 7·4 mm Hg. A greater fall in mean arterial pressure in response to 2 months' treatment with hydrochlorothiazide was seen in 21 heterozygous hypertension patients than in 37 wild-type homozygous hypertensive patients. The heterozygous patients had a mean decrease of 14·7 mm Hg, and the wild-type homozygous patients had a mean decrease of 6·8 mm Hg.

Conclusion.—A salt-sensitive form of essential hypertension is associated with α-adducin, according to the findings of significant linkage of the α-adducin locus to essential hypertension and greater sensitivity to changes in sodium balance among patients with the mutant allele. Hypertensive patients who will benefit from diuretic treatment or maneuvers to reduce total body sodium may be identified by the α-adducin polymorphism.

▶ The pathophysiology of human hypertension is complex and involves a number of regulatory factors. Genetic regulation of sodium absorption by the kidney plays a critical role in the regulation of volume and blood pressure. Liddle's syndrome is a hereditary disease caused by activating mutations in the β-subunit of the apical sodium channel of the distal nephron and hypertension. Also, primary aldosteronism, which stimulates salt absorption in the cortical collecting duct, also causes salt-dependent hypertension.

This study by Cusi et al., evaluated the impact of polymorphisms in the α-adducin gene in human hypertensives. α-Adducin is a heterodimeric protein that is thought to regulate cell signal transduction in part by changes in the actin cytoskeleton cells. Alterations in α-adducin could be manifest by increases in sodium potassium pump activity and therefore sodium reabsorption throughout the nephron.

The odds ratio for presence of hypertension associated with the presence of one or two mutant alleles of the α-adducin gene compared with homozygous for the wild-type gene was 1.6, and the odds ratio for hypertension in individuals homozygous or heterozygous for the mutant allele compared with a wild-type homozygous was 1.8. A striking finding was the observation that the decline in mean arterial blood pressure in response to acute salt sensitivity and chronic diuretic treatment was significantly greater in the patients heterozygous for the mutant type allele.

A major strength of this study is the large number of patients analyzed, including 137 hypertensive sibling pairs from 86 known hypertensive families. Although the clinical significance of α-adducin as an important factor in determining blood pressure regulation in essential hypertensives is not known, this interesting study sheds light on additional possible genetic causes of "essential" hypertension.

R.D. Toto, M.D.

α_1-Adrenergic Receptor Antibodies in Patients With Primary Hypertension

Luther H-P, Homuth V, Wallukat G (Humboldt Univ, Berlin)
Hypertension 29:678–682, 1997 3–6

Introduction.—Although in diseases such as lupus erythematous, systemic rheumatoid arthritis, and pernicious anemia, immune mechanisms are known to be important, they are not generally discussed in relation to hypertension. The initiation and maintenance of the hypertensive state may be somewhat linked to primary or secondary alterations in the function of the immune system. An elevated level of serum immunoglobulin is

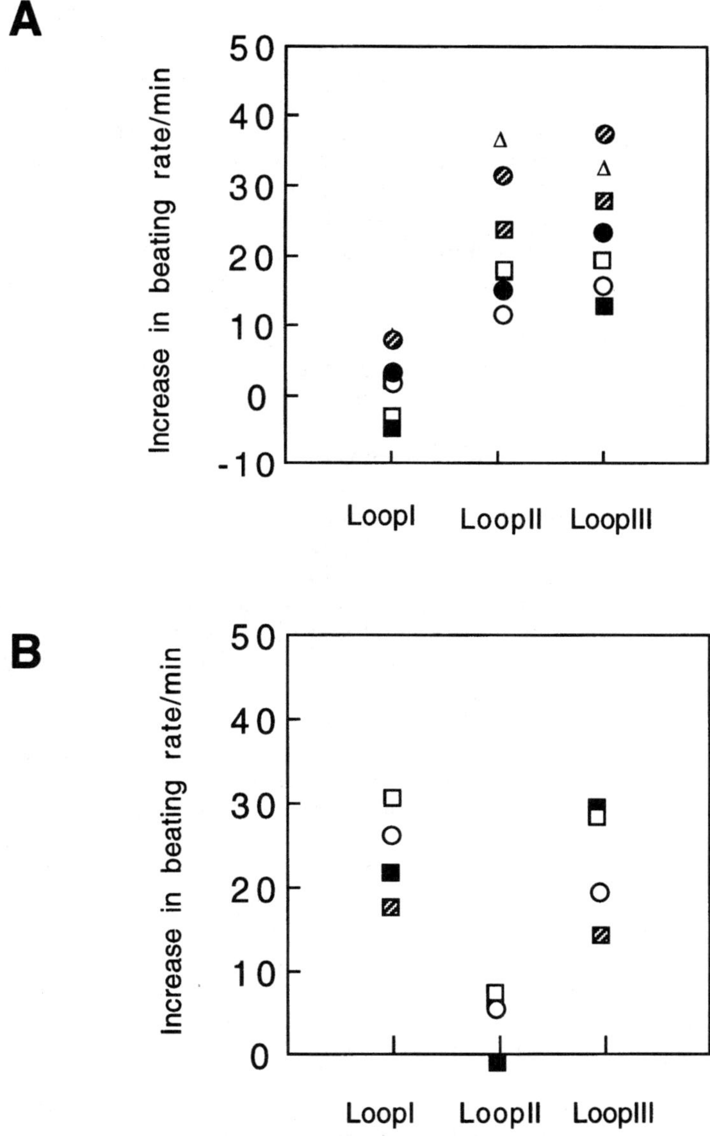

FIGURE 6.—Epitope analysis of immunoglobulin fractions from hypertensive patients. The immunoglobulin reaction (50 μL) was preincubated with peptides corresponding to the first (I), second (II), and third (III) extracellular loops of human α_1-adrenoreceptor in separate test tubes. Subsequent addition to the culture flask and measurement of the chronotropic effect are indicated. **A,** effect of immunoglobulin from hypertensive patients that contained autoantibodies against the first extracellular loop (I). These autoantibodies were inhibited by preincubation with peptides corresponding to the first loop. **B,** immunoglobulin from hypertensive patients with autoantibodies directed against the second extracellular loop. These autoantibodies were inhibited by preincubation with peptides corresponding to the second loop. The symbols indicated AAB from different patients. (Courtesy of Luther H-P, Homuth V, Wallukat G: α_1-Adrenergic receptor antibodies in patients with primary hypertension. *Hypertension* 29:678–682, 1997.)

seen in up to 40% of hypertensive patients compared with normotensive controls. In patients with essential hypertension, autoantibodies to nuclear structures and smooth muscle were found significantly more often than in normotensive controls. Previous studies with patients having malignant and secondary hypertension found autoantibodies against the α_1-adrenergic receptor. The incidence of agonistic α_1-adrenergic autoantibodies in the sera of patients with primary hypertension was determined, and their possible role in raising systemic arterial resistance was investigated.

Methods.—The immunoglobulin fractions of sera from 54 patients with primary hypertension and 26 normotensive controls were examined for the presence of autoantibodies against the α_1-adrenoreceptor to investigate the incidence of autoantibodies against the α_1-adrenoreceptor.

Results.—A positive response was found in the sera of 24 patients (44%) and 3 controls (12%). In two thirds of the positive responses, the antibodies were directed against the first extracellular loop of the α_1-adrenoreceptor. In one third of the positive responses, the antibodies were directed against the second extracellular loops, according to an epitope analysis of 16 autoantibody-positive immunoglobulin fractions (Fig 6). On isolated neonatal rat cardiomyocytes, the autoantibodies has a positive chronotropic effect, which was blocked by α_1-adrenergic antagonists.

Conclusion.—In patients with hypertension, the autoantibodies may play a role in elevating peripheral vascular resistance and promoting cardiac hypertrophy because their functional characteristics showed no desensitization phenomena.

► The immune system plays an important role in initiating and sustaining hypertension in a number of diseases. These include the production of autoantibodies in circulation as well as induction of inflammation in vascular tissues associated with vasculitides and chronic hypertension. In this interesting and provocative study by Luther et al., the authors demonstrate the presence of serum autoantibodies to α_1-adrenergic receptors in 44% of (selected) primary hypertensives. They also studied a small population of 26 control subjects in whom 3 were found to have such autoantibodies. The authors characterized the effect of these autoantibodies on the α_1-adrenergic receptor in cultured myocardial cells. Autoantibodies stimulated the α_1-adrenergic receptor similar to phenylephrine. Furthermore, the effect of the autoantibody could be prevented by preincubation with the α_1 agonist, prazosin. Moreover, they showed that the effect of the antibody could be abrogated by pretreating with peptide fractions corresponding to the first or second extracellular loop domains of the $alpha_1$ adrenoreceptor itself (see Fig 6).

The shortcomings of this study include the fact that the patient population was a selected primary hypertensive group, and it is not known whether the prevalence of these antibodies is as high as 40% in the general hypertensive population. Another shortcoming is the fact that 3 of the patients who were normotensive in the control group had antibodies and did not have evidence of increased blood pressure, or even resting tachycardia. Furthermore, a causal link between these antibodies and hypertension in humans was not demonstrated. For instance, infusion of such antibodies into normotensive humans or into normotensive animals was not conducted in the study. This would strengthen the association between the antibody and some pathogenetic role.

The results of this study suggest that autoantibodies to the α_1-adrenergic receptor may be responsible for sustaining hypertension or inducing acute hypertensive episodes in patients with malignant hypertension. Moreover, these results suggest the possibility that if these antibodies are pathogenetic, strategies designed to reduce antibody level or activity may be antihypertensive in patients.

Finally, the study raises the question of whether such antibodies might be present in patients with autoimmune disease who develop marked hypertension, for example, systemic lupus erythematosus and a progressive system of sclerosis. Further studies in this exciting and interesting area are awaited.

R.D. Toto, M.D.

Effect of Single-Drug Therapy on Reduction of Left Ventricular Mass in Mild to Moderate Hypertension: Comparison of Six Antihypertensive Agents

Gottdiener JS, for the Department of VA Cooperative Study Group on Antihypertensive Agents (Georgetown Univ, Washington, DC)

Circulation 95:2007–2014, 1997 3–7

Objective.—Antihypertensive drugs are not equally effective in reducing left ventricular (LV) mass. Covariates other than the drug also influence LV mass. Echocardiography was used to assess the response of LV mass and its structural components over a 1-year period of antihypertensive monotherapy.

Methods.—Echocardiograms were performed at baseline, at the end of the titration period, and at 1 year in 1,105 men, average age 58, with diastolic blood pressure 95–109 mm Hg, randomly assigned to receive either atenolol 25–100 mg daily (n = 178), captopril 12.5–50 mg twice daily (n = 188), clonidine 0.1–0.3 mg twice daily (n = 178), diltiazem-SR 60 to 180 mg twice daily (n = 185), prazosin 2–10 mg twice daily (n = 188), or hydrochlorothiazide 12.5–50 mg daily (n = 188). Patients who attained a diastolic blood pressure of less than 90 mm Hg for an 8-week titration period were treated for 1 year on a maintenance dose. Measurements of ventricular septum, LV cavity, and posterior wall dimensions were compared statistically by group.

Results.—There were 683 patients who completed the titration phase and 493 who completed the 1-year maintenance phase. Echocardiography data were available for 587 patients at baseline, 406 at 8 weeks, and 230 at the end of the maintenance phase. At baseline, blood pressure averaged 152.5 mm Hg, and LV mass averaged 327.3 g. When baseline LV mass was stratified into 3 groups, 275 g or less, 275–350 g, and greater than 350 g,

LV mass decrease at 1 year was significant for the highest tertile of hydrochlorothiazide patients (-42.9 g), captopril patients (-38.7 g), and atenolol patients (-28.1 g). Patients in the lowest tertile treated with diltiazem had an increase in LV mass.

Conclusion.—Hydrochlorothiazide, captopril, and atenolol reduced LV mass in men with mild to moderate hypertension. Diltiazem, clonidine, and prazosin did not.

► Left ventricular hypertrophy is commonly observed in hypertensives and is known to be an independent risk factor for sudden death in adult populations. Lowering blood pressure by pharmacologic or non-pharmacologic means has been shown to reduce LV wall mass, but the question remains as to whether this is in turn followed by a reduction in sudden death. An important question is whether any blood-pressure-lowering drug or method is sufficient to reduce LV wall mass. In this study, data on LV wall mass from a previously published trial on hypertension was analyzed to determine which of 6 different antihypertensive agents administered to mild-to-moderate hypertensives. As shown in the accompanying figure, captopril, hydrochlorothiazide, and atenolol all reduce LV mass at 1 year. Also, diltiazem lowered LV wall mass in those with the greatest degree of baseline LV mass. Of interest is the finding that neither prazosin nor clonidine, drugs that primarily reduce α-adrenergic activity, reduced LV mass. An unexplained finding is the apparent increase in LV wall mass in patients with the lowest baseline values. Blood pressure reduction was similar in all groups. An important aspect of this study is the finding that hydrochlorothiazide was found to reduce LV mass to the greatest extent as compared with the other antihypertensives. A shortcoming of this study was a relatively high dropout rate for lack of blood pressure control in some of the groups. Thiazides and β-blockers remain the only agents shown to lower cardiovascular mortality in hypertensive populations in long-term clinical trials. This study makes it tempting to speculate that perhaps the protective effects of these agents may be related in part to reduction in LV wall mass.

R.D. Toto, M.D.

Left Ventricular Hypertrophy Precedes Other Target-Organ Damage in Primary Aldosteronism

Shigematsu Y, Hamada M, Okayama H, et al (Ehim Univ, Japan)
Hypertension 29:723–727, 1997 3–8

Introduction.—Aldosterone regulates electrolyte transport in renal tubules and may also exert direct action on the heart. There is controversy about whether cardiac structural changes in the clinical setting result from long-term elevations in blood pressure or are a manifestation of nonhemodynamic factors acting on the myocardium. A study of 23 patients with aldosterone-producing adenoma (PA) and 116 with essential hypertension (EH) sought to assess the effects of prolonged aldosterone stimulation on the heart, brain, and kidneys; evaluate the progression of major target organ damage in PA; and compare target organ damage in PA and EH.

Methods.—To match left ventricular hypertrophy (LVH) between patients with PA and EH patients with LVH, participants were required to have an LV mass index of 140 g/m^2 or less. All had either never received hypertensive therapy or discontinued these agents at least 4 weeks before study entry. Echocardiographic studies provided data for calculation of the LV end-diastolic dimension index, LV mass index, and relative wall thickness. An ophthalmologist blinded to blood pressure levels and echocardiographic data assessed patients for hypertensive retinopathy. Blood and urine samples were obtained for determination of neurohumoral factors.

Results.—Relative wall pressure did not differ significantly among the PA, EH without LVH, and EH with LVH groups, but the LV end-diastolic dimension index was larger in PA patients than in both EH groups. When compared with the EH groups, PA patients had lower plasma renin activity and serum potassium concentrations and higher plasma aldosterone concentrations. Hypertensive retinopathy was most strongly concentrated in EH patients with LVH, and this group had the highest serum creatinine concentration. There was a strongly significant correlation between the degree of LV mass index and severity of hypertensive retinopathy and renal involvement independent of office blood pressure in EH. Despite mild extracardiac target organ damage, LVH markedly progressed in PA. Although the LV end-diastolic dimension index was significantly larger in the PA than in both EH groups, extracardiac target organ damage did not differ between 13 PA patients with eccentric LVH and 26 EH patients with eccentric LVH.

Discussion.—The progression of damage in 3 major target organs differs among PA and EH patients. Findings in this patient series suggest that predominantly volume load (of whatever cause) that results in eccentric LVH is less likely to lead extracardiac target organ damage than hemodynamic or nonhemodynamic mechanisms resulting in concentric LVH.

► Aldosterone has increasingly been reported as a cardiac and systemic vascular fibrosing factor. Studies in animals indicate that chronic aldosterone administration induces cardiac hypertrophy. Moreover, clinical trials suggest that elevated plasma aldosterone is associated with the pathogenesis and progression of chronic congestive heart failure. The authors in this study evaluated the changes in cardiac structure, renal function, and vascular disease in patients with primary aldosteronism as compared with essential hypertensives.

The key finding in the study was the observation that patients with primary aldosteronism had a high prevalence of eccentric LVH as compared with essential hypertensives. In addition, they found that the LVH appeared to precede evidence of renal dysfunction and retinopathy in these patients. Because hyperaldosteronism causes salt retention and volume expansion, they postulate that individuals with volume overload of hypertension have an additional mechanism of hypertrophy that reduces eccentric LVH, which is unclear in primary aldosteronism. Possible mechanisms include volume overload and hypokalemia. Chronic hypokalemia has been associated with fibrosis and myocytolysis in the heart and fibrosis and tubular atrophy in the kidney. In addition, hypokalemia has been reported to produce cysts in the kidney that may be reversible after correction of hypokalemia in patients with primary aldosteronism.

The implication of this study, if these findings hold true, is that aldosteronism antagonism may be a useful method for reducing target organ damage in patients with primary aldosteronism. Moreover, if secondary hyperaldosteronism in patients with heart failure is important in the pathogenesis of progressive heart failure, exploitation of aldosteronism antagonism could be useful in this situation as well.

Studies in patients with primary and secondary aldosteronism and hypertension or heart disease would be important for elucidating the role of aldosteronism in the pathogenesis of target organ damage. This article highlights the fact that increasing evidence points toward the hyperaldosterone state as an important independent pathogenetic factor of target organ damage in patients with chronic hypertension.

R.D. Toto, M.D.

Prevalence and Predictors of Renal Artery Stenosis in Patients With Myocardial Infarction

Uzu T, Inoue T, Fujii T, et al (Natl Cardiovascular Ctr, Osaka, Japan)

Am J Kidney Dis 29:733–738, 1997 3–9

Background.—Renal artery stenosis (RAS), an important cause of both end-stage renal disease and secondary hypertension, may be correctable. To determine the prevalence and predictors of RAS in the population of patients with atherosclerosis, autopsy data from patients older than 40 years who had evidence of myocardial infarction related to significant coronary artery disease were retrospectively examined.

Methods.—From 1981 to 1992, a total of 297 of 1,788 autopsy cases met inclusion criteria. Demographic data, smoking history, hypertension, hypercholesterolemia, diabetes, renal function, and proteinuria were determined from medical records. Coronary vessels were sectioned for examination of stenosis, which was characterized as to severity. Bilateral renal arteries were dissected to check for significant (≤75%) stenosis.

Results.—Renal insufficiency was noted in 23% of patients for whom data were available; proteinuria was noted in 32%. Thirty-five patients (12%) showed significant (≤75%) RAS. Infarct location did not differ between those with and without RAS. Prevalence of RAS varied with age, only 4% of patients younger than 60 years had significant RAS, compared to 14% of patients older than 60 years. Bilateral stenosis was found in 10 patients, all older than 60 years. Potential risk factors studied are shown in Fig 2. Renal artery stenosis was more common among patients with hypertension (19%, $P < 0.001$), proteinuria (39%, $P < 0.001$), and renal insufficiency (39%, $P < 0.001$). Extent of coronary artery occlusion was

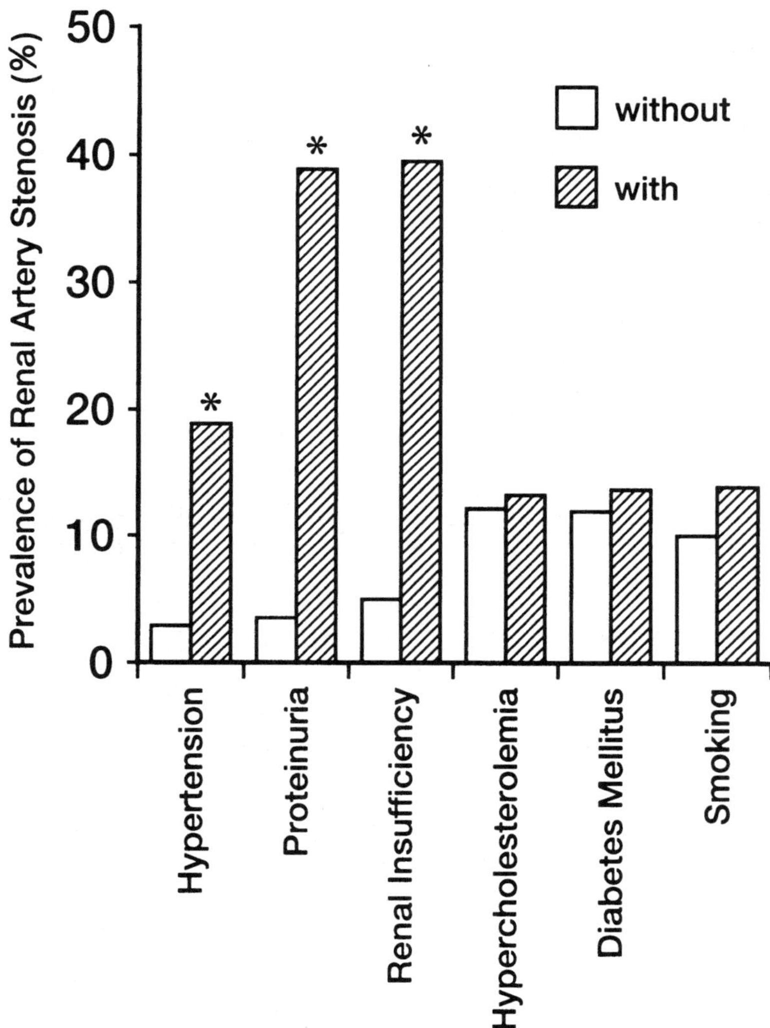

FIGURE 2.—The prevalence of renal artery stenosis in autopsy patients with myocardial infarction: comparison between 2 groups with and without clinical characteristics such as hypertension, proteinuria, renal insufficiency, hypercholesterolemia, diabetes mellitus, and smoking. $^*P < 0.001$. (Courtesy Uzu T, Inoue T, Fujii T, et al: Prevalence and predictors of renal artery stenosis in patients with myocardial infarction. *Am J Kidney Dis* 29:733–738, 1997.)

also related to RAS. As the number of coronary vessels with significant (≤75%) stenosis increased, so did likelihood of renal stenosis, and severity of occlusions in patients with 3-vessel disease showed a similar pattern. Hypertension, proteinuria, renal insufficiency, age, and number of significantly stenosed coronary arteries were found by multiple logistic regression to be independent predictors. Sex, hypercholesterolemia, diabetes, and smoking history were not.

Discussion.—From 5% to 22% of advanced renal failure in patients older than 50 years may be caused by RAS. Survival on dialysis is poor because of the high incidence of cardiovascular complications, but early RAS is potentially reversible by revascularization. A population potentially benefiting from intervention thus can be identified by the independent risk factors found in this study, which may be different from those in the general population. Conventional risk factors are not useful in examining the population with atherosclerosis of the coronary arteries.

▶ Renal artery stenosis is a common finding in patients with coronary artery disease and contributes to the development of hypertension as well as renal insufficiency. However, the factors that may predict whether patients with myocardial infarction are likely to have significant RAS have not been determined.

In this study by Uzu et al., autopsy-proven cases of RAS were monitored over a 12-year period. The authors used a strict criteria for the diagnosis of significant RAS, namely 75% or greater luminal area narrowing. They found that the presence of hypertension, proteinuria, and renal insufficiency were predictors of RAS in patients with documented acute myocardial infarction. Because the incidence of myocardial infarction is very high in patients with renal insufficiency, a finding known from previous clinical trials, it is conceivable that the development of myocardial infarction in the patient population is related to the underlying renal insufficiency.

As shown in Figure 2, the prevalence of RAS is much higher in hypertensive, proteinuric, and renal insufficiency patient groups. In contrast, diabetics, smokers and those with hypercholesterolemia had no significant increase in RAS prevalence.

Interestingly, the highest odds ratio for the development of RAS in patients with myocardial infarction was seen with proteinuria. This observation needs to be explored further. These factors for future trials may be an important way to screen for RAS and for possible intervention to prevent progressive renal disease.

R.D. Toto, M.D.

Patency of Percutaneous Transluminal Renal Angioplasty: A Prospective Sonographic Study

Baumgartner I, Triller J, Mahler F (Univ Hosp, Bern, Switzerland)

Kidney Int 51:798–803, 1997 3–10

Introduction.—Evaluation of the long-term results of percutaneous transluminal renal angioplasty (PTRA) is usually based on blood pressure measurements alone. A study of 50 consecutive patients treated by PTRA for suspected renovascular disease examined renal blood flow by color-coded duplex sonography (CCD). The aim of the prospective study was to systematically investigate the results of PTRA with regard to patency rate

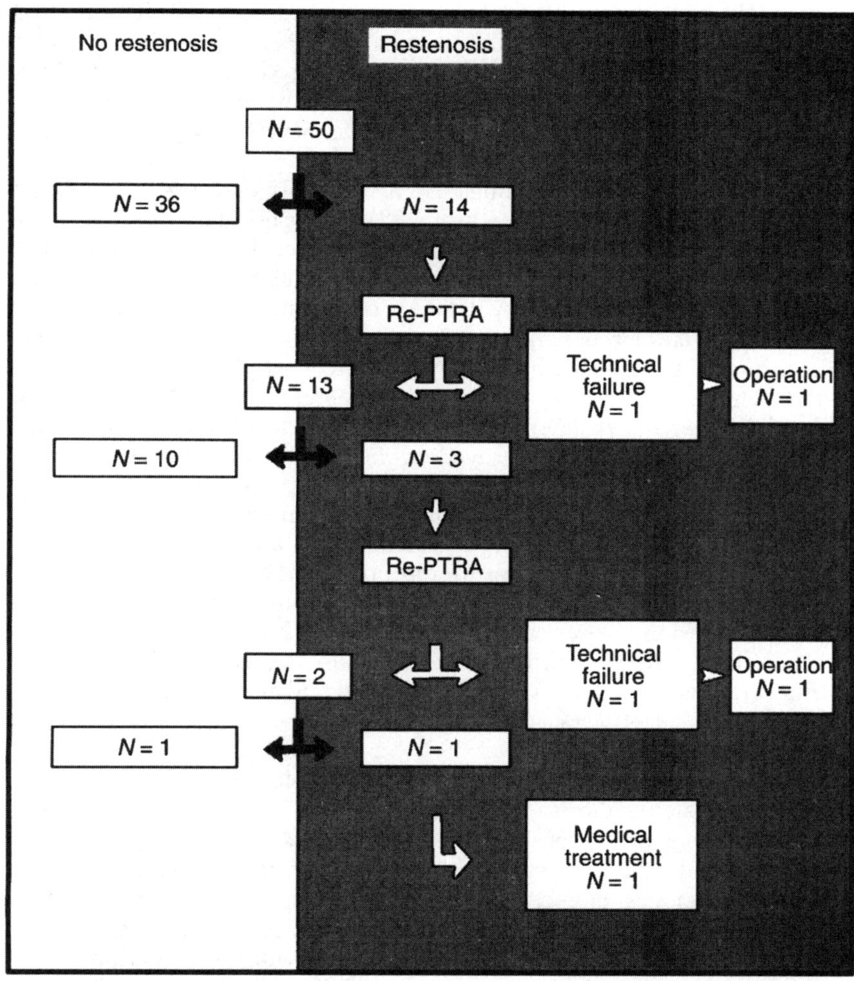

FIGURE 2.—Sequence of events in 50 patients of this series. *Abbreviation: PTRA,* percutaneous transluminal renal angioplasty. (Courtesy of Baumgartner I, Triller J, Mahler F: Patency of percutaneous renal angioplasty: A prospective sonographic study. *Kidney Int* 51[3]:798–803, 1997. Reprinted by permission of Blackwell Science, Inc.)

and to correlate sonographic and/or angiographic patency with effects on blood pressure and renal function.

Methods.—The patients were 26 women and 24 men with a mean age of 60. Forty-seven had 59 untreated renal artery lesions and 3 had a restenosis after angioplasty of 4 renal arteries. Renal artery obstruction was the result of atherosclerosis in 37 cases and fibromuscular dysplasia (FMD) in 13. During follow-up (average, 13 months), repeated PTRA was performed for 12 restenoses and 6 recurrent or re-restenoses in 63 renal arteries. Examinations with CCD were performed before PTRA and at 1 day, 3 months, 6 months, and 12 months after PTRA.

Results.—Of the 168 CCD follow-up investigations, 152 (90%) were estimated to be conclusive; nonconclusive studies were the result of obesity or excessive gas accumulation in the intestine. Seventy-five (93%) treated renal arteries could be assessed by CCD alone; 6 required intra-arterial angiography. Sonographic findings had a sensitivity of 100%, a specificity of 80%, and an overall accuracy of 93% for discrimination of 60% or greater restenosis. The primary patency rate after 12 months was 73%; inclusion of treated restenoses improved the rate to 94% overall. Two patients who failed secondary PTRAs of restenoses were successfully treated by an aortorenal bypass operation (Fig 2). Restenosis occurred more often in patients with mild residual stenosis identified 1 day after PTRA. The restenosis rate did not differ significantly between patients with atherosclerosis vs. FMD, nor between those with ostial vs. nonostial lesions. Hypertension was improved or cured in 85% of the patients with FMD and in 70% of those with atherosclerosis. Despite exclusion of 60% or greater restenosis at CCD and intra-arterial angiography, 12% of the patients had an increase in blood pressure. In 14% of the patients with restenosis, however, blood pressure did not increase.

Conclusion.—Consistent sonographic follow-up after PTRA and catheter reintervention for restenosis increased the 12-month patency rate to 94% in these patients with renovascular disease. Early CCD scanning allows early results of PTRA to be interpreted and aids in decision making.

► In this prospective study, renal US and color-coded Doppler were used to evaluate renal artery stenosis in patients referred for evaluation of renovascular hypertension and/or azotemia. Fifty patients underwent percutaneous transluminal angioplasty for renal artery stenosis. As shown in Figure 2, the primary patency rate at 1 year was 70%, whereas re-treatment of patients who had restenosis during the follow-up interval increased the patency (secondary patency) rate to 90%. This study included both patients with atherosclerotic renal artery disease and patients with FMD, and the results were similar between these two groups, including both ostial and nonostial lesions.

Additional important findings of note were, first, the authors found that among 22 patients with evidence of impaired renal function prior to PTRA, there was a significant reduction in serum creatinine within 3 months that persisted up to 12 months. Second, they found that blood pressure was not a sensitive indicator for the presence of restenosis. About 12% of the patients with recurrent hypertension had no significant restenosis, and 14% with restenosis had no recurrent increase in their blood pressure. Like others, these authors found that the cure rate of hypertension is extremely low (less than 10%). However, blood pressure improved or was unchanged in 40% of the patients with atherosclerotic renal artery disease.

This study also underscores the utility of using color-coded Doppler and US to assess both anatomy and function.

R.D. Toto, M.D.

Results of Percutaneous Transluminal Angioplasty for Atherosclerotic Renal Artery Stenosis: A Follow-up Study With Duplex Ultrasonography

Tullis MJ, Zierler RE, Glickerman DJ, et al (Univ of Washington, Seattle; Seattle Veterans Affairs Med Ctr)

J Vasc Surg 25:46–54, 1997 3–11

Objective.—There is little information about the short- and long-term anatomical outcomes after percutaneous transluminal renal angioplasty (PTRA). The anatomical results of PTRA were evaluated with serial duplex ultrasonographic studies.

Methods.—A total of 52 PTRA procedures were performed on 41 patients (15 women; average patient age, 65 years) with a greater than 60% diameter reduction of the renal arteries. Patients were followed by renal artery ultrasonic duplex scanning for an average of 34 months to classify the extent of disease.

Results.—Patients underwent 5 to 10 duplex examinations. Stents were placed in 12 arteries. Restenosis developed in 29 patients. The cumulative incidence of restenosis from normal to 60% was 13% at 1 year and 19% at 2 years. The cumulative incidence of restenosis from less than 60% to 60% or more was 44% at 1 year and 55% at 2 years. The difference in restenosis (normal vs. less than 60% stenosis) after 2 years was significant. Whereas 83% of stented arteries and 33% of unstented arteries were normal immediately after PTRA, 1 year later, 44% of stented arteries and 18% of unstented arteries had restenosed.

Conclusion.—Duplex ultrasonographic follow-up of PTRA shows that the initial anatomical result is predictive of restenosis. Although stenting gives superior improvement initially, arteries so treated show a high early restenosis rate.

▶ This study is a retrospective analysis of the outcome after PTRA in patients with known renal artery stenosis. The data are important because they illustrate the use of the duplex scan as a method for measurement, as well as monitoring of the outcome, of renal artery lesions. Although there are shortcomings in this technique—particularly dependence on the expertise of the technician performing the study—it may become a more important clinical tool for assessing atherosclerotic artery disease at baseline and in follow-up.

Whether the technique will replace renal arteriography for this purpose remains to be determined. However, future prospective studies should compare the technique with angiography. It may be the best test for screening and monitoring disease progress in the future.

R.D. Toto, M.D.

Short-term Effects of Blood Pressure Control and Antihypertensive Drug Regimen on Glomerular Filtration Rate: The African-American Study of Kidney Disease and Hypertension Pilot Study

Hall WD, Kusek JW, Kirk KA, et al (Natl Inst of Diabetes and Digestive and Kidney Diseases, NIH, Bethesda, Md)

Am J Kidney Dis 29:720–728, 1997 3–12

Introduction.—In blacks, hypertension occurs with greater frequency and severity than in other racial and ethnic groups. The level of blood pressure control and the use of a specific class of antihypertensive drugs with renoprotective properties are 2 factors that may be important in slowing the long-term decline in glomerular filtration rate in hypertensive blacks. A descriptive analysis was developed of the short-term changes in glomerular filtration rate after randomization to usual or low blood pressure goals and to 1 of 3 antihypertensive drugs in a nondiabetic, black, hypertensive population at high risk of progression to end-stage renal disease.

Methods.—There were 94 nondiabetic black men and women with a mean age of 53 years with presumed hypertensive nephrosclerosis and a mean glomerular filtration rate of 25–75 mL/min/per 1.73 m^2. Forty-six were were randomly assigned to blood pressure control at a usual mean arterial pressure goal of 102–107 mm Hg and 44 to a low mean arterial pressure goal of 92 mm Hg or less. There were 31 who received an antihypertensive drug regimen that included a beta-blocker (atenolol), 28 who received a calcium antagonist (amlodipine), and 31 who received an angiotensin-converting enzyme inhibitor (enalapril)

Results.—In participants assigned to the low mean arterial pressure group, the mean glomerular filtration rate was similar to the baseline levels, whereas for participants assigned to the usual mean arterial pressure group, the mean glomerular filtration rate increased by 3.9 mL/min/per 1.73 m^2. In participants assigned to the calcium channel blocker regimen, the mean glomerular filtration rate increased significantly. There were no changes in participants assigned to the angiotensin-converting enzyme inhibitor regimen or to the beta-blocker regimen. Among the 3 different groups, changes in glomerular filtration rates were significantly different at 3 months.

Conclusion.—When estimating sample size for clinical trials designed to evaluate the effects of interventions on long-term changes in the glomerular filtration rate slope, the magnitude of short-term effects of blood pressure control and antihypertensive drug regimens on glomerular filtration rate should be considered.

► The effects of blood pressure lowering and specific antihypertensive agents on renal function are incompletely understood. Moreover, there is very little information in the literature on the effects of various classes of antihypertensive agents on renal function in patients at risk for progressive renal disease. The Modification of Diet in Renal Disease Study showed that the short-term effects of blood pressure lowering have an important effect on glomerular filtration rate, which in turn has implications for interpreting long-term benefit of blood pressure lowering on renal outcome.

This article is an analysis of the blood pressure and renal function measurements made during the pilot phase of the NIH-sponsored multicenter clinical trial entitled "The African-American Study of Kidney Disease and Hypertension (AASK study)." In the pilot phase, participants were randomly assigned to a low blood pressure (BP) goal (mean arterial pressure (MAP) less than 92 mm Hg) or usual goal BP (MAP 102–107 mm Hg) and 1 of 3 drug regimens that included either an angiotensin-converting enzyme inhibitor, calcium channel blocker or a beta-blocker. Hall et al. report that after 3 months glomerular filtration rate (GFR) remained unchanged in the low BP goal but increased by about 4 mL/min/1.73 m^2 in the usual BP goal. There was a weak but positive correlation between change in BP and change in GFR at 3 months, indicating that a decrease in BP was associated with a decrease in GFR at 3 months. Despite similar BP control levels across the 3 antihypertensive regimens, there was a significant increase in GFR in amlodipine-treated participants regardless of MAP assignment. Overall, neither atenolol nor amlodipine resulted in significant changes in mean GFR, although there was a trend for a decrease in GFR in enalapril-treated participants assigned to the low MAP goal.

These findings are important for several reasons. First, they provide new information on the effects of commonly used antihypertensive agents in patients with renal disease. Second, the data are collected in a patient population at high risk for progressive renal disease attributed to hypertension, the second leading cause of end-stage renal disease in the United States. Third, the data support the findings in the modification of Diet in Renal Disease study that knowledge of the effects of BP lowering and varying effects of drug classes on GFR must be taken into consideration when designing and analyzing long-term clinical trials aimed at improving outcome in hypertensive patients with renal disease.

R.D. Toto, M.D.

Achievement and Safety of a Low Blood Pressure Goal in Chronic Renal Disease: The Modification of Diet in Renal Disease Study Group

Lazarus JM, Bourgoignie JJ, Buckalew VM, et al (Natl Inst of Diabetes and Digestive and Kidney Diseases, NIH, Bethesda, Md)

Hypertension 29:641–650, 1997 3–13

Introduction.—The incidence of cardiovascular and cerebrovascular disease can be decreased with treatment of hypertension. The rate of progression of chronic renal disease can also be slowed by reducing elevated blood pressure. The progression of renal disease has been beneficially affected by angiotensin-converting enzyme inhibitors. In patients with proteinuria, a previous study showed a beneficial effect of a lower-than-usual blood pressure goal on the progression of renal disease. The

TABLE.—Univariate Cox Regressions Relating Cumulative Mean Follow-up Blood Pressure Measurements to Frequency of Hospitalization

Predictor	Risk Ratio**	*P* value
First Hospitalization		
MAP	1.08	0.43
Systolic BP	1.17	0.001
Diastolic BP	0.83	0.07
First Hospitalization for Cardiovascular disease		
MAP	1.61	0.009
Systolic BP	1.35	0.001
Diastolic BP	1.11	0.6

(Adapted from (Lazarus JM, Bourgoignie JJ, Buckalew VM, et al: Achievement and safety of a low blood pressure goal in chronic renal disease: The modification of diet in renal disease study group. *Hypertension* 29:641–650, 1997.)

achievement of blood pressure goals and the safety of blood pressure interventions were assessed.

Methods.—There were 585 patients, few of which had a history of cardiovascular disease, who had a baseline glomerular filtration rate between 13 and 55 mL/min per 1.73 m^2 included in the study, and they were randomly assigned to either a low blood pressure goal of less than 92 mm Hg or a usual blood pressure goal of less than 107 mm Hg. Angiotensin-converting enzyme inhibitors with or without diuretics followed by calcium channel blockers were the preferred antihypertensive agents permitted, but all were allowed.

Results.—In the low blood pressure group, the mean arterial pressure was 93.0±7.3 mm Hg. In the usual blood pressure group, the mean arterial pressure was 97.7±7.7 mm Hg. In subgroups of patients with pre-existing hypertension, follow-up blood pressure was significantly higher. It was also higher in patients who had baseline mean arterial pressure greater than 92 mm Hg, baseline urinary protein excretion of greater than 1 g/day, 61 years or more, black race, and a diagnosis of polycystic kidney disease. In the low blood pressure group, the frequency of medication changes and incidence of symptoms of low blood pressure were greater. In the 2 groups, there were no differences between stop points, death, or hospitalizations Each 1-mm Hg increase in follow-up systolic blood pressure was associated with a 1.35-times greater risk of hospitalization for cardiovascular or cerebrovascular disease, when data from both groups were combined (see Table).

Conclusion.—In patients with chronic renal disease without cardiovascular disease, lower blood pressure than usually recommended for the prevention of cardiovascular disease is achievable by several medication regimens without serious adverse effects. Target blood pressure should be a mean arterial pressure of less than 92 mm Hg, equivalent to 125/75 mm Hg for patients with urinary protein excretion of more than 1 g/day.

► Optimal blood pressure lowering for renal protection is contentious and subject to serious debate. A major issue is whether lower than usual control of blood pressure (BP) is critical for preserving renal function in patients with renal diseases known to be progressive. A related and equally important issue is whether such lowering is safe, particularly in view of the high incidence of nonrenal cardiovascular complications in patients with renal disease, e.g., myocardial infarction.

In this article, Lazarus et al. report the experience of the Modification of Diet in Renal Disease study with these 2 important and related issues. First, they report that it is feasible to achieve and maintain a mean arterial pressure (MAP) less than 92 mm Hg (or less than 98 mm Hg for individuals older than 61 years) in patients with chronic renal disease and point out that this level of control is more effective at slowing progression of disease in patients with high-grade proteinuria (greater than 1 g/24 hr). Second, they found that although lowering BP to this level was associated with more frequent changes in BP medication and symptoms there was no increase in hospitalizations, stop points in the study, or deaths as compared to an MAP goal of 102–107 mm Hg. Finally, as shown in the table, they found that for each 1 mm Hg increase in follow-up systolic BP, there was a 1.35–times greater risk of hospitalization for cardiovascular or cerebrovascular disease and a 1.17–times greater risk of hospitalization for any cause. These findings are important because they illustrate the benefit/risk ratio of unconventional BP lowering (MAP less than 92 mm Hg or less than 98 mm Hg for patients older than 61 years) in a group of patients at high risk for nonrenal and renal complications. They also indicate that lowering blood pressure to 125/75 (or 135/80) mm Hg to preserve renal function in proteinuric patients is advisable, feasible, and relatively safe.

R.D. Toto, M.D.

Early Detection and Treatment of Renal Disease in Hospitalized Diabetic and Hypertensive Patients: Important Differences Between Practice and Published Guidelines

McClellan WM, Knight DF, Karp H, et al (Emory Univ, Atlanta, Ga; Georgia Med Care Found, Atlanta; St Louis Univ)

Am J Kidney Dis 29:368–375, 1997 3–14

Introduction.—In more than 60% of new patients with end-stage renal disease, diabetes or hypertension is the cause. Progressive kidney failure in diabetics and hypertensive patients with early renal disease can be delayed or prevented with effective treatment. Failure to identify and appropriately treat kidney disease among at-risk patients contributed to the increase in the occurrence of diabetic and hypertensive end-stage renal disease. The degree to which the care of hospitalized diabetic and hypertensive patients conforms to published guidelines for the detection and management of early renal disease was ascertained.

Methods.—A retrospective chart audit was conducted of 260 diabetic patients and 327 hypertensive patients who were Medicare beneficiaries

TABLE 5.—The Percentage of Diabetic Patients Discharged With Treatment According to the Degree of Proteinuria

Percentage of Patients at Discharge:	Degree of Proteinuria 1+	2+	3+	4+	Total
n	24	16	7	4	51
ACEI (%)	33.3	37	28	25	33
Protein restriction (%)	4.2	0	0	0	2
NSAIDS (%)	8.3	6	0	0	2
Acetamin (%)	8.3	18.8	14.3	25.0	
SBP (mm Hg)	140.6	142.0	133.3	137.0	
DBP (mm Hg)	70.7	70.4	74.1	72.8	

(Courtesy of McClellan WM, Knight DF, Karp H, et al: Early detection and treatment of renal disease in hospitalized diabetic and hypertensive patients: important differences between practice and published guidelines. *Am J Kidney Dis* 29:368–375, 1997.)

with a mean age of 65.9. Charts were reviewed for the first serum creatinine during the index hospitalization, any measurement for microalbuminuria, urinalysis, blood pressure at discharge, dietary restrictions, prescription of drugs, and diagnosis of renal disease or renal abnormalities in the discharge summary.

Results.—For 163 (62.7%) of the diabetic patients, a urinalysis was obtained, and of these, 31.3% had 1+ or greater dipstick proteinuria. For 298 (91%) of the hypertensive patients, a serum creatinine was obtained, and of these, 11.8% had a value of 1.5 mg/dL or greater. In the discharge summaries of 7.8% of the diabetics and in 11.4% of the hypertensives, abnormal renal function tests were recorded. Treatment with angiotensin-converting enzyme inhibitors was no more likely to occur for patients with abnormal renal function than for the other patients (Table 5). For 6% of the diabetics and for 8.8% of the hypertensives with abnormal renal function at discharge, nonsteroidal anti-inflammatory drugs were prescribed. An awareness of impaired renal function was not reflected in patient treatment plans at discharge.

Conclusion.—The medical records of these patients did not document awareness or appropriate management of the potential underlying kidney disease, despite the high prevalence of renal functional abnormalities detected by routine laboratory tests administered to elderly hospitalized diabetic and hypertensive patients. Among hospitalized diabetic and hypertensive patients, there was a low rate of screening for renal disease. Continuing medical education and quality improvement programs designed to improve the early detection and treatments of renal disease in these high-risk patients may be warranted in the hospital.

► Diabetes and hypertension account for two thirds of end-stage renal disease patients in the United States. Although prevention of the progression to end-stage renal disease has not been demonstrated consistently in either of these diseases, effective therapy can slow disease progression and, in some cases, stop it altogether. In this study, the authors report several remarkable findings concerning recognition and appropriate management of individuals less than age 75 hospitalized in 1994 with a primary or secondary diagnosis of hypertension or diabetes. First, they found that amongst the diabetic patients, one third did not have routine urinalysis performed.

Second, at discharge a high percentage of these patients did not have evidence of renal disease (that is, proteinuria, hypercreatinemia) addressed at the time of discharge. Moreover, despite the fact that published studies showing angiotensin converting enzyme (ACE) inhibitors slow the progression of diabetic nephropathy were available before 1994 (chart review for this study), only a third of proteinuric diabetics were prescribed ACE inhibitors at the time of discharge (see Table 5). This underscores the fact that translation of new clinical research to clinical practice and hospital management is very slow. This is an important study because it points out the fact that rapid and widespread dissemination of new and effective therapies for renal disease of hypertension and diabetes is needed. Closer communication between nephrologists and primary care physicians is an important future goal for preventing and treating these common and widespread renal diseases. Moreover, the application of other effective therapies, including protein restriction and possibly cholesterol lowering in these patient populations, needs to be advanced further.

R.D. Toto, M.D.

Kidney Vascular Damage and Cocaine

Di Paolo N, Fineschi V, Di Paolo M, et al (Univ of Siena, Italy; Dade County Med Examiner's Dept, Miami, Fla)

Clin Nephrol 47:298–303, 1997 3–15

Introduction.—Cocaine can cause vascular ischemia that can lead to cardiovascular damage, cerebral vasculitis, renal artery thrombosis, intestinal infarction, pneumothorax, and deep venous thrombosis of the peripheral circulation. Myocardial infarction and sudden death are the best known and examined pathologic conditions related to cocaine. Whether the same vascular changes are found in the kidneys of cocaine addicts as in the heart was determined via histologic examination of 40 kidney autopsy specimens classified as "cocaine-related deaths."

Methods.—Semiquantitative and quantitative morphometric analyses were performed on tissue preparations of kidneys from the 40 cocaine addicts and from 40 road-accident victims (controls).

Results.—The mean age of cocaine addicts was 35.1 years, and the mean age for controls was 36.2 years. The ratio of the number of glomeruli affected by hyalinosis to the total number of glomeruli, the degree of interstitial cellular infiltration, the degree of periglomerular fibrosis, and the presence of arterial sclerosis all were significantly higher in addicts than in controls. The ratio of glomeruli to tubular casts was similar in addicts and in controls. Medial thickening, luminal narrowing, and vessel obstruction were not observed in the control group. Greater lumen circumference, intima circumference, media circumference, intima area, intima thickness, and media thickness were significantly greater in cocaine addicts than in controls.

Conclusion.—Cocaine addiction usually manifests as toxic cardiopathy, but the severe damage observed in the renal arterioles definitely aggravates the hypertensive state caused by catecholamine stimulation.

▶ Cocaine abuse can cause widespread vascular damage, including strokes, acute myocardial infarction, and rhabdomyolysis with subsequent renal injury. However, few studies have addressed the question of whether cocaine abuse is associated with renovascular damage. This is an important issue because the incidence of hypertensive renal disease is high in inner city populations at risk for cocaine abuse.

Di Paolo et al. show that cocaine addicts have a very high incidence of renovascular damage. The kidney abnormalities found in these addicts are reported in patients with hypertensive nephrosclerosis, which is a progressive form of renal disease to which one third of end-stage renal disease cases have been attributed (in the U.S. population). The incidence of renovascular disease observed in these cases includes findings consistent with the ischemic injury, hyperplasia, and hypertrophy observed in hypertensive nephrosclerosis.

Although this study cannot confirm that cocaine was the responsible factor in the renovascular damage observed in these autopsy cases, it seems quite plausible. Cocaine abuse may engender and/or exacerbate renal damage in individuals with hypertension who are susceptible to renal injury. A prospective study examining the effects of cocaine in patients with hypertensive progressive kidney disease would be useful to confirm the findings in this interesting and provocative study.

R.D. Toto, M.D.

Genetic Susceptibility to Hypertension-induced Renal Damage in the Rat: Evidence Based on Kidney-specific Genome Transfer

Churchill PC, Churchill MC, Bidani AK, et al (Wayne State Univ, Detroit; Loyola Univ, Maywood, Ill; Czech Academy of Sciences, Prague, Czech Rebublic et al)

J Clin Invest 100:1373–1382, 1997 3–16

Introduction.—The question of genetic susceptibility to hypertension-induced renal damage has typically been addressed using a small number of blood pressure measures obtained with indirect methods over relatively brief periods of time. An experimental rat model was created in which 2 genetically different but histocompatible kidneys were simultaneously exposed on a long-term basis to the same blood pressure profile and metabolic environment within the same host.

Methods.—Kidneys from normotensive Brown Norway (BN) rats were transplanted into unilaterally nephrectomized spontaneously hypertensive

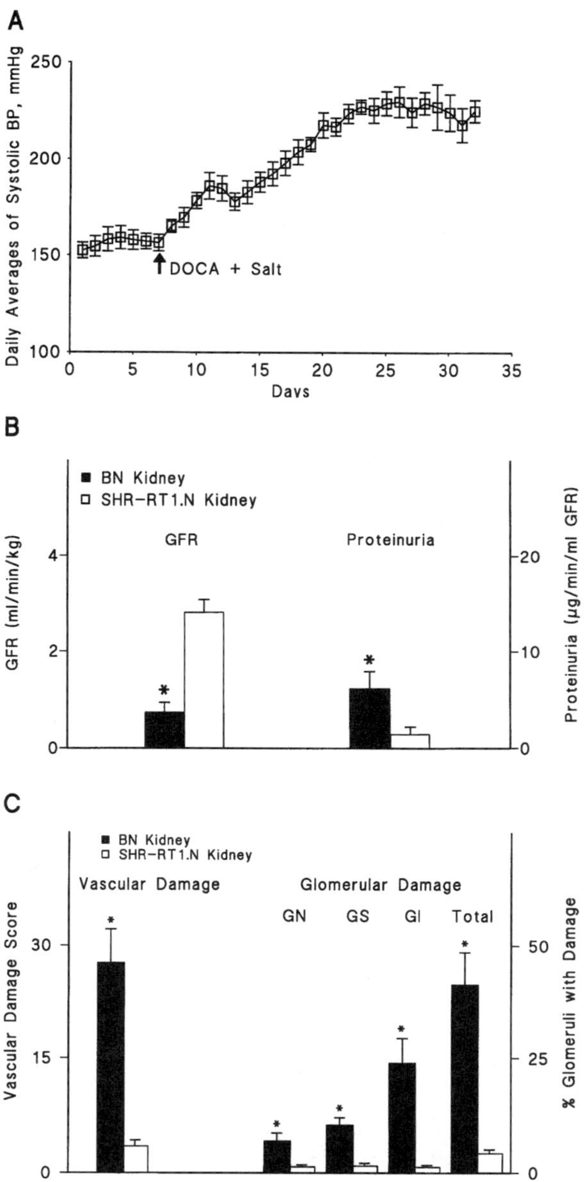

FIGURE 3.—Blood pressure, renal function, and renal histologic characteristics in unilaterally nephrectomized SHR-RT1.N recipients of BN donor kidneys (group 3; $n = 8$; 5 females and 3 males). **A,** daily averages of systolic blood pressure before and during administration of DOCA-salt. In each rat, systolic blood pressure was sampled for 5 sec every 10 minutes, 24 hr/day. **B,** glomerular filtration rates and protein excretion rates of transplanted and contralateral native BN kidneys. **C,** vascular and glomerular damage scores in transplanted and contralateral native BN kidneys. $^*P < 0.02$ maximum, BN kidney vs. SHR-RT1.N kidney. *Black bars,* BN kidney; *white bars,* SHR-RT1.N kidney. *Abbreviations: BN,* Brown Norway rat: *SHR,* spontaneously hypertensive rats; *BP,* blood pressure; *DOCA,* deoxycorticosterone acetate; *GFR,* glomerular filtration rate; *GN,* glomerular necrosis; *GS,* glomerular sclerosis; *GI,* glomerular ischemia; *total,* sum of the 3 individual glomerular damage scores. (Reproduced from *The Journal of Clinical Investigation* 100:1373–1382, 1997 by copyright permission of The Rockefeller University Press, from Churchill PC, Churchill MC, Bidani AK, et al: Genetic susceptibility to hypertension-induced renal damage in the rat: Evidence based on kidney-specific transfer.)

rats (SHR-RT1.N strain) (Fig 3). Recipient rats harbor the major histocompatibility complex of the BN strain. Rats were treated with deoxycorticosterone acetate (DOCA) via subcutaneous pellets and an oral salt solution to accelerate the development of hypertension and renal injury. The arterial blood pressure and heart rate were recorded, and split renal function studies were performed. The animals were killed, and the kidneys were examined histologically.

Results.—At 25 days after the induction of severe hypertension with DOCA and salt, proteinuria, an impaired glomerular filtration rate, and extensive vascular and glomerular injury were detected in the BN donor kidneys but not in the SHR-RT1.N kidneys. Control experiments showed that the strain differences in kidney damage could not be explained by the effects of transplantation-induced renal injury, immunologic rejection phenomena, or pre-existing strain differences in blood pressure.

Conclusion.—These findings show that the kidney of the normotensive BN rat is intrinsically much more susceptible to hypertension-induced damage than is the kidney of the SHR-RT1.N. The strain differences demonstrate the significance of genetics in hypertension.

▶ Hypertension is the attributed cause for nearly one third of the cases of end-stage renal disease in the United States, and a genetic predisposition to renal damage has been hypothesized in blacks, who bear a disproportionate burden of renal failure as a result of hypertension alone. The study is novel and, although not done in humans, provides compelling evidence for a genetic predisposition to hypertension.

In this cleverly designed study, Churchill et al. transplanted BN rat kidneys into SHR strains and measured blood pressure, renal function, glomerular filtration rate (GFR), proteinuria, and histologic characteristics.

As shown in Figure 3, prolonged hypertension reduced the GFR induced by a unilateral nephrectomy and administration of a DOCA–high salt diet in the transplanted BN kidney (black bars) but not in the native SHR kidney (white bars). Moreover, vascular damage was markedly increased in the BN rat kidney compared with the SHR kidney. Furthermore, evidence that genetic predisposition for renal injury comes from the fact that the maintenance of blood pressure at normal levels with antihypertensive agents before administration of DOCA–salt did not protect the BN kidney from subsequent hypertensive damage.

These data argue strongly that a genetic predisposition to hypertensive renal injury does indeed occur. Future studies looking for genetic hypertension in humans are needed to improve our ability to prevent hypertensive end-stage renal disease.

R.D. Toto, M.D.

Leukocyte Infiltration and ICAM-1 Expression in Two-Kidney One-Clip Hypertension

Haller H, Park J-K, Dragun D, et al (Humboldt Univ, Berlin)

Nephrol Dial Transplant 12:899–903, 1997 3–17

Introduction.—In a previous study, it was shown that in the rat, 2K 1C hypertension features interstitial infiltration of inflammatory leukocytes, proliferation of tubular epithelial cells, and matrix deposition. A tissue reaction generally associated with an inflammatory response was elicited with a marked increase in blood pressure. This process seems to involve vascular cell surface adhesion molecules because T lymphocytes and macrophages infiltrated the blood vessels to reach the interstitium. Early in the course of renal perfusion injury, the surface adhesion molecule ICAM-1 is expressed on the vascular endothelium. It is still not known how an increase in blood pressure induces hypertensive nephrosclerosis. This study tested the hypothesis that 2K 1C hypertension in the rat can induce ICAM-1 expression, which is associated with leukocyte infiltration in the kidney.

Methods.—Renal hypertension initiation was induced in rats by occluding the left renal artery with a silver clip and keeping the right kidney undisturbed. The clipped kidney was examined as a positive control. Sham operations were performed on control rats by making an incision in the flank following a 30-second interruption of the renal artery blood flow. Systolic blood pressure was measured 4 weeks after the clips, and then the animals were sacrificed. Immunohistochemistry and pathology were conducted, and the degree of leukocyte infiltration was determined.

Results.—In renovascular hypertensive rats, systolic blood pressure was significantly elevated in comparison with sham-operated controls after 4 weeks. The ICAM-1 expression on vascular endothelium and on tubular cells was significantly increased in unclipped kidneys compared with controls, according the quantitative densitometry measurements. Monocyte and granulocyte infiltration were also increased in the unclipped kidneys. In the clipped kidneys, the same variables were even more prominent.

Conclusion.—In unclipped kidneys exposed to hypertension as well as in clipped kidneys exposed to ischemia, ICAM-1 is expressed. An inflammatory adhesion molecule-mediate response and concomitant renal injury may be caused by mechanical injury induced by increased blood pressure.

► Hypertensive renal injury is a complex process involving a number of factors, including structural integrity of the vascular wall and endothelial injury. Both functional and anatomic studies indicate that increases in vascular resistance in kidneys, of hypertensives are associated with vascular remodeling. The mechanism by which hypertension induces remodeling within the vasculature, which contributes to the pathophysiology and pathogenesis of subsequent renal disease, remains unknown.

This experimental animal model of renovascular hypertension provides insight into pathogenesis of vascular injury. Intriguing data indicate that hypertensive response induces upregulation of intercellular adhesion molecules. Specifically, Haller et al. show that leukocyte infiltration is preceded with an increase in ICAM-1 expression in kidneys of hypertensive rats using the 2-kidney, 1-clip model. Their data strongly suggest that the vascular pathology is contributed to by the expression of specific surface adhesion molecules, which subsequently lead to attachment and infusion of inflammatory cells.

These findings are experimental, but they may be highly relevant to human disease in which similar pathological changes in the vessels occur. It seems not only plausible, but also highly likely, that hypertensive injury is one of many factors that leads to alterations in endothelial and smooth muscle cell function mediated by cytokines, adhesion molecules, and inflammatory cytokines.

R.D. Toto, M.D.

Left Ventricular Hypertrophy in Non–Insulin-dependent Diabetic Patients With and Without Diabetic Nephropathy

Nielsen FS, Ali S, Rossing P, et al (Steno Diabetes Ctr, Gentofte, Denmark; Rigshospitalet, Copenhagen; Naestved Hosp, Denmark)

Diabetic Med 14:538–546, 1997 3–18

Introduction.—The increased morbidity and mortality from cardiovascular disease seen in patients with non–insulin-dependent diabetes mellitus (NIDDM) compared with the general population cannot be completely explained by cardiovascular risk factors. Putative mechanisms of the increased cardiac morbidity and mortality in patients with NIDDM with and without diabetic nephropathy were assessed.

Methods.—Previous antihypertensive treatment was withdrawn 2 weeks before evaluation in 51 patients with NIDDM with diabetic nephropathy (group 1), 53 patients with NIDDM and normoalbuminuria (group 2), and 22 controls without diabetes (group 3). Patients underwent echocardiography to determine left ventricular mass index (LVMI) and systolic function.

Results.—The LVMI was elevated in group 1 and 2 compared with group 3 (157, 139, and 95 g/m2, respectively). The prevalence of left ventricular hypertrophy (LVH) was significantly higher for groups 1 and 2 compared with group 3 (75%, 51%, and 9%, respectively). Compared with group 3, groups 1 and 2 had a relatively reduced shortening fraction of the left ventricle (41.2%, 32.5%, and 33.4%, respectively) (Table 2). In a subgroup of 26 patients with NIDDM who had a normal amount of serum proteins in the urine and normal blood pressure, the LVMI was higher than in 14 controls without diabetes who had normal blood pressure (137 vs. 96 g/m2); the prevalence of LVH was 42% in the former group and 14% in the latter group.

Conclusion.—Patients with NIDDM with and without diabetic nephropathy who have normal blood pressure or hypertension commonly have

TABLE 2.—Echocardiographic Parameters in Patients With NIDDM With and Without Diabetic Nephropathy and in Control Research Subjects

	NIDDM patients with nephropathy	NIDDM patients with normoalbuminuria	Control subjects	p-value
LVDD (mm)	52.7 ± 1.0	51.8 ± 1.2	51.6 ± 1.3	NS
LVSD (mm)	35.8 ± 1.1	35.0 ± 1.3	30.5 ± 1.2	*,†
STD (mm)	13.6 ± 0.3	12.2 ± 0.3	9.2 ± 0.2	‡,§,‖
PWTD (mm)	10.7 ± 0.3	10.2 ± 0.3	8.1 ± 0.4	‡,§
PWTS (mm)	15.9 ± 0.4	15.4 ± 0.4	14.4 ± 0.4	NS
Left ventricular wall stress	90.9 ± 5.1	78.8 ± 5.2	67.5 ± 5.0	†
Shortening fraction of left ventricle (%)	32.5 ± 1.1	33.4 ± 1.1	41.2 ± 1.2	‡,§
Relative posterior wall thickness	0.42 ± 0.01	0.40 ± 0.01	0.32 ± 0.01	‡,§
LVM (g)	317 ± 14	277 ± 15	187 ± 11	‡,§,¶
LVMI (g m^{-2})	157 ± 6	139 ± 7	95 ± 5	‡,§,¶
Prevalence of left ventricular hypertrophy (%)	75 (60–86)	51 (37–65)	9 (1–29)	‡,§,**

Note: Data are mean plus or minus standard error.
*$P < 0.05$ comparing control research subjects and patients with NIDDM and normoalbuminuria.
†$P < 0.005$ comparing control research subjects with patients with NIDDM and nephropathy
‡$P < 0.001$ comparing control research subjects and patients with NIDDM and normoalbuminuria
§$P < 0.001$ comparing control research subjects with patients with NIDDM and nephropathy
‖$P < 0.005$ comparing patients with NIDDM with nephropathy and normoalbuminuria
¶$P = 0.05$ comparing patients with NIDDM with nephropathy and normoalbuminuria
**$P < 0.01$ comparing patients with NIDDM with nephropathy and normoalbuminuria.
Abbreviations: NIDDM, non–insulin dependent diabetes mellitus; *LVDD,* left ventricular end-diastolic diameter; *LVSD,* left ventricular end-systolic diameter; *STD,* ventricular septum thickness in diastole; *PWTD,* posterior wall thickness in diastole; *PWTS,* posterior wall thickness in systole; *LVM,* left ventricular mass; *LVMI,* left ventricular mass index.

(Courtesy of Nielsen FS, Ali S, Rossing P, et al: Left ventricular hypertrophy in non–insulin-dependent diabetic patients with and without diabetic nephropathy. *Diabetic Med* 14:538–546, 1997. © 1997 John Wiley & Sons, Ltd. Reprinted by permission of John Wiley & Sons, Ltd.)

LVH and relatively decreased systolic function, which can be independent risk factors for fatal and nonfatal cardiac events.

► Left ventricular hypertrophy is an independent risk factor for cardiovascular mortality. Moreover, the prevalence of LVH in patients with end-stage renal disease who start undergoing dialysis is as high as 75%. Also, patients with diabetes constitute the largest proportion of individuals entering the end-stage renal disease treatment environment in the United States.

In this study by Nielsen et al., the relationship between diabetes and diabetic nephropathy in patients wih NIDDM who have either normal blood pressure or hypertension is evaluated. The authors found that LVH was more severe in patients with nephropathy than in those without. Although the patients with nephropathy had albuminuria, the renal function was only mildly to moderately impaired. However, more interesting is the finding that even patients with type II diabetes with normal blood pressure but without albuminuria have increased left ventricular wall mass (see Table 2). As shown in Table 2, the LVMI is increased in patients with normoalbuminuria and diabetic nephropathy compared with controls. Furthermore, the left ventricular shortening fraction is impaired in the patients with diabetes.

Hypertension no doubt contributes to the magnitude of LVH in patients with nephropathy. However, it would appear from this cross-sectional study that some patients with NIDDM, of whom some fraction are expected to have nephropathy, have LVH for reasons unrelated to hypertension. Of note is the fact that ambulatory blood pressure measurements made in these patients showed that blood pressures were elevated in patients with nephropathy but not in patients with normoalbuminuria. This, again, suggests nonhypertensive factors—a mechanism of LVH in patients with NIDDM.

Concerning nonhemodynamic factors, this study did control for age, body mass index, salt intake, and blood viscosity. The factors or mechanisms responsible for inducing hypertrophy need to be evaluated further to develop strategies for reducing the likelihood of LVH, and thereby the cardiovascular mortality associated with this malady.

R.D. Toto, M.D.

Accuracy of the Diagnosis of Hypertensive Nephrosclerosis in African Americans: A Report From the African American Study of Kidney Disease (AASK) Trial

Fogo A, and the AASK Pilot Study Investigators (Vanderbilt Univ, Nashville, Tenn; Case Western Reserve Univ, Cleveland, Ohio; Morehouse School of Medicine, Atlanta, GA; et al)

Kidney Int 51:244–252, 1997 3–19

Background.—Compared to white Americans, African Americans have an excess of hypertension and end-stage renal disease presumably to be caused by hypertension. The African American Study of Kidney Disease (AASK) Trial assessed the effects of antihypertensive treatments and 2 levels of blood pressure control on the rate of decline of glomerular filtration rate in African Americans with presumed hypertensive renal disease.

Methods.—Eighty-eight eligible participants were assessed initially by renal biopsy to evaluate underlying lesions. The subjects were nondiabetic African Americans aged 18–70 years, with glomerular filtration rate between 25 and 70 mL/min/1.73 m^2 and with no marked proteinuria. Forty-three subjects did not undergo biopsy because of contraindications or refusal. Adequate renal biopsy specimens were acquired from 39 of the remaining 46 patients.

Findings.—Thirty-eight of the 39 biopsies showed arteriosclerosis and/or arteriolosclerosis. Both had a mean severity of 1.5 on a scale of 0–3+ scale. Moderate interstitial fibrosis was observed. Five biopsies showed segmental glomerulosclerosis. In 1 patient, biopsy and clinical findings suggested idiopathic focal segmental glomerulosclerosis. In addition, 1 patient had mesangiopathic glomerulonephritis; 1, basement membrane thickening suggesting diabetic nephropathy; and 2, cholesterol emboli. Arteriolar and arterial sclerosis were closely associated. It was also correlated with interstitial fibrosis and the reciprocal of serum creatinine. Global glomerulosclerosis involved an average of 43% of glomeruli. The extent of this lesion was unassociated with the degree of arteriolar and arterial thickening but was correlated with systolic blood pressure, the reciprocal of serum creatinine, serum cholesterol, and interstitial fibrosis.

Conclusions.—The clinical diagnosis of hypertensive nephrosclerosis, based on careful clinical and laboratory assessment, is very accurate. Renal biopsies in nondiabetic hypertensive African Americans with mild to moderate renal insufficiency in the absence of marked proteinuria are highly likely to show renal vascular lesions consistent with the clinical diagnosis of hypertensive neophrosclerosis.

▶ The diagnosis of hypertensive nephrosclerosis remains controversial. Although 29% of cases of end-stage renal disease are attributed to hypertension in the United States, most of these patients never undergo a kidney biopsy. Therefore, the diagnosis is based on clinical grounds and some have questioned whether kidney disease in these patients is attributable to systemic hypertension vs. a primary kidney disease. Although there are no pathognomonic changes of hypertensive nephrosclerosis, the finding of characteristic changes of hypertension is well known, including afferent arteriolar hyalinosis, glomerular sclerosis and ischemia, and interstitial nephritis.

In this article, Fogo et al. report the findings from kidney biopsies of 43 black hypertensive patients with chronic renal insufficiency enrolled in the African American Study of Kidney Disease and Hypertension pilot project. The African-American hypertensive population is at highest risk for end-stage renal disease and was the subject of this investigation. The key finding is that African Americans with hypertension who have no systemic disease and in whom urinalysis is remarkable only for mild proteinuria are highly likely to have changes consistent with hypertensive nephrosclerosis and not a primary glomerular disease. Other renal diseases (e.g. glomerulonephritis) were observed in only 2 patients. In other words, on clinical grounds, the diagnosis of hypertensive nephrosclerosis is generally solid.

The authors also found an association between higher serum cholesterol and global glomerular sclerosis. This finding suggests that hypercholesteremia plays a role in the renal damage observed with hypertensive sclerosis.

This study is an important study for physicians taking care of patients with hypertension and renal disease. The article does not prove that hypertension is the cause for renal disease for asymptomatic hypertensive patients. However, it indicates that in asymptomatic A-A hypertensive patients without signs of systemic disease, nephrotic syndrome or abnormal urinary sediment, hypertensive nephrosclerosis is the most likely renal disease.

R.D. Toto, M.D.

A Short-term Antihypertensive Treatment-induced Fall in Glomerular Filtration Rate Predicts Long-term Stability of Renal Function

Apperloo AJ, de Zeeuw D, de Jong PE (Univ Hosp Groningen, The Netherlands)

Kidney Int 51:793–797, 1997 3–20

Objective.—In patients with renal impairment, the initial fall in glomerular filtration rate (GFR) caused by antihypertensive treatment may lead to concern about progressive renal function loss. Because the fall in GFR may be the result of lowered intraglomerular pressure, it may indicate long-term effectiveness of treatment. Results of a prospective study of renal hemodynamic response in patients with varying degrees of renal function impairment before treatment, during treatment with either atenolol or enapril, and after withdrawal of treatment were presented.

Methods.—Mean arterial pressure, GFR, and effective renal plasma flow were measured before treatment, every 24 weeks during the 4-year treatment period, and 12 weeks after discontinuing therapy with either atenolol or enapril in 40 nondiabetic patients (19 female; average patient age, 49.3 years). Treatment effects were analyzed statistically.

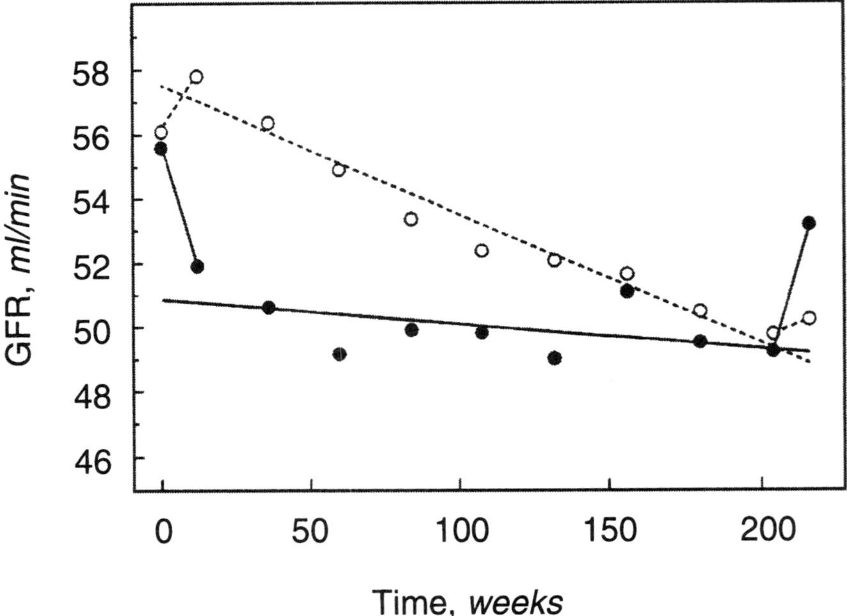

FIGURE 2.—Time course of glomerular filtration rate (GFR) before, during, and after withdrawal of antihypertensive treatment in group A and group B patients. Group A (*solid circle*) are patients who initially showed a distinct fall in GFR and group B (*open circle*) are patients in whom GFR did not fall after start of treatment. The change in GFR after start and withdrawal of treatment is indicated as well as the slope of GFR during treatment. (Reprinted by permission of Blackwell Science, Inc. from Apperloo AJ, de Zeeuw D, de Jong PE: A short-term antihypertensive treatment-induced fall in glomerular filtration rate predicts long-term stability of renal function. *Kidney Int* 51[3]:793–797, 1997.)

Results.—Blood pressure fell during treatment but returned to pretreatment levels after therapy was discontinued. Whereas the initial change in GFR varied from −11 to 11 mL/min, GFR decreased slowly but significantly during the 4-year follow-up period. After therapy was discontinued, GFR rose an average of 2.2 mL/min. The initial fall and subsequent rise after withdrawal of GFR were correlated. Patients with a steeper GFR fall had a more stable course during the follow-up period. Patients were divided into 2 groups, group A had a fall in GFR initially whereas group B had a stable GFR initially. Initially, group A had a fall in filtration fraction, whereas group B did not (Fig 2). Posttreatment GFR was significantly different from baseline in group B but not in group A because of the rise in GFR in group A.

Conclusion.—Glomerular filtration rate was more stable in the long run in patients who experienced an initial fall in GFR during treatment with antihypertensive drugs.

► In experimental animal models of hypertension and chronic renal failure, lowering blood pressure with angiotensin converting enzyme (ACE) inhibitors decreases glomerular capillary pressure, single nephron glomerular filtration rate, proteinuria, and glomerulosclerosis. Angiotensin converting enzyme inhibitors also reduce the risk of progressive renal failure in patients with nondiabetic and diabetic nephropathy. It is inferred that this protective effect is caused, in part, by a reduction in glomerular capillary pressure. Because glomerular capillary pressure cannot be measured in humans, it is unknown whether lowering blood pressure by any means, including ACE inhibitors, lowers glomerular capillary pressure to any extent.

In this report, Apperloo et al. studied a population of nondiabetic patients with progressive renal disease. Patients were administered either atenelol or enalapril in a randomized fashion with additional antihypertensive agents, including hydrochlorothide, clonidine, and calcium channel blockers as needed to maintain a diastolic blood pressure of less than 95 mm Hg.

Twenty patients who had a distinct decrease in GFR within the first 3 months of therapy had a slow overall decline in GFR during the following 45 months. In contrast, 20 patients who did not have a distinct lowering of GFR (in fact, their GFR increased) had a faster decline in GFR over the same period. Moreover, the authors found that withdrawal of antihypertensive therapy was associated with a rebound in GFR in those patients who initially had a decline in GFR, whereas there was no rebound in GFR in those who did not have the initial decrease. The authors concluded that an acute but reversible decline in GFR in response to antihypertensives identifies patients who are likely to benefit most in the long term.

Although the study is interesting and is consistent with reports from animal literature, there are several notes of caution. First, the 2 groups were identified retrospectively based on decline in GFR, not during prospective evaluation. Second, it is important to note that the group with the more rapidly declining GFR had a much higher average protein excretion rate at baseline. In fact, the mean protein excretion rate at baseline was 1.38 g/day vs. 0.4 g/day for the other group. Proteinuria is a well-known risk factor for rapid progression of renal disease and has been cited as a reason for intensifying blood pressure control to reduce the risk of progressive renal failure in patients with both nondiabetic and diabetic renal disease. Moreover, because the slopes of the 2 groups cross over at the end of the 4-year period, it is not known whether the changes in renal function would have continued the change shown on the initial slope in Figure 2. In conclusion, this study is interesting from the standpoint of mechanism. It is possible that the more sharp rates of decline are not related to effects of blood pressure control on GFR, but are caused by underlying renal disease, namely higher grade proteinuria.

R.D. Toto, M.D.

Differences Between Nisoldipine and Lisinopril on Glomerular Filtration Rates and Albuminuria in Hypertensive IDDM Patients With Diabetic Nephropathy During the First Year of Treatment

Rossing P, Tarnow L, Boelskifte S, et al (Steno Diabetes Ctr, Gentofte, Denmark)

Diabetes 46:481–487, 1997 3–21

Introduction.—Persistent albuminuria, a relentless decline in glomerular filtration rate (GFR) and increased arterial blood pressure, are characteristic of the clinical syndrome of diabetic nephropathy. An alternative hypertensive treatment in patients with diabetic nephropathy may be calcium antagonists. Previous studies have examined short-acting first-generation dihydropyridine calcium antagonists or have used few patients, mixed study populations, or uncontrolled designs. The change in kidney function during treatment with the second-generation long-acting dihydropyridine calcium antagonist nisoldipine or the angiotensin converting enzyme (ACE) inhibitor lisinopril was examined in hypertensive IDDM (insulin-dependent diabetes mellitus) patients with diabetic nephropathy.

Methods.—In 52 hypertensive IDDM patients with diabetic nephropathy, a 1-year double-blind, double-dummy, randomized controlled study was performed that compared nisoldipine (20–40 mg once daily) with lisinopril (10–20 mg once daily). Ten nisoldipine- and 8 lisinopril-treated patients required diuretics. Measurements were taken of albuminuria in three 24-hour samples with enzyme immunoassay and 24-hour ambulatory blood pressure every 3 months. Every 6 months, recordings were taken of GFR.

Results.—In the lisinopril group, mean arterial blood pressure decreased from a mean of 108 ± 3 mm Hg at baseline to 101 ± 2 during treatment (Fig 1). In the nisoldipine group, mean arterial blood pressure decreased from a mean of 105 ± 2 to 103 ± 2 mm Hg. In the lisinopril group, albuminuria was reduced 47% whereas in the nisoldipine group, albuminuria increased by 11%. In the lisinopril group, fractional albumin clearance was reduced by 37%, and in the nisoldipine group, there was an

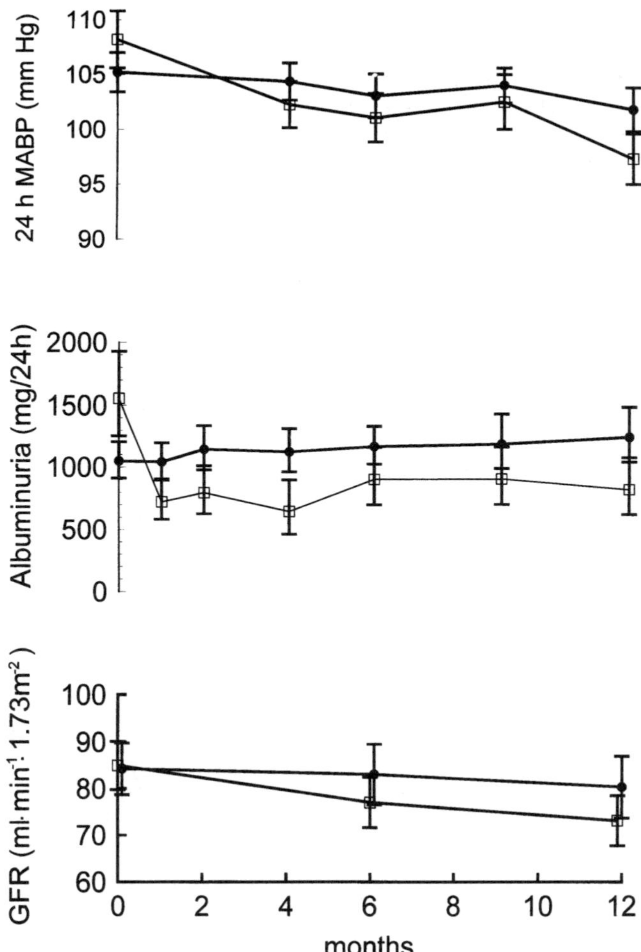

FIGURE 1.—Mean course of 24–h ambulatory mean arterial blood pressure (MABP), albuminuria, and GFR in hypertensive IDDM patients before and during antihypertensive treatment with lisinopril (*open circle*, n = 24) or nisoldipine (*closed circle*, n =25). Analysis of repeated measurements evaluating arterial blood pressure and albuminuria revealed a significant effect of time (P less than 0.01) but not of treatment group. There was a significant interaction between time and treatment group when evaluating albuminuria (P = 0.001). The decline in GFR after 12 months was greater in the lisinopril versus nisoldipine group (P less than 0.01). Bars represent standard error (Albuminuria: geometric mean ×/÷ antilog standard error). (Courtesy of Rossing P, Tarnow L, Boelskifte S, et al: Differences between nisoldipine and lisinopril on glomerular filtration rates and albuminuria in hypertensive IDDM patients with diabetic nephropathy during the first year of treatment. *Diabetes* 46:481–487, 1997.)

increase of 35% of fractional albumin clearance. In the lisinopril group, GFR decreased from 85 ± 5 ml · min-1 · 1.73 m^{-2} to 73 ± 5. In the nisoldipine group, GFR decreased from 84 ± 6 to 80 ± 7. Changes in systemic blood pressure and baseline variables in multiple regression analyses were independent of the effect of study medication on albuminuria and GFR.

Conclusion.—In hypertensive IDDM patients with diabetic nephropathy during the first year of treatment, lisinopril reduced albuminuria and glomerular filtration rate to a greater extent than did nisoldipine. To clarify whether these drugs have different renoprotective effects, longer follow-up is required.

▶ Diabetic nephropathy is the number one cause of end-stage renal disease in the United States. Approximately one third of patients with end-stage renal disease resulting from diabetes are type I diabetics, and approximately one third of type I diabetics will develop progressive renal disease. Microalbuminuria followed by overt proteinuria is a marker of insidious diabetic nephropathy in Type I diabetics. In recent years, a number of studies have shown that at similar levels of blood pressure, control-converting enzyme inhibitors are more effective than dihydropyridine calcium channel blockers for reducing proteinuria and preserving renal function. In this study by Rossing et al., the effects of once-daily lisinopril were compared with once daily nisoldipine on ambulatory blood pressure, albuminuria, and glomerular filtration rate on 52 hypertensive type I diabetics with established diabetic nephropathy (overt proteinuria greater than 300 mg/day). Patients from this population were randomized to either lisinopril or the nisoldipine in a double-blind fashion and maintained on a standard type I diabetes diet with moderate salt restriction for 12 months. The remarkable finding was that GFR was better preserved in the nisoldipine group despite similar blood pressure level and sodium excretion. However, a decline in GFR with lisinopril (see Fig 1) was greater during the first 6 months, and the rate of change from 6 to 12 months between the two groups seemed to be similar. This is in keeping with the concept that the renal protective effect of ACE inhibition is in part the result of acute lowering of GFR, followed by preservation of GFR over the long-term period. As expected, proteinuria was reduced more in the lisonipril group compared with the nisoldipine group. Of great interest is the fact that a high percentage of patients, 50% in lisinopril and 64% in nisoldipine group, had white coat hypertension as evidenced by comparison of office blood pressure to ambulatory blood pressure.

Further long-term studies comparing nisoldipine and lisinopril will be important to determine whether blood pressure control, per se, vs. specific antihypertensive agent used is the most important factor for preserving renal function in diabetic nephropathy.

R.D. Toto, M.D.

Effect of Calcium Channel or β-Blockade on the Progression of Diabetic Nephropathy in African Americans

Bakris GL, Mangrum A, Copley JB, et al (Ochsner Clinic, New Orleans, La; Rush Univ, Chicago)

Hypertension 29:744–750, 1997 3–22

Introduction.—The highest percentage of new patients starting dialysis in the United States are accounted for by African Americans, and the primary causes of renal failure are diabetes and hypertension. It is not known whether a certain class of antihypertensive drug offers an advantage in slowing renal disease progression in African Americans. The risk of cardiovascular event through a reduction in heart rate has been shown to be reduced with β-blockers. In African Americans with established nephropathy from non–insulin-dependent diabetes mellitus, the effects on the progression of diabetic renal disease were examined of 2 different classes of antihypertensive medications that lower heart rate.

Methods.—A randomized study that compared the effects of a heart rate-lowering calcium channel blocker, sustained-release verapamil, with those of a β-blocker, atenolol, were compared to examine whether different effects on proteinuria affect the progression of diabetic nephropathy. There were 34 African Americans who had serum creatinine greater than 1.4 mg/dL, proteinuria greater than 1500 mg/d, longer than a 5-year

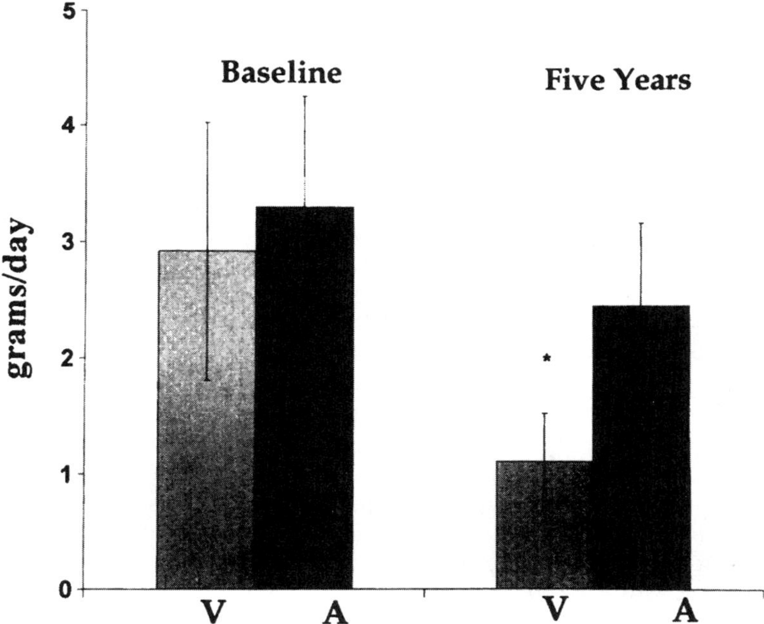

FIGURE 5.—Mean reduction in proteinuria at 54 months in each group of participants receiving sustained-release verapamil (V) or atenolol (A). *$P < 0.01$ vs. atenolol. (Courtesy of Bakris GL, Mangrum A, Copley JB, et al: Effect of calcium channel or β-blockade on the progression of diabetic nephropathy in African Americans. *Hypertension* 29:744–750, 1997.)

history of non–insulin-dependent diabetes mellitus and hypertension, and exclusion of other renal diseases. To help achieve the blood pressure goal of less than 140/90 mm Hg, all patients received loop diuretic as second line agents. At 6-month intervals, measurements were taken of 24-hour urinary protein and sodium excretions and creatinine clearance.

Results.—A slower rate of decline in creatinine clearance and a greater reduction in proteinuria was seen in the calcium channel blocker group than in the atenolol group after a mean follow up of 54 ± 6 months (Fig 5). The creatinine clearance was from -1.7 ± 0.9 in the calcium channel blocker group, and it was -3.7 ± 1.4 mL/min per year per 1.73 m^2 in the atenolol group. A 50% or more increase in serum creatinine was seen in a greater proportion of the atenolol group compared with the verapamil group with 32 ± 9% for the atenolol group vs. 16 ± 7% for the verapamil group. Differences in blood pressure control could not explain these between-group differences.

Conclusion.—In African Americans, the progression of diabetic renal disease is slowed to a greater extent by antihypertensive agents that persistently maintain reductions in arterial pressure and proteinuria than those agents without these effects.

► Diabetic nephropathy is the most common cause of end-stage renal disease in the United States, and one half of such cases are Type II diabetes. Long-term prospective trials in the patient population comparing blood pressure control level and different antihypertensives have not been carried out.

This is a new and important study that addresses this issue. As Bakris et al. demonstrate in this article, administration of verapamil as compared to atenolol in a small group of African Americans with Type II diabetes and overt nephropathy (urine protein excretion greater than 1500 mg/day and reduced creatinine clearance) results in a greater reduction in proteinuria and greater decrease in deterioration of renal function in the verapamil-treated group. This was carried out over a period of 54 months. The blood pressure control level achieved in the 2 groups was virtually identical over the follow-up period. Therefore, the improved outcome in renal function could not be attributed to the lowering per se. The reduction in proteinuria was substantially greater in the verapamil treated group (see Fig 5), comparing the baseline to five-year follow-up average values.

These results support the notion that the non-dihydropyridine calcium channel blockers are similar to angiotensin converting enzyme inhibitors in providing renal protection in some diabetic populations. Because the African-American population has a very high incidence ratio of end-stage renal disease due to diabetes (predominantly Type II diabetics) compared with non-African Americans, this paper provides evidence of preferential treatment with these agents over β-blockers. Moreover, when one reviews the adverse side effect profile in these two patient groups, it is clear that sustained release verapamil is superior to atenolol in many respects, including reduced incidence of impotence, lethargy, and exercise intolerance.

R.D. Toto, M.D.

Ritodrine- and Terbutaline-induced Hypokalemia in Preterm Labor: Mechanisms and Consequences

Braden GL, von Oeyen PT, Germain MJ, et al (Baystate Med Ctr, Springfield, Mass; Tufts Univ, Boston)

Kidney Int 51:1867–1875, 1997 3–23

Introduction.—The 2 β-adrenergic drugs most commonly used in the United States to inhibit preterm labor are ritodrine hydrochloride and terbutaline sulfate. Their use results in uterine and bronchiole smooth muscle relaxation. Both drugs may induce profound hypokalemia, but consequences of hypokalemia have not been fully studied. To date, changes in blood glucose and insulin during terbutaline and ritodrine administration have been the only factors studied to explain the hypokalemia induced by these drugs. In women treated with these drugs, therapy has been complicated by lactic acidosis, pulmonary edema, and tachyarrhythmias. The drugs may also cause significant renal sodium and water retention. In women being treated with ritodrine and terbutaline for preterm labor, the effects of these agents on potassium homeostasis, urinary electrolyte excretion, renal function, and cardiac rhythm were examined to better delineate the mechanisms for hypokalemia induced by these drugs.

Methods.—Five women given ritodrine and 5 given terbutaline had blood and urine samples obtained for 2 hours before and during 6 hours

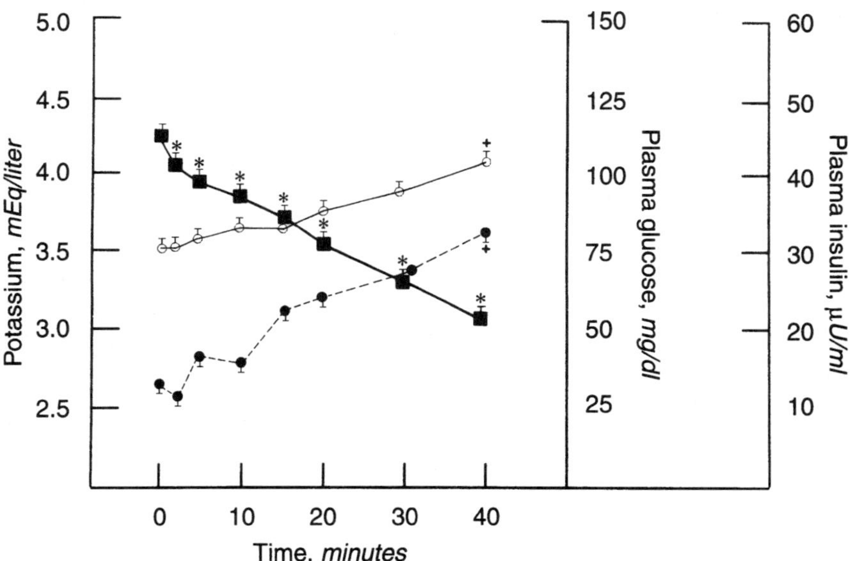

FIGURE 3.—The early effects of intravenous ritodrine and terbutaline on plasma potassium (*black square*), glucose (*white circle*) and insulin (*black circle*). Data are expressed mean ± standard error. *$P < 0.05$ potassium versus time 0; ^{+}P less than 0.05 glucose or insulin vs. time 0. (Courtesy of Braden GL, von Oeyen PT, Germain MJ, et al: Ritodrine- and terbutaline-induced hypokalemia in preterm labor: mechanisms and consequences. *Kidney Int* 51[6]:1867–1875, 1997. Reprinted by permission of Blackwell Science, Inc.)

of administration of the drug to determine the effects of the drugs on potassium and acid-base homeostasis and renal function. There were 42 women with preterm labor randomly assigned to ritodrine and 41 to terbutaline who were examined for plasma potassium and glucose homeostasis. Fourteen women receiving either ritodrine or terbutaline were studied for cardiac rhythm and compared to 12 women treated with saline and morphine.

Results.—These drugs showed no differences in any parameters affecting renal function or potassium homeostasis. After 30 minutes of drug infusion, a decrease in mean plasma potassium of 0.9 mean-liter was seen before any significant changes in plasma glucose or plasma insulin occurred. After 4 hours of drug infusion, the mean plasma potassium was 2.5 plus or minus 0.1 mEq-liter (Fig 3). After 60 minutes of drug therapy, plasma insulin rose to a level known to induce cellular potassium uptake (39.2 ± 7.7 mU/mL) and remained at this level for 4 hours. At 4 hours, hyperlactatemia occurred and plasma lactate/pyruvate ratio increased in a 10:1 ratio. Glomerular filtration rate, sodium, potassium, and chloride excretion and urinary flow rate were significantly reduced by both drugs. Ritodrine- or terbutaline-induced hypokalemia were not affected by changes in acid-base homeostasis, plasma aldosterone, or renal potassium excretion. The maximum decrease in plasma potassium occurred after 6 hours of drug infusion in the women randomly assigned to one of the drugs. Symptomatic cardiac arrhythmias at the lowest plasma potassium developed in 3 of 14 women treated with ritodrine or terbutaline. Cardiac arrhythmias were not seen in any of the women treated with saline and morphine.

Conclusion.—By stimulating cellular potassium uptake, ritodrine and terbutaline induce profound hypokalemia. Significant renal sodium and fluid retention and cardiac arrhythmias are caused by both drugs. During tocolytic therapy with ritodrine or terbutaline, careful monitoring of electrolytes, fluid balance, and cardiac rhythm should occur.

► It has been well demonstrated that β_2-adrenergic stimulation causes hypokalemia by increasing cellular uptake potassium. This is mediated by activation of adenylcyclases with subsequent increase in intracellular cyclic adenosine monophosphate and stimulates Na^+-K^+ATPase activity. The occurrence of this phenomenon has been noted during the use of these agents as tocolytics in preterm labor. However, the mechanism of hypokalemia in this situation has not been carefully evaluated. In this elegant study, Braden et al. show that ritodrine or terbutaline cause profound hypokalemia in preterm women when administered at routine clinical doses. Moreover, they show that the hypokalemic response is in part due to β-adrenergic stimulation, and in part to increase in plasma insulin levels (see Fig 3).

The authors also measured glomerular filtration (creatinine clearance) and urinary excretion of potassium and sodium. They found that these two adrenergic agonists actually reduce glomerular filtration rate and potassium and sodium excretion. Therefore, hypokalemia is apparently due to transcellular shifts only and not to renal loss of potassium. This is an important finding because it indicates that there is no net loss of potassium as a result of the administration of these agents. However, the magnitude of the hypokalemia is remarkable. Indeed, several patients in this study developed arrhythmias during therapy. This finding underscores the importance of careful monitoring of such patients and the requirement for subsequent potassium infusion in order to mitigate the cardiac arrhythmias that may develop.

An additional interesting finding in the study was β_2-agonist induced hyperlactatemia without a change in blood pH. This observation indicates that increased production of lactic acid and primary respiratory alkalosis occur together and offset change in blood pH. It was not feasible in this experimental setting, but it would have been interesting to glucose clamp these individuals to determine whether the subsequent changes in plasma and potassium were caused by hyperinsulinemia or an independent effect of the β-adrenergic agonist.

This study underscores the fact that profound hypokalemia (serum potassium less than 2.5mEq/L) is a relatively common routine tocolytic dose of β-adrenergic agonists. Furthermore, it will initiate future studies to determine the dose of potassium required to maintain normal serum potassium concentration and therefore prevent potentially life-threatening arrhythmias.

R.D. Toto, M.D.

Additive Effects of Losartan and Enalapril on Blood Pressure and Plasma Active Renin

Azizi M, Guyene T-T, Chatellier G, et al (Institut National de la Santé et de la Recherche Médicale, et Assistance Publique des Hôpitaux de Paris)

Hypertension 29:634–640, 1997 3–24

Introduction.—It would be worthwhile to have more complete blockage of the hemodynamic and tissue effects of angiotensin II than what is offered with the usual doses of angiotensin-I–converting enzyme (ACE) inhibitors. In individuals with sodium depletion and normal blood pressure, single oral doses of captopril (an ACE inhibitor) and losartan (a type 1 angiotensin II receptor antagonist) have additive effects on blood pressure fall and renin release. The magnitude of the hemodynamic and hormonal consequences of renin–angiotensin system blockage was assessed in a single-dose, double-blind, randomized, 3-way crossover trial comparing the ACE inhibitor enalapril alone with that of enalapril and losartan combined.

Methods.—Twelve research subjects with sodium depletion and normal blood pressure were randomized to receive either 10 mg enalapril, 20 mg enalapril, or 50 mg losartan and 10 mg enalapril. The mean blood pressure (MBP) and heart rate were monitored before and 2, 4, 6, 9, 12, and 24 hours after dosing. Serum samples were taken at the same intervals for determination of plasma active and total renin, ACE activity, and levels of aldosterone and cortisol.

Results.—The area under the curve (AUC) from 0 to 24 hours (AUC_{0-24}) of the MBP fall after the combined drugs was significantly greater than that of either 10 or 20 mg of enalapril. Compared with both enalapril doses, the combination significantly increased the AUC_{0-24} of plasma active renin but had no additive effect on the decrease in the level of plasma aldosterone.

Conclusion.—Losartan and enalapril combined is more effective in reducing blood pressure and increasing plasma active renin than doubling the dose of enalapril.

▶ Angiotensin-converting enzyme inhibitors lower blood pressure by blocking the production of angiotensin II. In some patients, an escape of the blood pressure response to ACE inhibitors occurs because angiotensin II levels tend to revert toward normal within 24 hours. This effect may begin to occur on a long-term basis and may mitigate some of the dose-limiting effects. Furthermore, it is known that the non–ACE-dependent production of angiotensin II occurs in humans. This provides a rationale for study of the effects of combined angiotensin II receptor blockade and ACE inhibition.

Azizi et al. have shown in a population with salt depletion and normal blood pressure that the combination of 50 mg losartan and 10 mg enalapril has a greater hypotensive effect than enalapril in doses of 10–20 mg/day alone. Although this study was not performed in a population with hypertension, the triple crossover study design using patients as their own controls indicates that the effect of blocking the angiotensin II receptor in conjunction with reduction of angiotensin II levels is more effective for blood pressure lowering than is an ACE inhibitor at higher doses alone.

Similar studies in populations with hypertension and acute and chronic blood pressure measurements are needed to confirm the observations by Azizi et al. The fact that plasma renin activity is raised further by the combination of the angiotensin receptor blocker and the ACE inhibitor suggests that the differential pharmacologic action of these agents on the angiotensin II–aldosterone axis is a potent way of controlling blood pressure in patients with long-term hypertension.

R.D. Toto, M.D.

4 Renal Injury and Chronic Renal Failure

Mediators and Therapies

Role of Glomerular Mechanical Strain in the Pathogenesis of Diabetic Nephropathy

Cortes P, Zhao X, Riser BL, et al (Henry Ford Hosp, Detroit)

Kidney Int 51:57–68, 1997 4–1

Introduction.—Basement membrane thickening and early and progressive expansion of the mesangial areas caused by the deposition of extracellular matrix material characterizes the glomerular injury of diabetes. The glomerular expansion and mesangial cell stretch induced by variations in intracapillary pressure is limited by glomerular rigidity. By modulating the glomerular distention and mesangial cell stretch associated with glomerular hypertension, altered glomerular rigidity in diabetes may influence extracellular matrix components accumulation. After short- and long-term diabetes, the biomechanical properties of glomeruli were characterized. Under conditions of high and normal extracellular glucose concentrations, collagen metabolism in cultured mesangial cells subjected to stretch was also characterized.

Methods.—At 4 days, 5 weeks, and 6 months after induction of diabetes, compliance was measured in isolated perfused glomeruli from steptozotocin-injected rats. In mesangial cells cultured in 8 and 35 mmol/L of glucose, collagen metabolism induced by stretch was investigated.

Results.—In 5-week rats, glomerular compliance was normal. In 4-day (16%) and 6-month (14%) rats, glomerular compliance was moderately increased. Total collagen synthesis and catabolism were increased by mesangial cell stretch, compared with static cultures. In 35 mmol/L stretched cultures, the fraction of newly formed collagen being catabolized was unchanged, but it was increased in 8 mmol/L-stretched cultures. There was a marked increase in the net collagen accumulated in the incubation medium and in the cell layer.

Conclusions.—The largely unaltered glomerular stiffness renders hypertension-induced mesangial cell stretch unopposed in diabetes. In a milieu of high glucose concentration, the accumulation of extracellular matrix components caused by any degree of mechanical strain is greatly aggravated. In the development of diabetic glomerulosclerosis, the interplay of mechanical forces and metabolic alterations as pathogenetic factors are better understood.

Tyrosine Kinase Dependent Expression of TGF-β Induced by Stretch in Mesangial Cells

Hirakata M, Kaname S, Chung U-G, et al (Univ of Tokyo)
Kidney Int 51:1028–1036, 1997 4–2

Introduction.—After subtotal nephrectomy, increased glomerular hydraulic pressure is often observed and has been suggested as a major factor in the development of glomerular sclerosis. The magnitude of mechanical stretch to mesangial cells is increased by the elevation of glomerular pressure. A multifunctional regulator of cell proliferation and differentiation, transforming growth factor-β has been shown to contribute to the accumulation of extracellular matrix proteins by stimulating their synthesis and/or decreasing the activities of some extracellular proteases. The effect of mechanical stretch on expression of transforming growth factor-β and extracellular matrix components in cultured rat mesangial cells was investigated.

Methods.—By culturing glomeruli isolated from kidneys of rats, mesangial cells were obtained. They were subjected to mechanical stretch with Flexercell Strain Unit FX-2000. Northern blot analysis was performed as well as bioassay for transforming growth factor-β activities.

Results.—In a time-dependent manner, mechanical stretch stimulated mRNA expression for transforming growth factor-β 1 and transforming growth factor-β 3. Substantial amounts of transforming growth factor-β proteins were stimulated by mesangial cells in response to stretch. For collagen types I and IV, and fibronectin, major components of mesangial extracellular matrix, stretch was also shown to stimulate mRNA expression. Neutralizing antibody to transforming growth factor-β inhibited the stretch-induced mRNA expression for extracellular matrix components. Tyrosine kinase inhibitors, genistein or herbimycin A, inhibited stretch-induced mRNA expression of transforming growth factor-β. Calcium channel blockers nitrendipine or $Gd^{3}+$ and inhibitors for protein kinase A or C had no effect on the expression of transforming growth factor-β.

Conclusions.—Transforming growth factor-β mRNA was induced by stretch primarily through tyrosine kinase–dependent mechanisms in cultured rat mesangial cells. For the stretch-induced expression of extracellular matrix proteins, the secreted transforming growth factor-β may play a significant role. In the progression of glomerular sclerosis, stretch-induced transforming growth factor-β of mesangial cells might be a mediator as an autocrine-paracrine factor.

► Increases in mesangial matrix production caused by stretching these cells in vitro have been previously demonstrated by Cortes' group and others (Abstract 4–1). The present studies demonstrate additional findings related to this phenomenon. Specifically, measuring the compliance of diabetic glomeruli from diabetic animals revealed a modest increase in their compliance, meaning that they would stretch to a somewhat greater degree for any given degree of increase in intraglomerular pressure. This finding suggests that diabetic glomeruli may be quite distended because pressures are elevated within them. Secondly, the inclusion of high glucose concentrations in the media further enhanced collagen synthesis in vitro. Thus, the stretching and high glucose concentrations may be key stimuli to matrix production by mesangial cells.

The mechanism whereby stretching would increase mesangial matrix components receives investigation in the study by Hirakata et al. (Abstract 4–2). In these investigations, again mesangial cells were stretched on a pliable matrix in vitro. The stretching induced formation of transforming growth factor-β (TGF-β) and the tyrosine kinase pathway was apparently responsible for this TGF-β production. The authors imply that TGF-β produced by the mesangial cells might work in some paracrine fashion to autostimulate matrix production or perhaps decrease the matrix production by other elements of the kidney. Putting it all together, increased pressure plus increased compliance lead to increased TGF-β and matrix production. Glucose amplifies the process.

T.H. Hostetter, M.D.

Endothelin-1 Transgenic Mice Develop Glomerulosclerosis, Interstitial Fibrosis, and Renal Cysts but not Hypertension

Hocher B, Thöne-Reineke C, Rohmeiss P, et al (Humboldt Univ of Berlin; Free Univ of Berlin; Univ of Heidelberg, Mannheim, Germany; et al)

J Clin Invest 99:1380–1389, 1997 4–3

Introduction.—Endothelins have vasoconstrictive abilities and also cause a variety of biological activities in nonvascular tissues. To determine whether an endogenous activation of the paracrine endothelin system is a cause or a consequence of glomerular injury, the human endothelin-1 (ET-1) gene was transferred into the germline of mice.

Methods.—Human ET-1 transgenic mice were produced by microinjection of linear human ET-1 genomic DNA fragments into 1-cell embryos obtained from hormone-primed NMRI females mated the night before injection with NMRI males. Viable eggs were transferred to the oviducts of pseudopregnant NMRI mice. Southern blot analysis and polymerase chain reaction (PCR) of tail biopsy specimens were used to identify transgenic mice. Three independent transgenic lines (238, 260, and 856) were established; lines 238 and 856 were selected for further analysis.

Results.—Northern blot analysis identified transgene expression in the brain, lungs, and kidneys of both transgenic mouse lines in equal amounts.

With the more sensitive reverse transcriptase–PCR (RT-PCR), lower levels of transgenic expression were detected in other organs. None of the transgenic littermates exhibited transgene expression. Renal overexpression of ET-1 was associated with an age-dependent development of renal cysts and renal fibrosis without hypertension. In both transgenic mouse lines, pronounced renal fibrosis led to a significantly decreased glomerular filtration rate leading to fatal kidney disease.

Conclusions.—The transgenic lines produced here provide a new animal model of ET-1–induced renal pathology leading to renal fibrosis and fatal kidney disease. This process was not related to systemic hypertension, suggesting that an activated renal-ET system is a blood-pressure independent factor for the progression of renal fibrosis to end-stage renal disease.

Effect of a Specific Endothelin Receptor A Antagonist and an Angiotensin-converting Enzyme Inhibitor on Glomerular mRNA Levels for Extracellular Matrix Components, Metalloproteinases (MMP) and a Tissue Inhibitor of MMP in Aminonucleoside Nephrosis

Ebihara I, Nakamura T, Tomino Y, et al (Koto Hosp, Tokyo; Juntendo Univ, Tokyo)

Nephrol Dial Transplant 12:1001–1006, 1997 4–4

Introduction.—Angiotensin-converting enzyme (ACE) inhibitors have been shown to prevent systemic hypertension, lower urinary protein excretion, and preserve glomerular structure in various models of renal disease. The upregulated mRNA expression of endothelin-1 and extracellular matrix components in diabetic glomeruli was effectively reduced by enalapril in a previous study. Endothelin-1 may be a mediator of renal injury. In a remnant kidney model, an endothelin receptor A antagonist attenuated renal injuries. Using the rat model of puromycin aminonucleoside nephrosis, it was determined whether a specific endothelin receptor A antagonist or ACE inhibitor (enalapril) modulated glomerular expression of mRNA for extracellular matrix components, endothelin-1, metalloproteinases, and a tissue inhibitor of metalloproteinases.

Methods.—The rats were divided into 6 groups: rats injected with puromycin aminonucleoside and given no treatment; rats injected with puromycin aminonucleoside and given enalapril, 35 mg/L in their drinking water; rats injected with puromycin aminonucleoside and given an intraperitoneal injection of FR139317, a specific endothelin receptor A antagonist; rats injected with saline and given no treatment; rats injected with saline and given enalapril in their drinking water; and rats injected with saline and given FR139317. Northern blot analysis and glomerular RNA were performed.

Results.—At the peak of proteinuria on day 8, glomerular mRNA levels for $\alpha 1$ (IV) collagen chain, B1 and B2 chains, endothelin-1, metalloproteinases-2, and tissue inhibitor of metalloproteinase-1 increased. By day 20, they decreased to the control level. Throughout the experimental periods, those for α1 (I) and α1 (III) collagen chains, metalloproteinase-1, metalloproteinase-3, and GAPDH showed little change. On day 8, mRNA levels for heparan sulphate proteoglycan decreased and then increased to the control level by day 20. For α1 (IV) collagen chain, laminin chains, and endothelin-1, enalapril and FR139317 attenuated the increases in mRNA levels. The agents attenuated the decreases in mRNA levels for heparan sulphate proteoglycan in glomeruli of rats injected with puromycin aminonucleoside. For metalloproteinases-2 and tissue inhibitor of metalloproteinase-1 in puromycin aminonucleoside nephrosis, enalapril had little effect on increased glomerular mRNA levels. In glomerular mRNA levels for metalloproteinase-2 and tissue inhibitor of metalloproteinase-1, FR139317 attenuated the increases.

Conclusions.—Modulation of glomerular mRNA expression of extracellular matrix components and endothelin-1 may be related to the beneficial effects of enalapril and FR139317. In regulating the glomerular mRNA expression for metalloproteinases-1 and tissue inhibitor of metalloproteinases-1 in puromycin aminonucleoside nephrosis, these agents may follow a different mechanism.

Quinapril Decreases Renal Endothelin-1 Expression and Synthesis in a Normotensive Model of Immune-Complex Nephritis

Ruiz-Ortega M, Gómez-Garre D, Liu XH, et al (Universidad Autónoma, Madrid; Universidad Complutense, Madrid)

J Am Soc Nephrol 8:756–768, 1997 4–5

Introduction.—In the pathogenesis of renal damage, it is suggested that the renin-angiotensin system is involved. Proteinuria and sclerosis were reduced in experimental models of renal injury by treatment with angiotensin-converting enzyme. In the regulation of renal hemodynamics in physiologic and pathophysiologic conditions, endothelin-1 (ET-1) plays an important role as well. The effect of the angiotensin-converting enzyme (ACE) inhibitor quinapril on preproET-1 and ET_A receptor mRNA expression, and on endothelin-1 protein levels was studied in a normotensive model of immune-complex nephritis, in which there exists an increase in renal ACE activity.

Methods.—Immune-complex nephritis was induced in normotensive rats. After proteinuria reached 20–50 mg/day, the rats were divided into 2 groups: an untreated group and the quinapril-treated group at a concentration of 100 mg/L added to the drinking water and replaced every 48 hours. The rats were euthanized 3 weeks after the onset of proteinuria. Blood pressure was measured and kidney tissue and blood were processed. Endothelin was measured in plasma. Angiotensin-converting enzyme was measured in serum and renal tissue. There was RNA extraction and reverse transcription, polymerase chain reaction and analysis of its products, renal histopathologic studies with light microscopy, and in situ hybridization and tissue localization of endothelin-like immunoreactivity.

Results.—In renal cortex and medulla, nephritic rats showed an increase in preproET-1 and ET_A receptor gene expression, in relation to controls This coincided with the maximal renal ACE activity. In glomerular capillary walls, mesangial and glomerular epithelial cells, in the brush border of some proximal tubules, and in small vessels, preproET-1 mRNA and ET-1 protein were localized. In all of these areas, there was an increase in preproET-1 mRNA levels and ET-1 protein in nephritic rats, without modification of their distribution. There was a decrease in proteinuria and morphologic lesions, preproET-1 gene transcription, and ET-1 protein levels, as well as ET_A receptor mRNA, with the administration of the ACE inhibitor quinapril.

Conclusions.—In several structures of the kidney, there was an overexpression of ET-1 in a normotensive model of immune-complex nephritis, that was downregulated by quinapril administration. The modulation of local production of angiotensin II and ET-1 may be the cause of the beneficial effect of ACE inhibitors.

► It has been about 7 years since the reports by Remuzzi and colleagues incriminating endothelin in the pathogenesis of the remnant kidney model. These studies (Abstracts 4–3, 4–4, and 4–5) continue to investigate the relation of endothelin to progressive renal disease, and all suggest that endothelin is not necessarily leading to injury through effects on blood pressure. Studies with transgenic mice overexpressing endothelin clearly show progressive fibrotic renal pathology and declines in function. However, there is no detectable arterial hypertension and no notable proteinuria in the animals. The studies with the endothelin receptor A antagonist target a model of nephrotic syndrome and progressive sclerosis and demonstrate, with a number of biochemical measures, diminution in the fibrosing process. This effect seems to be independent of arterial pressure because the model is normotensive and no effects on blood pressure were detected. This lack of dependence of endothelin's actions on arterial pressure is further demonstrated by studies in the immune-complex model of nephritis. Previously, other investigators have shown that interruptions in the renin-angiotensin system may reduce endothelin expression, and they have argued that this may be a mechanism by which drugs such as ACE inhibitors exert their beneficial effects. The studies by Ruiz-Ortega et al. seem consistent with that notion.

Many remaining questions exist in this area including exactly which receptor is best for targeting; some studies have found that nonspecific targeting of both A and B endothelin receptors is particularly useful. In addition, determining whether endothelin blockers are clinically useful may be difficult for a number of reasons. If ACE inhibitors interrupt endothelin action, endothelin blockers simply may not be of much additional use. Because these rat studies suggest that they could be useful without affecting blood pressure and perhaps even without detectable changes in proteinuria, clinical studies of these would necessarily rest on long-term changes in glomerular filtration rate or perhaps other end points. Thus, the development of these drugs as clinically useful agents for renal disease seems a bit problematic.

T.H. Hostetter, M.D.

Effect of Vitamin E on Antioxidant Enzymes, Lipid Peroxidation Products and Glomerulosclerosis in the Rat Remnant Kidney

Van den Branden C, Verelst R, Vamecq J, et al (Vrije Universiteit Brussel, Belgium; INSERM, Villeneuve d'Ascq, France)

Nephron 76:77–81, 1997 4–6

Background.—Small-molecule antioxidants such as vitamin E play a key role in antioxidant defense systems, especially in the extracellular space, where antioxidant enzymes may be absent. Antioxidant vitamins may reduce tissue damage by trapping organic free radicals or deactivating excited oxygen molecules. Renal vitamin E activity was studied in a rat remnant kidney (RK) model.

Methods.—Five-sixth nephrectomy was performed in male Wistar rats to produce an RK; this is a commonly used model of chronic renal failure. For 11 or 16 weeks after reduction of nephron number, some rats were treated with vitamin E (α-tocopherol). The effects of this treatment on deterioration of renal function and on glomerulosclerosis in particular were investigated.

Results.—Vitamin E treatment made no difference in catalase activity or H_2O_2 production in the remnant kidney cortex. However, by 16 weeks, glutathione peroxidase activity was increased by up to 140% and superoxide dismutase activity by up to 180% in the vitamin E group. Both the renal cortex and urine from vitamin-E-treated animals showed decreased lipid peroxidation, as reflected by malonaldehyde and 4-hydroxynonenal concentrations. At both 11 and 16 weeks, vitamin E treatment was associated with a greater than 50% reduction in glomerulosclerosis.

Conclusions.—In this rat RK model, vitamin E appears to have little effect on antioxidant enzyme levels or lipid peroxidation. However, it is associated with an important reduction in glomerulosclerosis. In pharmacologic doses, vitamin E may add a supplementary increase to the natural upregulation of the cytosolic antioxidant enzymes glutathione peroxidase and superoxide dismutase.

Aggravation of Polycystic Kidney Disease in Han:SPRD Rats by Buthionine Sulfoximine

Torres VE, Bengal RJ, Litwiller RD, et al (Mayo Clinic and Found, Rochester, Minn)

J Am Soc Nephrol 8:1283–1291, 1997 4–7

Introduction.—The Han:SPRD rat provides a useful model for the study of autosomal dominant polycystic kidney disease (PKD). The course of disease in this model is significantly altered by treatment with ammonium chloride, sodium bicarbonate, or potassium bicarbonate. The observed effects of acidification and alkalinization could be mediated by alterations in redox metabolism of the proximal tubular epithelial cells. Glutathione is a key cellular thiol and scavenger of reactive oxygen species. This article studies the effects of glutathione depletion on the development of PKD in Han:SPRD rats.

Methods.—Homozygous normal and heterozygous diseased Han:SPRD rats were divided into several groups. One group received L-buthionine(S,R)-sulfoximine (BSO), which specifically inhibits γ-glutamylcysteine synthetase, the rate-limiting enzyme for glutathione synthesis. Another group received glutathione monoethyl ester (GME), which increases intracellular glutathione levels. A third group received both BSO and GME. Treatment continued from age 3 weeks to 6 or 8 weeks, at which time the animals were killed for examination. The effects of changing redox metabolism on the development of PKD were evaluated.

Results.—The heterozygous diseased rats had higher renal levels of oxidized glutathione than the homozygous normal rats, although levels of reduced glutathione were comparable. Rats treated with BSO showed markedly reduced glutathione levels. Those receiving GME showed a significant increase in glutathione level within 2 hours, but no increase by 12 hours. Animals receiving both BSO and GME had a lesser increase in renal glutathione level after GME administration. This suggested that at least part of the increased glutathione level resulted from de novo synthesis. Disease development—as indicated by renal weights, histologic scores, and plasma urea concentrations—was exacerbated by BSO-induced glutathione depletion. Animals receiving GME in addition to BSO showed no reduction in cystic disease and no reversal of the effects of BSO.

Conclusions.—In the Han:SPRD rat model of PKD, alterations in redox metabolism influence the development of disease. The mechanism of this effect is unknown. Administration of BSO, a glutathione inhibitor, enhances the development of PKD. Its effects are not reversed by administration of the glutathione promoter GME, probably because of the transient effect of GME administration and the accompanying increases in cysteine and oxidized glutathione.

Dietary Antioxidant Inhibits Lipoprotein Oxidation and Renal Injury in Experimental Focal Segmental Glomerulosclerosis

Lee HS, Jeong JY, Kim BC, et al (Seoul Natl Univ, Korea)

Kidney Int 51:1151–1159, 1997 4–8

Objective.—The pathogenesis of human focal segmental glomerulosclerosis (FSGS) remains uncertain. The finding of lipid deposits and foam cells in FSGS lesions, as in atherosclerosis, suggests a common mechanism, possibly involving lipid peroxidation. A rat model of focal segmental glomerulosclerosis was used to test whether lipid-soluble antioxidants could prevent renal injury.

Methods.—The experimental model used Sprague-Dawley rats with chronic puromycin aminonucleoside (PA) nephrosis and dietary hypercholesterolemia. In addition to a high-cholesterol diet, 1 group of animals received treatment with lipid-soluble antioxidants, either 1% probucol or vitamin E, 100 IU/kg. Other animals underwent PA nephrosis but were given a normal diet, while still others received saline rather than PA injections and a high-cholesterol diet, with or without antioxidants. After 32 weeks, the effects of protecting lipoproteins from oxidation on renal injury were analyzed.

Results.—Untreated rats with PA showed proteinuria, FSGS, and tubulointerstitial lesions. These changes were present whether or not the animals received a high-cholesterol diet, although they were of greater magnitude in the high-cholesterol group. Beginning at week 16, PA rats receiving a normal diet were no longer hypercholesterolemic. The PA rats on a high-cholesterol diet had elevated renal cortical malondialdehyde (MDA) levels and had greater susceptibility of plasma very-low-density (VLDL) + low-density lipoprotein (LDL) to copper-mediated oxidation, compared to PA rats on a normal diet or control rats on a high-cholesterol diet.

In PA rats receiving a high-cholesterol diet, treatment with probucol or vitamin E was associated with lower susceptibility of plasma VLDL + LDL to in vitro oxidation. Treated rats also had a lower renal cortical MDA level, less proteinuria, reduced mesangial volume density, and reduced magnitude of FSGS and interstitial lesions. Immunohistochemical examination of glomeruli from PA rats receiving a high-cholesterol diet revealed oxidized LDL in a focal segmental distribution. This finding was reduced in animals receiving probucol or vitamin E. Untreated PA rats receiving a high-cholesterol diet had a greater prevalence of infiltrating glomerular macrophages than PA rats receiving a normal diet or control rats receiving a high-cholesterol diet.

Conclusions.—In hypercholesterolemic PA rats, antioxidant treatment with probucol or vitamin E leads to significant reductions in number of glomerular macrophages. In animals with chronic PA nephrosis, a high-cholesterol diet appears to exacerbate the renal damage associated with increased renal lipid peroxide levels. This renal injury is reduced by probucol or vitamin E administration, perhaps by making lipoproteins oxidation resistant and by inhibiting intraglomerular macrophage infiltration.

Prevention of Glomerular Dysfunction in Diabetic Rats by Treatment With d-α-Tocopherol

Koya D, Lee I-K, Ishii H, et al (Harvard Med School, Boston; Sapporo Med Univ, Japan)

J Am Soc Nephrol 8:426–435, 1997 4–9

Purpose.—Hyperglycemia and angiotensin activity have been identified as causes of diabetic nephropathy; glycemic control reduces the onset and progression of nephropathy and other microvascular complications of diabetes. Previous studies have shown that d-α-tocopherol (vitamin E) can reduce diacylglycerol (DAG) levels and prevent protein kinase C (PKC) activation, which have been linked to retinal and renal complications. The effects of d-α-tocopherol treatment on glomerular hyperfiltration, albuminuria, and PKC activity were studied in rats with streptozocin-induced diabetes.

Methods.—Diabetes was induced in Sprague-Dawley rats by a single intraperitoneal injection of streptozocin. One group of animals was treated with d-α-tocopherol, 40 mg/kg by intraperitoneal injection, every other day. The effects of treatment on activation of DAG-PKC pathways and on the onset of early renal dysfunction were analyzed. The mechanism by which d-α-tocopherol affects the DAG-PKC pathway was analyzed by measuring activity and protein levels of DAG kinase α and γ, which are responsible for metabolizing DAG to phosphatidic acid.

Results.—Within 2 weeks, the diabetic rats showed a 106% increase in total DAG content and a 66% increase in PKC activity in glomeruli, compared with control animals. These increases were inhibited by treatment with d-α-tocopherol. Both glomerular filtration rate and filtration fraction were significantly increased in diabetic rats; both hemodynamic changes were normalized by d-α-tocopherol treatment. By 10 weeks, the diabetic rats showed significantly increased albuminuria, compared with control rats; this effect was nearly normalized by d-α-tocopherol treatment (Fig 4, **A**).

d-α-Tocopherol treatment increased glomerular DAG kinase activity by 23% in control rats and 29% in diabetic rats. Baseline DAG kinase activity was similar in the 2 groups. Immunoblotting found no difference in protein levels of DAG kinase α and γ, suggesting that d-α-tocopherol was influencing the enzyme kinetics of DAG kinase.

Conclusions.—The glomerular hyperfiltration and increased albuminuria associated with diabetes may involve increases in the DAG-PKC pathway, these findings indicate. Treatment with d-α-tocopherol can normalize the increases of DAG and PKC levels in glomerular cells, perhaps helping to prevent the early changes associated with diabetic renal dysfunction. More animal and human studies are needed to help determine the mechanism of action of d-α-tocopherol and its treatment potential in preventing renal dysfunction in diabetes.

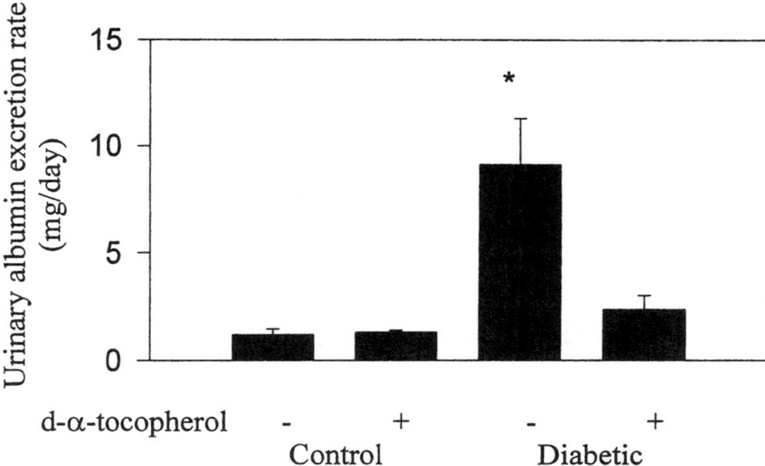

FIGURE 4, A.—Effect of 10 weeks of treatment with d-α-tocopherol on urinary albumin excretion rate in glomeruli from control and diabetic rats. Urinary albumin concentration was determined by enzyme-linked immunosorbent assay. Twenty-four-hour urine collection from each group was performed on 2 consecutive days in metabolic cages. Results were shown as mean ± SE. N = control; 14, control + d-α-tocopherol; 4, diabetic; 14, diabetic + d-α-tocopherol; 10. *$P < 0.05$ versus other groups. (Courtesy of Koya D, Lee I-K, Ishii H, et al: Prevention of glomerular dysfunction in diabetic rats by treatment with d-α-tocopherol. *J Am Soc Nephrol* 8[3]:426–435, 1997.)

► Chronic oxidant damage has received considerable attention as a "final common pathway" of progressive renal disease. These 4 papers test this in 4 interesting and separate models of progressive renal disease (Abstracts 4–6 through 4–9). They approach the question by attempting to provide oxidant scavengers vitamin E (which is synonymous with α-tocopheral) or probucol and by alternatively depleting natural endogenous scavengers such as glutathione by blockers of its synthesis. Broadly, these papers are all consistent in finding beneficial effects of enhancing antioxidant defenses and deleterious effects of reducing native scavengers. The mechanisms whereby these oxidant effects enhance the underlying tissue injury likely vary between the models. For example, in the model studied by Lee and coworkers of progressive sclerosis with nephrotic syndrome (Abstract 4–8), the effect may be on reducing the oxidation of lipids trapped within the glomerulus and their downstream effects. On the other hand, in the diabetes studies by Koya et al, (Abstract 4–9), the effects may have rather more precise origins by a tendency of α-tocopheral to inhibit 1 of the apparently key second messenger pathways generating diabetic nephropathy, namely protein kinase C activation. Yet other mechanisms may underlie the effects in the remnant kidney model and in the polycystic kidney disease model. Hopefully, we will soon be seeing small- and large-scale clinical trials seeking to assess the value of these therapies in clinical renal disease.

T.H. Hostetter, M.D.

Low-dosage Ibopamine Treatment in Progressive Renal Failure: A Long-term Multicentre Trial

Stefoni S, Mosconi G, La Manna G, et al (Univ of Bologna, Italy; Ancona Gen Hosp, Italy; Cesena Gen Hosp, Italy; et al)

Am J Nephrol 16:489–499, 1996 4–10

Objective.—A variety of therapies are used to slow the progression of chronic kidney failure. Whereas dopamine has been used successfully to prevent and treat acute renal impairment, the fact that it must be administered intravenously limits its long-term clinical utility. Oral dopamine-like drugs, such as ibopamine, may slow the progression of renal failure. The safety and efficacy of ibopamine in preventing or slowing progression of renal failure were tested in a randomized, long-term multicenter trial.

Methods.—For 2 years, 189 patients, aged 18–70, with mild- to-moderate renal failure (creatinine levels 1.5–4.0 mg/dL), recruited from 11 renal centers around Italy, were given ibopamine 100 mg/day (n = 96, 31 females) or placebo (n = 93, 31 females). All patients were given a low protein diet (0.8 g/kg) with a daily caloric intake of 30–35 kcal/day. Clinical and laboratory examinations were performed at 3-month intervals. Renal function indices were analyzed using multiple regression techniques.

Results.—There were 176 patints who completed the first year and 147 the second year. The 4 drug-related adverse events resulting in dropouts included 3 epigastralgias and 1 tachycardia. Over the study period, the decrease in creatinine clearance was significantly slower (1.8 times) for the treated group (39.8–38.1 mg/dL) than for the control group (41.7–36.2 mg/dL). Renal function survival curves (non-worsening) showed a significant difference between the treated group and controls both at the 20% and 40% levels. Mean plasma creatinine levels rose by 36% in controls and 17% in the treated group. Ibopamine appears to stimulate dopaminergic receptors resulting in an increase in renal plasma flow and dilation of the afferent and efferent arterioles with little or no increase in intraglomerular pressure.

Conclusion.—Long-term low-dose administration of ibopamine to patients with mild-to-moderate renal failure retards progress in a safe and effective manner.

▶ The role of dopamine and the dopaminergic system in renal disease remain elusive. This study has the intriguing result of a modest slowing of progression of renal disease occurring with an oral dopamine agonist. No effects on blood pressure or proteinuria were detectable, but a slowing of decline in creatinine clearance was reported. Although the effect was not dramatic, the patients were not very proteinuric. A subgroup analysis of more proteinuric patients would have been of interest, but this was not provided. Furthermore, since the majority of patients did not have glomerular pathology as their primary disease, the trial involved a group of patients with renal insufficiency in whom it is particularly difficult to demonstrate the efficacy of any therapy. The authors are circumspect in their discussion of the mechanisms of this effect, but a potential means for reducing progression of this drug might be suppression of the renin-angiotensin-aldosterone system.

T.H. Hostetter, M.D.

Exercise Training and the Progression of Chronic Renal Failure

Eidemak I, Haaber AB, Feldt-Rasmussen B, et al (Herlev Hosp, Denmark)
Nephron 75:36–40, 1997 4–11

Objective.—Regular physical exercise slows progress of chronic renal failure (CRF) in rats. A prospective randomized controlled study was undertaken to examine the possible beneficial effects of regular physical exercise on progression of CRF.

Methods.—Thirty nondiabetic patients with moderate progressive CRF (glomerular filtration rate [GFR] median = 25 mL/min·1.73 min^2) were randomly assigned to a daily 30-minute program of increasing exercise duration and intensity (n = 15, 8 women), aged 22–70 years or to a control group (n = 15, 5 women), age 28–65. Patients were followed for a minimum of 1.5 years or to dialysis or kidney transplantation. Rate of progression was determined by following the rate of change of glomerular filtration rate (GFR) over time.

Results.—During the study, 3 exercise patients and 2 control patients died. One control patient died of unknown causes, and 1 patient terminated the study. Whereas maximal aerobic work capacity increased significantly in the exercise group but not in the control group, median loss of GFR was similar in both groups (−0.27 vs. −0.28 mL/(min·month).

Conclusion.—Regular exercise does not appear to have a beneficial effect on progression of CRF.

▶ Studies in rats have shown slowing of progression of renal disease with imposition of increased exercise. The present article shows that in patients with renal disease, there was no benefit to an exercise program carried out over 20 months. However, because there was a preponderance of patients with cystic disease, tubulointerstitial, and vascular disease and few with glomerular disease, the comparison to the animal studies is difficult because the animal studies were conducted in the remnant kidney with progressive proteinuric glomerulosclerosis. In any case, the studies, while negative with regard to progression, show on the other hand that there is no overt disadvantage to exercise in patients with renal insufficiency. This point is of some value as exercise even in normal individuals does cause transient falls in renal blood flow, elevations in blood pressure, mild proteinuria, and urinary sediment abnormalities. As always, more extensive studies across a wider range of disease would be interesting, but this one serves at least to suggest that no exercise is safe in patients with renal insufficiency.

T.H. Hostetter, M.D.

Protein Intake in Renal Disease

Pollock CA, Ibels LS, Zhu F-Y, et al (Royal North Shore Hosp, New South Wales, Australia)

J Am Soc Nephrol 8:777–783, 1997 4–12

Objective.—Whereas dietary protein restriction is recommended for slowing progression of renal disease, a high dietary protein level is desirable after dialysis is established. Adaptation to such a dietary change is sometimes difficult and results in suboptimal protein stores within the first 6 months. Dietary protein intake was studied in patients with normal kidney function and varying degrees of renal dysfunction.

Methods.—Dietary protein intake (DPI) was established using urea nitrogen appearance (24-hour urinary urea nitrogen [UUN] appearance) in 565 patients (239 female), average age 51.7, with a serum creatinine less than 0.12 mmol/L, and 201 patients (90 female), average age 61.9, with a serum creatinine greater than 0.12 mmol/L. There were 180 patients in the first group and 148 patients in the second group who were advised to follow a low-protein diet.

Results.—Overall DPI was significantly and most strongly correlated with creatinine clearance (level of renal function) regardless of diet and was also correlated with body mass index and serum albumin level (Fig 1). DPI was significantly and inversely correlated with age and levels of plasma cholesterol, triglycerides, and blood sugar. Patients on a low-protein diet with normal serum creatinine had a significantly lower DPI

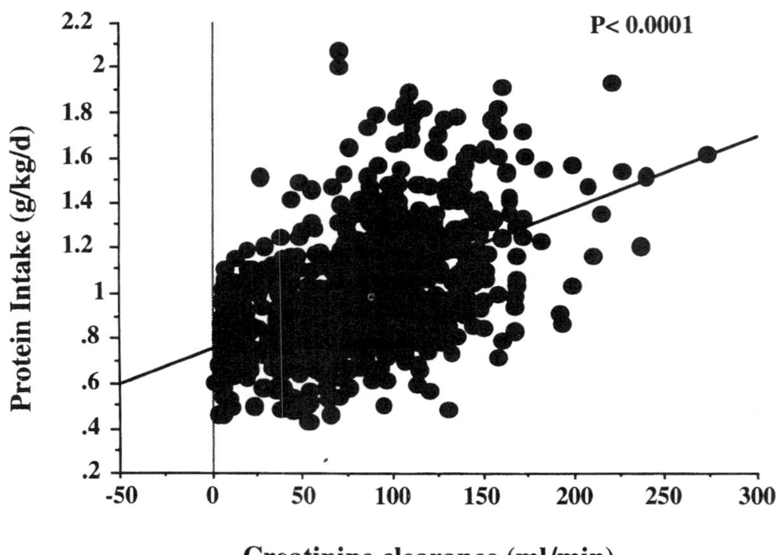

FIGURE 1.—Correlation between dietary protein intake and renal function, measured by creatinine clearance rate. (Courtesy of Pollock CA, Ibels LS, Zhu F-Y, et al: Protein intake in renal disease. *J Am Soc Nephrol* 8[5]:777–783, 1997)

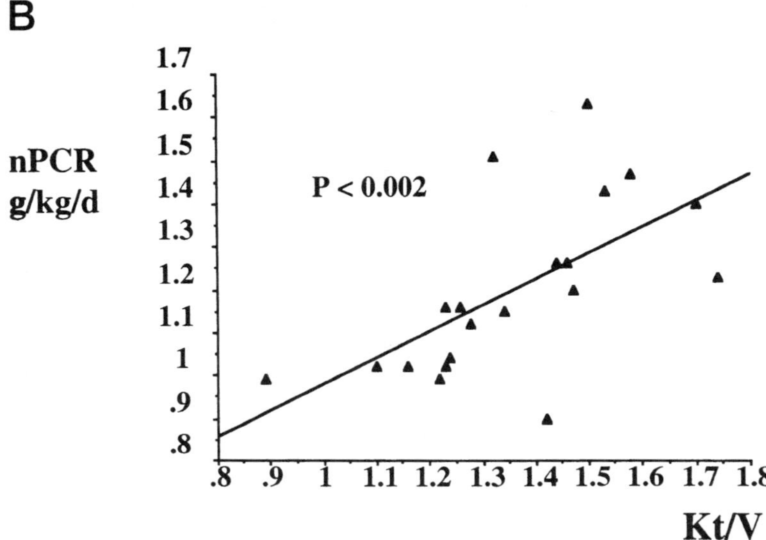

FIGURE 3, B.—Kt/V vs. nPCR in hemodialysis patients 6 to 9 months after commencing dialysis (Kt/V expressed per dialysis treatment). (Courtesy of Pollock CA, Ibels LS, Zhu F-Y, et al: Protein intake in renal disease. *J Am Soc Nephrol* 8[5]:777–783, 1997).

than did patients with normal serum creatinine on an unrestricted diet (0.96 versus 1.08 g/kg/day). Patients with abnormal serum creatinine on a low protein diet had a lower DPI than did patients with abnormal serum creatinine on an unrestricted diet (0.87 vs. 0.93 g/kg/day). There were 52 patients evaluated 3 months prior to dialysis and 49 evaluated 6–11 weeks after dialysis began. Mean DPI had not increased significantly in this group compared with baseline (0.82 vs. 0.79 g/kg/day). Within 6–9 months, protein intake had increased significantly to 1.04 g/kg/day. There was a significant correlation between Kt/V and protein intake (Fig 3).

Conclusion.—Low DPI in patients with renal impairment occurs whether or not they are on a protein-restricted diet. Attempts to increase DPI during the first 3 months of dialysis were unsuccessful. Protein intake increased significantly 6–9 months after commencement of dialysis.

► Relations between protein intake and creatinine clearance must be interpreted carefully to assess which is causal. Specifically, does an increased protein intake drive an increase in creatinine clearance in the higher ranges of creatinine clearance? On the other hand, does a lower creatinine clearance lead to anorexia for protein on the lower end of creatinine clearances? Both of these effects could account for the correlation observed in the overall population. The correlation between protein intake and dialysis delivery, measured as KT/V, suggests that renal function may determine protein appetite even when that function is replaced artificially. The lag phase (more than 2 months) in re-establishing higher protein intakes after institution of dialysis is mysterious. Do diet suppressing factors linger so long or is it a more general return of well being that allows for a higher protein intake?

T.H. Hostetter, M.D.

Effect of Renal-Artery Stenting on Progression of Renovascular Renal Failure

Harden PN, MacLeod MJ, Rodger RSC, et al (Western Infirmary, Glasgow, Scotland)

Lancet 349:1133–1136, 1997 4–13

Objective.—For patients with atherosclerotic renovascular disease, progression to renal failure is likely unless the condition is treated. Renal artery stenting has a high technical success rate for patients with this condition. However, little is known about its impact on renal outcome. Renal function was studied before and after renal artery stenting in a group of patients with renovascular renal failure.

Methods.—The prospective study included patients with renal impairment and underlying renovascular disease identified by digital renal angiography. Serial serum creatinine studies were performed before and after renal stent placement. Most of the stents were placed for ostial stenoses that had recoiled during percutaneous renal artery angioplasty. In 23 patients, the reciprocal slopes of serum creatinine were compared with time plots made before and after stenting to analyze the effect of the intervention on progression of renal failure.

Results.—A total of 33 stents were placed, with an immediate patency rate of 100%. The 6-month angiographic restenosis rate was 12%. There was 1 death from procedure-related hemorrhage. The median diastolic blood pressure decreased from 95 mm Hg before stenting to 87 mm Hg afterward. There was no change in the requirement for antihypertensive drugs, however. Sixty-nine percent of patients had improvement or stabilization of renal function. Stenting significantly slowed the progression of renal failure, decreasing the mean of the slopes of reciprocal serum creatinine values from −4.34 to −0.55 μmol/L/day.

Conclusion.—For some patients with atherosclerotic renal disease, renal artery stenting can significantly slow the progression of renovascular renal failure. This study finds a one fourth reduction in the mean rate of progression from before to after interventions. For these aging patients, renal stent placement may delay the need for renal replacement therapy.

► Renal artery stenosis is a common problem in the aging population. Its therapy remains a major dilemma. This study suggests that the introduction of vascular stents may be technically successful without real clinical benefit. Immediate patency was achieved in all of the patients and an apparent reduction in the rate of decline in glomerular filtration rate was noted. However, survivals were still rather dismal over a longer term follow-up and likely reflected the relatively advanced average age (67 years) of the patients and the well-known multiorgan nature of atherosclerosis. Also, we must carefully interpret the apparent slowing of the progression of renal disease as this was an uncontrolled study, and patients aggressively treated with medical therapy, for example, might have done just as well.

Interestingly, the number of antihypertensive medications could not be reduced, even though the diastolic pressure was somewhat reduced after the procedure. Thus, this technique represents a modest step forward; however, it may suffice in the patient for whom there is true concern that ischemic, progressive renal disease is occurring but in whom major surgery is highly risky.

T.H. Hostetter, M.D.

Transforming Growth Factor β1 and Renal Injury Following Subtotal Nephrectomy in the Rat: Role of the Renin-Angiotensin System

Wu LL, Cox A, Roe CJ, et al (Repatriation Med Centre, Heidelberg, Victoria, Australia; Univ of Melbourne, Victoria, Australia)

Kidney Int 51:1553–1567, 1997 4–14

Objective.—Although transforming growth factors have been implicated in the progression of renal diseases, the mechanism leading to glomerular and interstitial fibrosis and the timing of altered gene regulation are unknown. Transforming growth factor-β1 (TGF-β1) gene regulation in both glomeruli and tubulointerstitium following subtotal nephrectomy (STNx) and the renoprotective effects of angiotensin-converting enzyme (ACE) inhibition and angiotensin II (Ang II) receptor blockade were studied in the rat.

Methods.—Male Sprague-Dawley rats were randomly allocated to undergo subtotal nephrectomy (STNx) (n = 30) or partial nephrectomy (PNx) (n = 30) to study the timing of altered gene regulation over time. Male Sprague-Dawley rats were sham operated (SHAM) (n = 10), given STNx only (n = 10), given STNx plus the ACE inhibitor ramipril (3 mg/L drinking water) (n = 10), or given STNx plus the receptor blocker valsartan (30 mg/kg/d by gavage) (n = 10) for 12 weeks. Body weight, systolic blood pressure, plasma urea, glomerular filtration rate (GFR), and creatinine were determined. Tubulointerstitial and glomerular morphology were performed. Mononuclear leukocytes were determined immunohistochemically. The TGF-β1 levels were measured using Northern blot analysis.

Results.—Hypertension, proteinuria, renal impairment glomerulosclerosis, tubulointerstitial fibrosis, and mononuclear cell infiltration developed in rats that had undergone STNx. Ramipril greatly lowered hypertension, and valsartan lowered hypertension to some extent in STNx rats, improved proteinuria, and reduced glomerular. Plasma renin activity increased, demonstrating blockade of the renin-angiotensin system by both drugs. Over the 16-week study period, TGF-β1 gene expression increased by a factor of 2.5. TGF-β1 was found on sclerotic glomeruli, tubulointerstitial injury, and sites of mononuclear cell infiltration. Ramipril and valsartan significantly decreased glomerular and tubulointerstitial injury and reduced the infiltration similarly.

Conclusion.—Transforming growth factor-β1 gene transcription increased significantly in rats after STNx. Both ramipril and valsartan improved the damage caused by TGF-β1 overexpression by reducing TGF-β1 overexpression.

The Renoprotective Properties of Angiotensin-converting Enzyme Inhibitors in a Chronic Model of Membranous Nephropathy Are Solely Due to the Inhibition of Angiotensin II: Evidence Based on Comparative Studies With a Receptor Antagonist

Zoja C, Donadelli R, Corna D, et al (Mario Negri Inst for Pharmacological Research, Bergamo, Italy; Ospedali Riuniti di Bergamo, Italy)

Am J Kidney Dis 29:254–264, 1997 4–15

Objective.—Angiotensin-converting enzyme (ACE) inhibitors reduce proteinuria and control glomerulosclerosis. Whether these results are due to the inhibition of angiotensin II (Ang II) synthesis or inhibiting breakdown of bradykinin is not known. The effects of ACE inhibition in rats with passive Heymann nephritis (PHN) were compared with those of an Ang II receptor blocker, L-158,809, highly selective of Ang II type I receptors, and the influence of both molecules on renal gene expression of TGF-β and extracellular matrix proteins were investigated.

Methods.—Passive Heymann nephritis was induced in 24 male Sprague-Dawley rats with 0.5 mL/100 g of rabbit anti-Fx1A antibody. For 12 months, 8 rats received lisinopril (40 mg/L of drinking water), 8 rats received L-158,809 (100 mg/L of drinking water for 6 months and 50 mg/L of drinking water for 6 months), and 8 control animals received no treatment. Renal morphology was evaluated in all animals. Changes in renal gene expression of TGF-β and extracellular protein was determined at 2, 4, and 8 months after induction of PHN. Systolic blood pressure, renal excretion, and urinary protein excretion were monitored. Kidney fragments were examined using light microscopy and electron microscopy. Ribonucleic acid was isolated and analyzed to determine glyceraldehyde-3 messenger ribonucleic acid renal expression.

Results.—At 6 months PHN rats had a significant increase in systolic blood pressure compared with normal rats (160 vs. 132 mm Hg). Lisinopril- or L-158,809-treated PHN rats had significantly lower systolic blood pressures than did untreated rats at 12 months (110 vs. 111 vs. 160 mm Hg). At 12 months untreated PHN rats had significantly higher proteinuria compared with control animals (702 vs. 79 mg/day). Rats treated with lisinopril or L-158,809 had significantly lower protein excretion values than untreated rats at 12 months (149 vs. 52 mg/day) with proteinuria values of L-158,809-treated rats becoming significantly lower than values for lisinopril-treated rats at 6 and 8 months. Glomerular filtration rate

(GFR) decreased significantly in untreated rats compared with control (1.18 versus 2.49). Lisinopril- and L-158,809-treatment significantly prevented a decrease in GFR (1.76 and 1.67 mL/min) and significantly decreased renal gene expression of TGF-β and extracellular matrix protein.

Conclusion.—The ACE inhibitors and Ang II receptor antagonists were equally effective in preventing renal disease progression.

► In a complementary study of the remnant kidney model (Abstract 4–14), Wu and colleagues confirm earlier reports that an ACE inhibitor and angiotensin receptor blocker both mitigate injury in this model. As with the study of membranous nephropathy, TGF-β expression was also blunted by these drugs.

The ACE inhibitors have been remarkably effective at lessening injury in various models of progressive renal disease in rats. The question has sporadically risen as to whether these effects are purely through blockade of angiotensin II generation or through some other effect such as accumulation of bradykinin by reducing its degradation. Prior studies in other models have suggested that blockade of angiotensin II is a sufficient explanation. In this study (Abstract 4–15), using a model of membranous nephropathy, the authors come to the same conclusion. That is, similar results were obtained with a converting enzyme inhibitor, lisinopril, as with an angiotensin II receptor blocker, the L-158,809 agent. Furthermore, preliminary studies by others using different models have suggested that the combination of these agents may not be any better than each agent alone although this issue remains incompletely tested. However, this study also has the interesting finding that both the methods of reducing activity of the renin-angiotensin system lead to lower levels of TGF-β. This theme of TGF-β as one of a limited number of final local scarring factors is becoming increasingly pervasive.

T.H. Hostetter, M.D.

Inappropriately High Plasma Renin Activity Accompanies Chronic Loss of Renal Function

Yeyati NL, Adrogué HJ (Universidad de Buenos Aires, Argentina; Dept of Veterans Affairs Med Ctr, Houston)

Am J Nephrol 16:471–477, 1996 4–16

Objective.—Abnormally high production of renin and angiotensin contributes to the histologic damage observed in chronic renal disease (CRD). To date, however, evidence for excessive activation of the renin-angiotensin system (RAS) has not been demonstrated. Plasma renin activity (PRA), glomerular filtration rate (GFR), and sodium excretion were examined in a control group and in patients with CRD.

Methods.—Plasma renin activity, serum electrolytes, and GFR were measured in 9 patients (3 female), age 38–67, with CRD who had a creatinine clearance of less than 30 mL/min, and in 9 age- and sex-matched controls.

Results.—Controls had significantly higher mean GFR, 24-hour sodium excretion, and PRA than study patients (105.2 vs. 9.2 mL/min, 293 vs. 143 mmol/day, 3.24 vs. 1.63 ng/mL/hr, respectively) and significantly lower fractional excretion of sodium and PRA/GFR (1.49 vs. 11.11 %) and 3.02 versus 28.46 ng/mL/hr/100 mL GFR, respectively. Plasma renin activity is abnormally elevated in patients with CRD. When PRA/GFR ratio is calculated to correct for the level of nephrons remaining, it becomes apparent that the RAS is abnormally activated. This explains the significant reduction in GFR when angiotensin-converting enzyme inhibitors are administered and the dramatic rise in salt excretion per nephron.

Conclusion.—Patients with CRD have elevated levels of PRA resulting from stimulation of the RAS as an adaptation to progressive renal damage and nephron loss.

▶ The operation of the renin cascade in chronic renal disease has been studied for more than 20 years. In general, but not uniformly, an inappropriate elevation of renin has been reported in patients with mixed chronic renal disease. Often, the absolute plasma renin activities are low, but when considered in terms of nephron mass and sodium intake, abnormalities have often been detected. The present study normalizes plasma renin activity for GFR as a means of estimating the renin secretion per residual nephron and arrives at a very large number for that normalized parameter. Even more perplexing, however, is the perverse relationship to sodium intake with higher renin values noted at higher sodium intake. The stimuli to this persistent renin release and its disregulation are not investigated. These studies again give evidence for the notion that some unusual control of this system erupts during renal insufficiency and may account for the apparent beneficial effects of drugs blocking this hormonal pathway in progressive renal injury.

T.H. Hostetter, M.D.

Glomerular Disease

A Reevaluation of Routine Electron Microscopy in the Examination of Native Renal Biopsies

Haas M (Univ of Chicago)

J Am Soc Nephrol 8:70–76, 1997 4–17

Introduction.—Electron microscopy is a routine part of the biopsy evaluation of native kidneys. Its use is based on several older studies, the largest of which suggests that electron microscopy is needed to make the correct diagnosis in more than 10% of cases, and to confirm the diagnosis or provide additional information in another third. Since that time, immunofluorescent studies have become available and new glomerular diseases and variants have been described. The authors reevaluate the need for electron microscopy in native renal biopsies.

Methods.—The study included 288 native renal biopsies evaluated over a 6-month period in 1996. Of these, 233 underwent study of 5 or more glomeruli by light microscopy, 2 or more glomeruli by immunofluorescence, and at least 1 glomerulus by electron microscopy, not including glomeruli with global scarring. Within 48 hours, each specimen was studied by light microscopy and immunofluorescence, and a preliminary diagnosis was made. This was followed by electron microscopy, after which the final diagnosis was made. The effects of electron microscopic examination on the final diagnosis were analyzed.

Results.—The final diagnosis required electron microscopy in 50 cases (21%). This included 48 cases in which no preliminary diagnosis was reached and 2 in which the preliminary diagnosis was wrong. Although the preliminary diagnosis was correct in the remaining cases, the information provided by ultrastructural examination was deemed important for confirmatory purposes in 21%. In another 3% of cases, electron microscopy provided information on another, unrelated diagnosis.

Several diagnoses frequently could not be made without the use of electron microscopy, including minimal change nephropathy, early diabetic nephropathy, membranous lupus nephritis, membranoproliferative glomerulonephritis, postinfectious glomerulonephritis, thin basement membrane nephropathy, and HIV-associated nephropathy. Electron microscopy was also needed to rule out thin basement membrane nephropathy in patients with unexplained hematuria, and to rule out HIV nephropathy in patients with collapsing glomerulopathy. Other diagnoses could be made without electron microscopy, such as IgA nephropathy, diffuse proliferative lupus nephritis, focal segment glomerulosclerosis, pauci-immune crescentic glomerulonephritis, acute interstitial nephritis, and amyloid nephropathy.

Conclusions.—Electron microscopy still appears to be necessary for the diagnosis of native renal biopsies. In nearly half of cases, it is necessary for either diagnosis or confirmatory purposes. Electron microscopy should be performed on a routine basis for evaluation of native renal biopsies; if it cannot be done, some tissue should be reserved for later ultrastructural examination.

▶ Although the conclusion is generally the same as that reached several decades ago, this revisit to the topic of the utility of electron microscopy is timely for 2 reasons. First, the spectrum of diagnoses has changed. Some of the new ones, such as collapsing glomerulopathy, appear not to require electron microscopy for diagnosis in most cases, whereas other new entities such as thin basement membrane disease and HIV nephropathy do usually profit by it. Secondly, with the continuous and often unsupported attempts to reduce the cost, every procedure is under question in the present climate. Electron microscopy should still be done.

T.H. Hostetter, M.D.

Sickle Cell Anemia Causes a Distinct Pattern of Glomerular Dysfunction
Guasch A, Cua M, You W, et al (Emory Univ, Atlanta, Ga)
Kidney Int 51:826–833, 1997 4–18

Background.—Renal findings in patients with sickle cell anemia (SSA) include hematuria, inability to concentrate urine, tubular defects, and papillary necrosis. Some patients develop glomerulopathy leading to end-stage renal disease; the prevalence of renal failure among adult patients with SSA has been estimated at 4%. However, glomerular involvement may be more common than suspected, and could become clinically more important as patients with SSA survive longer. Glomerular function was studied in patients with SSA, including those with and without renal insufficiency.

Methods.—Two groups of adult patients with SSA were studied: 12 with normal renal function (SSA-controls) and 15 with renal insufficiency (SSA-CRF). A group of healthy controls were studied as well. In the SSA controls, the glomerular hemodynamic and capillary wall function findings were analyzed to determine the possible mechanisms of glomerular injury. The nature of glomerular dysfunction accompanying SSA-CRF was studied to assess the mechanisms of proteinuria and the pattern of glomerular injury.

Results.—The 2 groups had comparable glomerular filtration rates (GFRs), but the SSA-control group had higher renal plasma flow. Albumin and IgG excretion were increased in the SSA-CRF group. For all dextran sizes, from 26 to 64 Å, fractional clearances were significantly elevated in both SSA groups, compared with healthy controls. Fractional clearance of dextrans larger than 58 Å was elevated in the SSA-CRF group. According to an isoporous + shunt model, mean restrictive pore radius was 5 Å greater for both SSA groups, compared with healthy controls. The SSA-CRF group had greater than a 70% reduction in total membrane pore number, with a doubling of the shunt parameter—a parameter reflecting fraction of filtrate passing through "shunts" lacking any effective restriction.

Conclusions.—A particular variety of glomerular dysfunction is observed in patients with SSA. This pattern includes a generalized increase in dextran permeability, resulting from an increased pore radius. The development of CRF is associated with a reduced number of membrane pores, resulting in a size-selectivity defect. Neither hemodynamic alterations nor modulators of membrane porosity can account for the change in dextran permeability. Thus the glomerular pathology of SSA appears to have a unique mechanism.

► Renal insufficiency is a moderately common complication of sickle cell anemia, and as patients live longer with this disorder it becomes even more commonly observed. The renal histology was described in detail recently and consists of early glomerular hypertrophy followed by segmental and global glomerulosclerosis.[1] The study by Guasch and colleagues demonstrates that early microalbuminuria is also common in patients with sickle cell disease who have normal GFRs but glomerular hyperperfusion. At this stage, the permselectivity effects were already detectable by dextran sieving and with overt reductions in GFR additional defects interpreted as increases in the size of large abnormal pores in the glomerulus appeared. Although histologic correlates were not a feature of this study, the large selective defects have been viewed by others as a loss of epithelial processes in small focal areas. These intriguing studies call forth a number of questions in pathophysiology and therapy. Do changes in hematocrit influence these physiologic abnormalities? Will other presently available therapies for other microalbuminuric states, specifically ACE inhibition in diabetes, be effective in blunting in a renal disease in patients with sickle cell anemia? What are the cellular and physiologic mechanisms leading to this early permeability defect in late sclerosis? One suspects that this group of investigators will considerably illuminate our understanding of this disease, whose natural history is likely to continue to change in the era of gene therapy.

T.H. Hostetter, M.D.

Reference

1. Falk RJ, Scheinman J, Phillips G, et al: Prevalence and pathologic features of sickle cell nephropathy and response to inhibition of angiotensin-converting enzyme. *N Engl J Med* 326:910–915, 1992.

Idiopathic Membranous Nephropathy in the Elderly: A Comparative Study

Zent R, Nagai R, Cattran DC (Metropolitan Toronto Glomerulonephritis Registry)

Am J Kidney Dis 29:200–206, 1997 4–19

Objective.—Even in older adults, the main renal cause of nephrotic syndrome is idiopathic membranous nephropathy. This condition often has a benign course, although renal insufficiency develops in about 30% of patients. It has been suggested that older patients have a poorer outcome. This study compares the outcomes of idiopathic membranous nephropathy in patients older and younger than 60 years.

Methods.—The retrospective study included 323 patients treated for idiopathic membranous nephropathy over a 19-year period. Of these, 74 (23% of the total) were 60 years old or older. Their characteristics and outcomes were compared with those of the remaining, younger patients. The study definition of chronic renal insufficiency was a creatine clearance of less than 50 mL/min. The rate of change in renal function was measured in terms of the time to doubling of baseline creatinine.

Findings.—Mean patient age was 67 years in the elderly group versus 41 years in the younger group. At presentation, median serum creatinine was 1.3 mg/dL in the elderly group versus 1.0 mg/dL in the younger group.

Adjusted creatinine clearance, with correction for age, weight, and sex, was 55 versus 95 mL/min, respectively. At a mean follow-up of 47 months, the incidence of chronic renal insufficiency was 59% in the elderly group versus 25% in the younger group. However, the 2 groups had a similar incidence of end-stage renal failure, 18% versus 12%. There were no significant differences in the rate of change in renal function or the complete remission rate. In the elderly group, 46% of patients were treated. Treatment consisted of steroids alone in 76% of patients, immunosuppressive agents alone in 9%, or a combination of these in 15%. Treatment did not appear to change the complete remission rate or incidence of chronic renal insufficiency.

Conclusions.—Among patients with idiopathic membranous nephropathy, the likelihood of chronic renal insufficiency appears to be higher in the elderly. However, since there is no difference in the rate of decline of renal function, the difference appears to be related to age and decreased functional reserve. Serum creatinine gives an inadequate picture of renal function in elderly patients; an estimated or calculated creatinine clearance should be used. Prednisone treatment does not appear to improve patient outcome, and so should not be offered on a routine basis to elderly patients.

▶ Viewed from almost every angle, membranous nephropathy is a clinical and therapeutic enigma. This particular paper holds that it has the same roughly similar course but ambiguous response to therapy in older patients as it does in younger patients. The authors suggest that steroid therapy be reserved in the elderly for those with high risk as defined in their earlier publication.[1] By their criteria, the high-risk patients would be those with more than 8 g of protein per day for more than 6 months or those who are rapidly progressing toward renal failure. Given the probably greater risk of steroid therapy in the elderly, one might use even a lighter hand in doling out treatment in this age group.

T.H. Hostetter, M.D.

Reference

1. Pei Y, Cattran D, Greenwood C: Predicting chronic renal insufficiency in idiopathic membranous glomerulonephritis. *Kidney Int* 42:960–966, 1992.

Treatment of Lupus Nephritis: A Meta-Analysis of Clinical Trials

Bansal VK, Beto JA (Loyola Univ, Maywood, Ill)

Am J Kidney Dis 29:193–199, 1997 4–20

Purpose.—Lupus nephritis may be the most important prognostic factor in patients with systemic lupus erythematosus (SLE). There is continued debate over the best treatment for lupus nephritis, largely because of the lack of controlled trials of adequate size. This meta-analysis compares the various treatments for lupus nephritis, using the end points of end-stage renal disease (ESRD) and total mortality.

Methods.—The meta-analysis included 19 prospective, controlled trials of treatment for lupus nephritis. All assigned treatment by either randomization or consecutive enrollment. All followed the American Rheumatism Association criteria for diagnosis of SLE and required clinical or biopsy evidence of lupus nephritis. The trial included a total of 440 patients. The treatments assessed were oral prednisone alone, azathioprine with and without prednisone, oral cyclophosphamide with prednisone, azathioprine and oral cyclophosphamide with prednisone, and IV cyclophosphamide with prednisone. The analysis included both pooled data on crude risk and adjusted pooled risk using a random effect model. Absolute risk differences and number needed to treat were used to compare treatments for clinical effectiveness. The analysis compared treatment efficacy of oral prednisone with that of all other immunosuppressive agents with prednisone, and compared all treatment groups with each other.

Results.—Immunosuppressive agents plus oral prednisone were significantly more effective than prednisone alone in terms of both total mortality and ESRD—for both outcomes, absolute risk differences were around 13%. Intravenous cyclophosphamide plus oral prednisone was significantly more effective than oral prednisone alone, with a 20% risk difference in total mortality and a 16% difference in ESRD. With azathioprine plus oral cyclophosphamide plus oral prednisone, given simultaneously, the incidence of ESRD was 17% lower than with oral prednisone alone. However, these data—which included only 30 patients from 2 trials—showed no difference in total mortality. In terms of total mortality or ESRD, no immunosuppressive agent proved more effective than another.

Conclusions.—Meta-analysis of the existing data cannot identify any definitive treatment for lupus nephritis. However, immunosuppressive therapy with simultaneous oral prednisone appears to be more effective than prednisone alone. There is no evidence to support the use of one immunosuppressive agent over another, or the use of IV versus oral administration. Thus the best approach to immunosuppressive therapy may be the one with the fewest side effects. Randomized, clinical trials of treatment for lupus nephritis, with clear end-points and uniform comparative data, are needed.

▶ This meta-analysis supports the use of an immunosuppressive with prednisone in patients targeted for treatment of lupus nephritis. Interestingly, no difference could be found, however, whether the additional immunosuppressive was oral azathioprine or cyclophosphamide or intravenous cyclophosphamides. As usual, with this frustrating topic, the authors call for more prospective studies. Surely these could be useful, but one has the feeling that whereas the treatment of these patients has improved incrementally, both better prospective clinical trials and more effective mechanistically targeted therapies are desperately needed. At present, we seem to be attempting to find the optimal arrangement for relatively crude weaponry.

T.H. Hostetter, M.D.

Nephropathy in Human Immunodeficiency Virus-1 Transgenic Mice Is Due to Renal Transgene Expression

Bruggeman LA, Dikman S, Meng C, et al (Mount Sinai Med Ctr, NY; Yale Univ, New Haven, Conn; Duke Univ, Durham, NC)

J Clin Invest 100:84–92, 1997 4–21

Background.—Human immunodeficiency virus-associated nephropathy (HIVAN), a progressive glomerular and tubular disease, is increasingly common in patients with AIDS. It is one of the major causes of end-stage renal disease in African Americans. It is unknown whether the disease is caused by renal cell infection or a "bystander" phenomenon mediated by systemically dysregulated cytokines. This issue was addressed in a murine model.

Methods and Findings.—Two experimental approaches and an HIV-1 transgenic mouse line that develops a progressive renal disease histologically similar to HIVAN in humans were used. Kidney tissue expresses the transgene in the murine model. In heterozygous adults, renal disease develops shortly thereafter. With the use of a terminal deoxynucleotide transferase-mediated dUTP-biotin nick-end labeling assay, apoptosis of renal tubular epithelial cells was found to be a component of the molecular pathogenesis, similar to the disease in humans. To determine whether apoptosis is caused by transgene expression or environmental factors, fetal kidney explants were treated with ultraviolet light to induce transgene expression. Apoptosis was noted in transgenic mice but not in normal littermates after stimulation of transgene expression. Kidneys were then transplanted between normal and transgenic mice to confirm a direct effect of HIV expression on the production of HIVAN. The disease developed in the transgenic kidneys transplanted into nontransgenic littermates. However, normal kidneys transplanted into transgenic littermates remained free of disease.

Conclusions.—These experiments show that transgene expression has a direct effect on the development of HIVAN in the mouse. Thus, in humans, a direct effect of HIV-1 expression, rather than an indirect effect of cytokine dysregulation, is probably the essential cause of HIVAN.

Effect of Angiotensin-converting Enzyme Inhibition in HIV-associated Nephropathy

Burns GC, Paul SK, Toth IR, et al (St Vincent's Hosp, New York; New York Med College)

J Am Soc Nephrol 8:1140–1146, 1997 4–22

Background.—Angiotensin-converting enzyme inhibition (ACEI) has been shown to delay the progression of renal disease in diabetic and nondiabetic patients. The effect of oral fosinopril in patients with HIV-associated nephropathy was investigated.

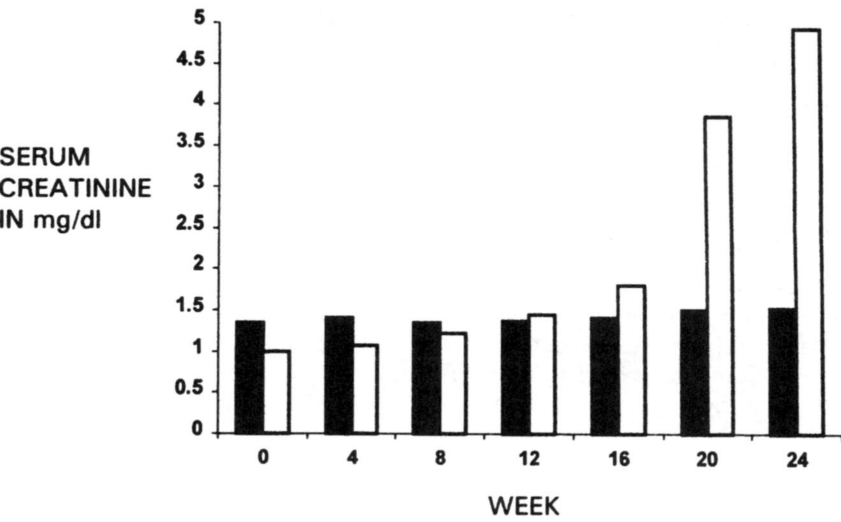

FIGURE 1.—Mean serum creatinine (in mg/dL) of patients with non–nephrotic-range proteinuria treated with (*filled bars*) and without (*open bars*) fosinopril, 10 mg by mouth daily for 24 weeks. Differences are significant at 24 weeks ($P = 0.006$). (Courtesy of Burns GC, Paul SK, Toth IR, et al: Effect of angiotensin-converting enzyme inhibition in HIV-associated nephropathy. *J Am Soc Nephrol* 8[7]:1140–1146, 1997.)

Methods and Findings.—Eleven patients with non–nephrotic-range proteinuria and 9 with nephrotic-range proteinuria were included in the study. Seven patients in the former group received 10 mg of fosinopril daily, and 4 did not. The mean baseline creatinine for treated and untreated patients

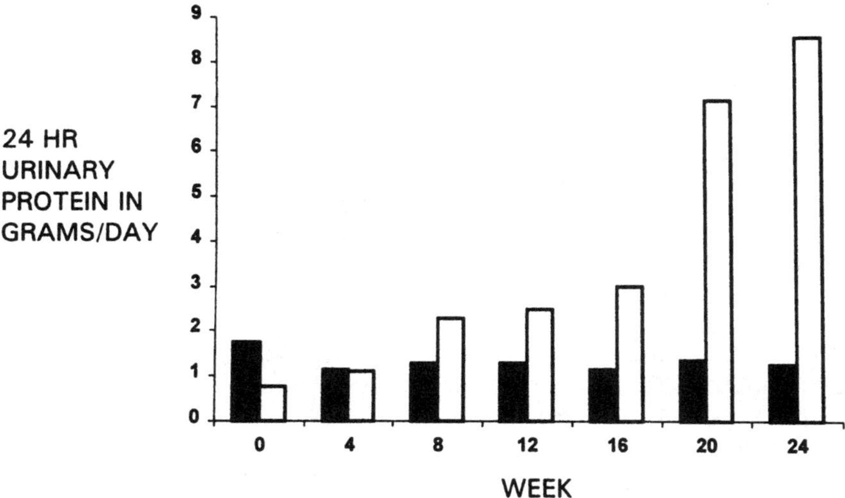

FIGURE 2.—Mean 24-hour urinary protein excretion (in g/day) in patients with non–nephrotic-range proteinuria treated with (*filled bars*) and without (*open* bars) fosinopril, 10 mg by mouth daily for 24 weeks. Differences are significant at 24 weeks ($P = 0.006$). (Courtesy of Burns GC, Paul SK, Toth IR, et al: Effect of angiotensin-converting enzyme inhibition in HIV-associated nephropathy. *J Am Soc Nephrol* 8[7]:1140–1146, 1997.)

was 1.3 and 1 mg/dL, respectively. At 24 weeks, these levels were 1.5 and 4.9 mg/dL, respectively. Mean baseline 24-hour urine protein excretion in treated and untreated patients was 1.6 and 0.78 g/day, compared to 1.25 and 8.5 g/day, respectively, at 24 weeks. In the nephrotic-range proteinuria group, 5 were treated and 4 were not. Treated and untreated patients had mean baseline creatinine levels of 1.7 and 1.9 mg/dL, respectively. At 12 weeks, these values were 2 and 9.2 mg/dL, respectively. Twenty-four-hour protein excretion levels were 5.4 and 5.2 g/day in treated and untreated patients, respectively, at baseline, compared to 2.8 and 10.5 g/day at 12 weeks (Figs 1 and 2).

Conclusions.—Treatment with ACEI may stabilize serum creatinine and 24-hour protein excretion for up to 24 weeks in patients with non–nephrotic-range proteinuria and for up to 12 weeks in paients with nephrotic-range proteinuria with initial serum creatinine of 2 mg/dL or less. Also, the renin-angiotensin system may play a role in HIV-associated nephropathy. Early ACEI treatment may be beneficial in such patients.

Renal TGF-β in HIV-associated Kidney Diseases

Bódi I, Kimmel PL, Abraham AA, et al (George Washington Univ, Washington, DC; Duke Univ, Chapel Hill, NC; Mount Sinai School of Med, New York, et al)

Kidney Int 51:1568–1577, 1997 4–23

Objective.—An HIV-associated nephropathy develops in about 10% of HIV-positive patients who also have increased levels of TGF-β1. Renal TGF-β1 and TGF-β3 appear to increase in HIV-transgenic mice as renal damage progresses. Renal tissue from patients with and without HIV infection was examined to assess levels of TGF-β.

Methods.—Biopsy and autopsy renal tissue from 71 patients (n = 36 HIV-positive), were examined for accumulation of TGF-β1 and TGF-β3 and extent of interstitial fibrosis and interstitial CD45-positive cellular infiltrate using immunohistochemistry.

Results.—Extracellular TGF-β1/β3 was found in the cortical interstitium of diseased kidneys, particularly in areas with fibrotic material, and was highest in HIV-positive patients and patients with crescentic glomerulonephritis. Significant correlations were found between fibrosis score and interstitial TGF-β1/β3 score (r = 0.79), fibrosis score and CD45 score (r = 0.70), and CD45 score and TGF-β1/β3 score (r = 0.60). Compared with patients without HIV infection, HIV-positive patients had a significantly higher CD45 score (1.4 vs. 2.7) and a borderline increased TGF-β1/β3 score (1.5 vs. 2.2). Fibrosis scores were similar between uninfected and infected patients (1.6 vs. 2.2). In patients with focal segmental glomerulosclerosis (FSGS), patients with HIV had significantly higher CD45 scores than did noninfected patients (2.6 vs. 1.3), borderline higher TGF-β1/β3 score (2.3 vs. 1.3), and similar fibrosis scores (2.4 vs. 1.7). There were significant correlations in HIV-positive patients between interstitial fibrosis and CD45RO scores (r = 0.85), OPD4 scores (r = 0.71), and macrophage scores (r = 0.79). Intracellular TGF-β1/β3 was localized to tubular epithelial cells, extraglomerular crescents, and intraglomerular cells and interstitial cells, with TGF-β3 also found on arteriolar walls and interstitial mononuclear cells. Intracellular TGF-β3 was found in glomerular cells only in HIV-positive patients.

Conclusion.—Significantly increased levels of TGF-β were found in renal tissue of HIV-positive patients, and intermediate levels were found in renal tissue of patients with other progressive glomerular diseases. Fibrosis scores were significantly correlated with CD45, OPD4, and CD68 macrophage scores in HIV-positive patients but not in patients with FSGS.

▶ An animal model of HIV nephropathy, the transgenic mouse studied by Bruggeman and colleagues (Abstract 4–21), strongly suggests that HIV expression in the kidney itself is the source of renal injury rather than the injury arising as a consequence of systemic infections and circulating inflammatory mediators. Furthermore, the data suggest that the production of this virus in the renal tubule epithelium is sufficient for even glomerular injury. Indeed, epithelial-directed interstitial injury is intuitively appealing and various kinds of evidence, including the present data, suggest that the epithelial cells may elaborate substances in response to viral infection, particularly TGF-β that, in turn, cause tubulointerstitial and glomerular injury. Indeed, the clinical correlations adduced by Bodi et al. (Abstract 4–23) highlight TGF-β as a potential mediator of HIV nephropathy.

The study by Burns (Abstract 4–22) of angiotensin-converting enzyme inhibition is therapeutically exciting, even though the study is not a randomized or controlled one. The dramatic differences between proteinuria and serum creatinine in patients taking a converting enzyme inhibitor and those not so treated compel a formal study of this promising result.

T.H. Hostetter, M.D.

Thin GBM Nephropathy: Premature Glomerular Obsolescence Is Associated With Hypertension and Late Onset Renal Failure

Nieuwhof CMG, de Heer F, de Leeuw P, et al (Univ Hosp Maastricht, The Netherlands; Maasland Hosp, Sittard, The Netherlands)

Kidney Int 51:1596–1601, 1997 4–24

Background.—Thin glomerular basement membrane (GBM) nephropathy is diagnosed by the finding of a uniform thinning of the lamina densa of the GBMs. The condition, also called familial benign hematuria, affects both sexes equally and generally has an excellent renal prognosis. A recent report of a missense mutation in collagen type IV raises the possibility that thin GBM nephropathy is an atypical form of Alport syndrome, a progressive renal hereditary disorder. A prospective epidemiologic study sought to discern early Alport syndrome from thin GBM nephropathy.

Patients and Methods.—Patients were participants in a study of idiopathic glomerular disease conducted between 1978 and 1984. Renal biopsy specimens were taken from patients aged 16–65 years who had no systemic extrarenal disease or known familial renal disorders. Included in the study were 27 patients with primary IgA nephropathy, 24 with normal renal tissue, and 19 with thin GBM nephropathy. Patients were followed up for a median of 12 years for signs of disease progression: development of hypertension, increase in proteinuria, or development of uremia.

Results.—Family research conducted during follow-up revealed that 9 patients with thin GBM nephropathy had relatives with hematuria, proteinuria, and/or impaired renal function. Within 4 families, 6 elderly members had end-stage renal disease requiring dialysis. The mode of inheritance in these families appeared to be autosomal dominant. None of the 24 patients with normal renal tissue had family members with renal insufficiency. Renal biopsy specimens taken at study entry showed an increased incidence of focal global glomerulosclerosis in the GBM group compared with normal and IgA nephropathy groups. The presence of Alport syndrome was clinically ruled out because none of the patients had hearing loss or visual abnormalities. At the end of follow-up, the incidence of hypertension in thin GBM nephropathy (7 of 18) was greater than that in healthy controls (2 of 24). Although the incidences of hypertension and increased proteinuria were comparable in thin GBM and IgA nephropathy groups, 3 patients with IgA nephropathy had progressed to renal failure.

Conclusions.—Patients with thin GBM nephropathy are significantly more likely than those with idiopathic IgA nephropathy or normal renal tissue to have an increased incidence of focal global glomerulosclerosis and renal insufficiency in first-degree relatives. Thin GBM nephropathy, although clinically different from Alport syndrome, predisposes to premature glomerular obsolescence, hypertension, and an increased incidence of late-onset renal insufficiency. Both disorders appear to result from defects in collagen type IV coding genes.

► Familial hematuria caused by thin basement membrane has generally been viewed as a benign process. Cases of progression have been noted, and this survey suggests that the more adverse outcome may be more common than thought. The authors carefully define the cases by standard morphometric techniques and have the advantage of follow-up in these subjects. Furthermore, they take pains to distinguish them from Alport syndrome. Thin basement membrane disease likely represents another defect in collagen synthesis, and the authors suggest we will soon see molecular studies of the familial basis of this entity.

T.H. Hostetter, M.D.

Inhibitory Effect of *Tripterygium wilfordii* Multiglycoside on Increased Glomerular Albumin Permeability *In Vitro*

Sharma M, Li JZ, Sharma R, et al (Med College of Wisconsin, Milwaukee; Beijing Med Univ, People's Republic of China; Univ of Trieste, Italy)
Nephrol Dial Transplant 12:2064–2068, 1997 4–25

Background.—*Tripterygium wilfordii* multiglycoside (TWG) is an extract of a widely used Chinese medicinal plant, *T. wilfordii* Hook F. In China, TWG is used to treat rheumatoid arthritis and glomerular nephritis, and as an immunosuppressive and antifertility agent. Studies of nephrosis or nephritis in animals and humans have suggested that TWG can reduce proteinuria. The effects of TWG on glomerular albumin permeability ($P_{albumin}$) were studied in vitro.

Methods.—The investigators isolated rat glomeruli and then incubated them with protamine, human recombinant tumor necrosis factor (TNF)-α, superoxide, or serum from a patient with focal segmental glomerular sclerosis (FSGS). In parallel tubes, TWG in a dose of 1 mg/mL was added to investigate the effects on $P_{albumin}$. Identical incubation conditions, without TWG, were used in control glomeruli. The change in glomerular volume in response to an applied oncotic gradient was used to calculate the albumin reflection coefficient ($\sigma_{albumin}$). The equation for $P_{albumin}$ was calculated as $1 - \sigma_{albumin}$.

Results.—Protamine and TNF-α each significantly increased glomerular $P_{albumin}$, compared with control specimens. Incubation with xanthine and xanthine oxidase—resulting in superoxide production—and with FSGS serum also increased $P_{albumin}$ of glomeruli. All of these effects were blocked by TWG, which itself had no effect on $P_{albumin}$.

Conclusion.—In this in vitro study, TWG was found to block increased glomerular albumin permeability mediated by protamine, TNF-α, superoxide, or FSGS serum. The ability of TWG to reduce proteinuria in various types of glomerular disease may result from protection of the glomerular filtration barrier. It remains to be seen whether the compound responsible for this effect is the same as that responsible for the immunosuppressive properties of TWG.

► Not all Chinese herbal medicines are nephrotoxic. These studies employ the very useful technique, pioneered by Dr. Savin, one of the authors of this study, to examine glomerular permeability to proteins in vitro. By this technique, the effects of various glomerular toxins—such as TNF-α, complement, and reactive oxygen species have been shown to increase glomerular permeability. Whether obtainable levels of this herbal extract would actually protect the glomerulus in vivo seems unclear. However, these fascinating in vitro studies should push efforts to ascertain the in vivo effects, and if they are in some toxic range, further drug exploration for nontoxic analogues would be useful. It would be refreshing, to say the least, to have something other than the current steroid, immunosuppression and—failing these—

angiotensin-converting enzyme inhibitor and low protein diet approaches to proteinuria that we now use.

T.H. Hostetter, M.D.

Relationships Between Arterial Hypertension and Renal Allograft Survival in African-American Patients

Cosio FG, Falkenhain ME, Pesavento TE, et al (Ohio State Univ, Columbus)
Am J Kidney Dis 29:419–427, 1997 4–26

Introduction.—In renal transplant recipients, arterial hypertension is a common and multifactorial complication with an important impact on morbidity and mortality. For African-American kidney allograft recipients, the development of arterial hypertension within 6 months after transplantation has been linked to high graft loss rates. African-American renal allograft recipients were studied to determine the effects of pretransplant blood pressure (preBP) and early posttransplant blood pressure (postBP) on graft function and survival.

Patients.—The retrospective study included 116 African-American patients receiving their first cadaveric renal allograft. The mean follow-up was 64 months. Seventy-eight percent of patients received antihypertensive drugs before transplantation. Blood pressure was poorly controlled in 59% of patients, with an average mean arterial pressure of 107 mm Hg or greater. Particularly in patients with poorly controlled PreBP, blood pressure rose significantly in the first month after transplantation. Ninety-five percent of patients required antihypertensive drug treatment in the first 6 months after transplantation. After transplantation, the patients' need for and dosages of antihypertensive medications increased significantly. Thirty-eight patients continued to have high blood pressure despite antihypertensive therapy.

Findings.—Posttransplant blood pressure was significantly correlated with pretransplant patient weight and blood pressure. One-month postBP was significantly correlated with preBP, with 70% of patients with poorly controlled postBP having had uncontrolled preBP. The graft survival rate was significantly reduced for patients with poorly controlled preBP. For patients with high postBP, graft survival was reduced and serum creatinine values at 10 days and 6 months after transplantation were significantly elevated, compared with patients with well-controlled postBP (Fig 3). Patient compliance was not significantly related to control of postBP.

Conclusions.—In African-American renal allograft recipients, high postBP has a significant impact on graft survival. Information on preBP may be used to predict which patients will have severe postBP and which will be at risk for graft failure. Possible causes of poor preBP control should be investigated carefully, with close monitoring of blood pressure levels and antihypertensive treatment immediately after transplantation.

► Hypertension is bad for the kidneys and bad kidneys cause hypertension. This vicious circle has classically been difficult to resolve into a clear-cut

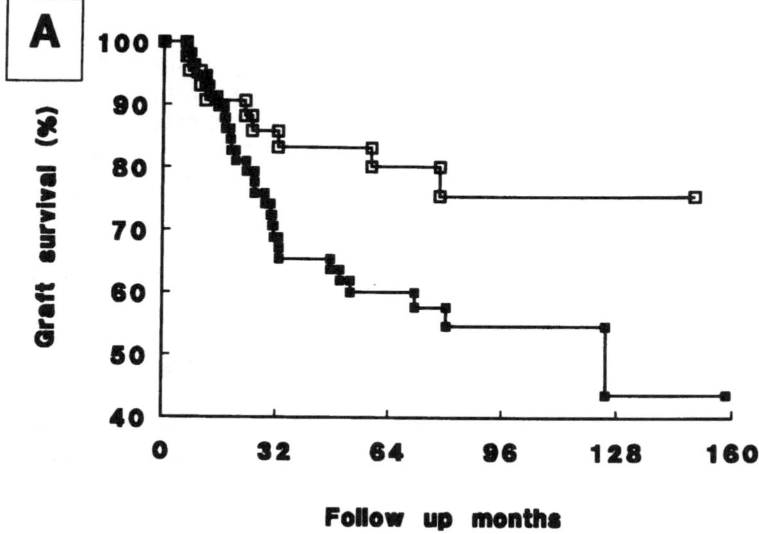

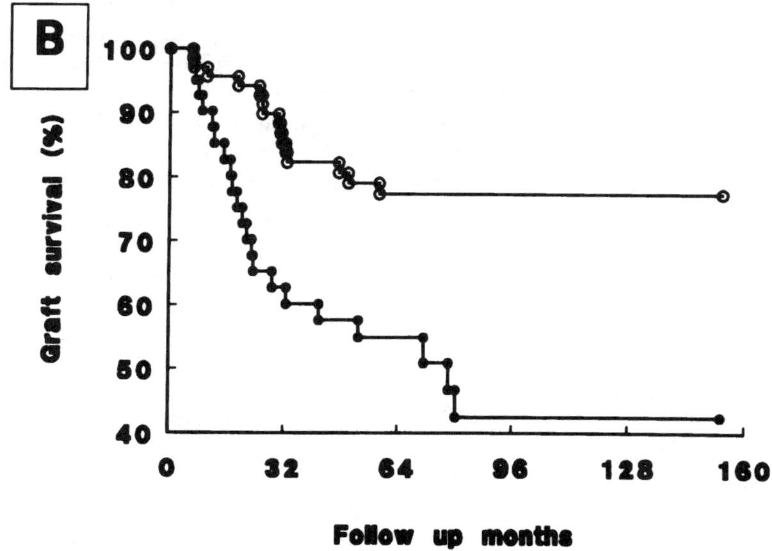

FIGURE 3.—Kaplan-Meier graft survival plots for patients divided according to blood pressure levels. **A**, patients divided according to pretransplant blood pressure. *Open squares* mean arterial pressure (MAP) less than 107 mm Hg; *solid squares*, MAP 107 mm Hg or greater (P = 0.03, Cox). **B**, patients divided according to posttransplant blood pressure. *Open circles*, MAP less than 107 mm Hg; *solid circles*, MAP 107 mm Hg or greater (P = 0.0006, Cox regression). (Courtesy of Cosio FG, Falkenhain ME, Pesavento TE, et al: Relationships between arterial hypertension and renal allograft survival in African-American patients. *Am J Kidney Dis* 29:419–427, 1997.)

linear relationship. The increasing focus on hypertension in renal transplantation is, however, a welcome chapter in care of the transplant patient. Although the present studies do not tell us whether poor graft function leads to hypertension or vice versa, they do clearly indicate that hypertension is a risk factor for the development of bad renal function, even when the hypertension occurs before transplant. The correlational studies are so strong, and the results of antihypertensive therapy in native renal disease so clear, that it seems long past the time for major trials of antihypertensive therapy in slowing renal injury post transplantation.

T.H. Hostetter, M.D.

Tubulo-interstitial Disease

Interstitial Myofibroblasts: Predictors of Progression in Membranous Nephropathy

Roberts ISD, Burrows C, Shanks JH, et al (Univ of Manchester, England; Royal Liverpool Hosp, England; The Univ Hosp of Southern Manchester, England)

J Clin Pathol 50:123–127, 1997 4–27

Objective.—Membranous nephropathy can lead to progressive kidney failure through a thickening of the glomerular capillary walls and inflammation of the tubulointerstitial compartment. Because the interstitial changes correlate with outcome, it is important to study the impact of interstitial inflammation and fibrosis to identify effective treatments. Results of a retrospective study of the function of interstitial myofibroblasts (IMF) in the progression of membranous nephropathy and the value of quantifying IMF in predicting long-term outcome are discussed.

Methods.—Renal biopsy samples obtained at University Hospital of South Manchester, Manchester, England, between 1984 and 1987, from 26 patients with membranous nephropathy were examined histologically to determine interstitial volume and morphologically to identify numbers of myofibroblasts. Patients were followed for 7 or 8 years or to death or dialysis. Serum creatinine and creatinine clearance were determined.

Results.—Creatinine clearance was significantly associated with age and with creatinine clearance at baseline. The number of IMF was increased in 21 specimens. The numbers of IMF and interstitial volume were significantly correlated with serum creatinine at biopsy or follow-up and were inversely correlated with creatinine clearance. There was no significant correlation between renal function at biopsy or followup and percentage of sclerosed glomeruli, stage of glomerular disease determined by electron microscopy, or lack of chronic inflammation of the interstitial compartment. Fifteen specimens contained little or no evidence of interstitial fibrosis, but 4 had a substantial increase in numbers of IMF. At follow-up, 3 of these patients had died of their disease and 1 was on dialysis. Of the remaining 11 patients with lower increases in numbers of IMF, 3 progressed to renal failure.

Conclusion.—In this small study, patients with no or mild interstitial fibrosis but a substantially increased number of IMF progressed to chronic renal failure.

Myofibroblasts and the Progression of Diabetic Nephropathy

Essawy M, Soylemezoglu O, Muchaneta-Kubara EC, et al (Northern General Hosp NHS Trust, Sheffield, England)

Nephrol Dial Transplant 12:43–50, 1997 4–28

Objective.—Diabetic nephropathy is one of the most common causes of end-stage renal failure. Myofibroblasts are thought to be involved in renal fibrosis and therefore may play a role in the progression of diabetic nephropathy. The distribution of myofibroblasts and their associated cytoskeletal proteins in the kidneys of patients with progressive diabetic nephropathy were retrospectively examined.

Methods.—Using immunohistochemistry, cytoskeletal proteins (α-smooth-muscle actin (α-SMA), vimentin, and desmin) were identified in renal biopsies from 25 patients (14 with insulin-dependent diabetes mellitus and 11 with non–insulin dependent diabetes mellitus), aged 17–78, with moderate to severe renal impairment and 5 with glomerulonephritis. Clinical, biochemical, and histological parameters were evaluated. Renal function was evaluated over a 6-month to 8-year follow-up period. Results were compared with those from patients with minimal change nephropathy and healthy specimens from patients with hypernephroma. Rate of decline of renal function was measured as 1/serum creatinine (Cr) slope.

Results.—Severity of tubular atrophy was correlated with rate of progression of renal insufficiency and was significantly predictive of 1/Cr slope. Whereas α-SMA was found in the media of the arteries and arterioles in healthy patients, α-SMA staining was seen in some glomeruli, tubules, and interstitium in diabetic patients. Vimentin was found in the glomeruli of normal kidneys Vimentin level in kidneys of diabetic patients decreased as glomerulosclerosis progressed, appeared in tubules and interstitium, and was essentially absent in diabetic patients with severe glomerular hyalinosis and sclerosis. Desmin was not detected in either healthy or diabetic kidneys. Interstitial α-SMA immunostain and rate of progression of renal failure were correlated. Interstitial α-SMA levels were the best predictors of the rate of decline in renal function.

Conclusion.—Myofibroblastic cells appear to be involved in progressive diabetic renal fibrosis and are markers of rate of decline of renal function.

▶ Interstitial disease has been recognized as a powerful correlate of function in chronic progressive disease for a long time. These two articles (Abstracts 4–27 and 4–28) demonstrate that the character of the interstitial fibroblast is a particularly important marker for progression. Specifically, the transformation to a myofibroblast, meaning that it expresses smooth muscle actin, is predictive of a more rapid course in diabetic nephropathy and in membranous nephropathy. Whether these myofibroblasts have especially adverse effects themselves or simply reflect ongoing active scarring is not addressed. However, as discussed in some detail in the paper by Essawy et al., TGF-β (may be an important signal for this switch from quiescent fibroblast to more active myofibroblast. Thus this immunohistochemical examination for smooth muscle actin may be indirectly examining the activity of the TGF-β (system. In any case, this assessment might add further prognostic power to the renal biopsy. It will be of great interest to determine the general applicability of this finding across other glomerular and interstitial diseases.

T.H. Hostetter, M.D.

SPARC Is Expressed in Renal Interstitial Fibrosis and in Renal Vascular Injury

Pichler RH, Hugo C, Shankland SJ, et al (Univ of Washington, Seattle; Oregon Health Sciences Univ, Portland)

Kidney Int 50:1978–1989, 1996 4–29

Introduction.—In a broad variety of renal diseases, the extent of chronic tubulointerstitial damage has been the best histologic correlate of the decline in renal function and the best predictor of long-term renal outcome. Secreted *p*rotein *a*cidic and *r*ich in *c*ysteine SPARC has been demonstrated to regulate angiogenesis, affect cellular interaction with matrix proteins, modulate cell proliferation, and bind to and/or inhibit growth factors such as platelet-derived growth factor. In the development of interstitial fibrosis, the role of SPARC was investigated in a variety of models of renal disease that are characterized by interstitial fibrosis.

Methods.—Using immunohistochemistry and in situ hybridization in experimental models characterized by tubulointerstitial fibrosis and matrix expansion in rats, the expression of SPARC was investigated. Four models were used with rats: passive Heyman nephritis, an experimental model of membranous nephropathy; experimental cyclosporine nephropathy; remnant kidney model; and angiotensin II infusion model.

Results.—In the remnant kidney model, chronic cyclosporine A nephropathy, and in passive Heyman nephritis, interstitial expression of SPARC was most prominent (Fig 1). To a lesser extent, it was seen in angiotensin II–infused animals. At sites of tubulointerstitial fibrosis/matrix expansion, SPARC protein and mRNA were substantially increased. SPARC protein was expressed by interstitial fibroblasts that also produced α-smooth muscle actin and correlated spatially and temporally with sites of type I collagen deposition in the passive Heyman nephritis model. The development of interstitial fibrosis was preceded by interstitial cell proliferation. The initial decline in interstitial proliferation coincided with maximal SPARC expression. An increase in SPARC protein and mRNA was seen in

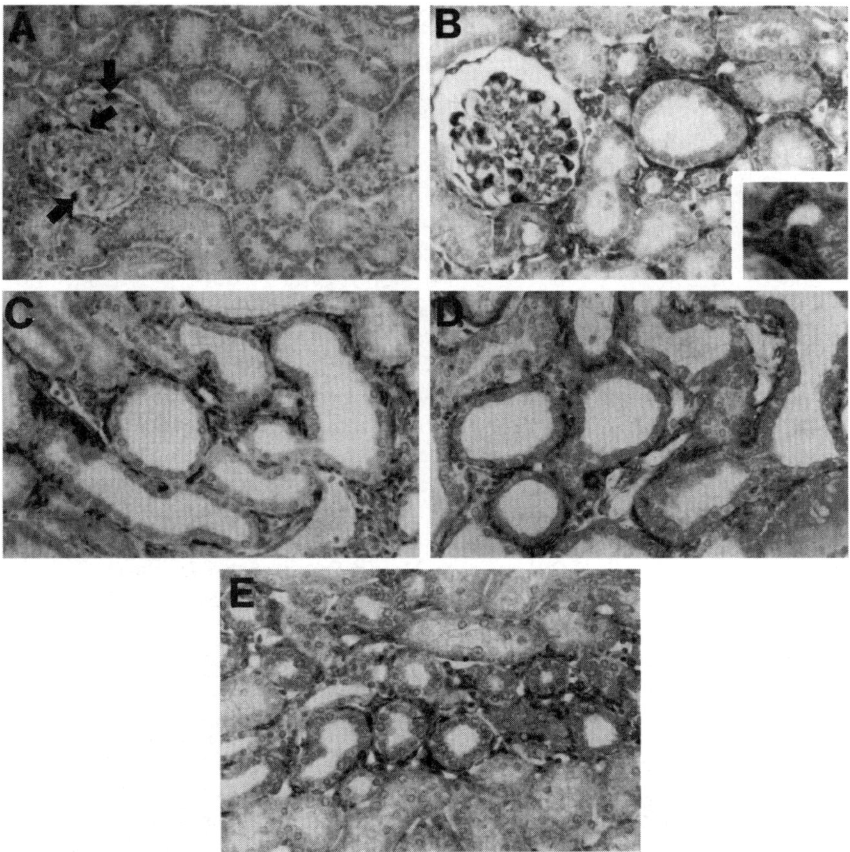

FIGURE 1.—SPARC (*s*ecreted *p*rotein *a*cidic and *r*ich in *c*ysteine) is expressed in areas of tubulointerstitial fibrosis. In normal rats (**A**), SPARC was expressed by visceral glomerular epithelial cells (*arrows*) in the glomeruli but was absent from the tubulointerstitium. SPARC was increased in glomerular epithelial cells and in interstitial fibroblasts in passive Heyman nephritis (**B**) at day 10. In experimental cyclosporine nephropathy (**C**), SPARC was expressed by interstitial cells around dilated and atrophic tubules at day 35. In the remnant kidney model (**D**) (4 weeks), SPARC was also expressed in the tubulointerstitium, in large part by interstitial fibroblasts. In the angiotensin II–infusion model (day 14) (**E**), SPARC was also present in the tubulointerstitium. (Courtesy of Pichler RH, Hugo C, Shankland SJ, et al: SPARC is expressed in renal interstitial fibrosis and in renal vascular injury. *Kidney Int* 50[6]:1978–1989, 1996. Reprinted by permission of Blackwell Science, Inc.)

injured blood vessels in the angiotensin II–infusion model, which is characterized by arteriolopathy and tubulointerstitial injury. Vascular smooth muscle cells and cells in the adventitia of hypertrophied arteries expressed SPARC.

Conclusions.—SPARC was expressed transiently by interstitial fibroblast at sites of tubulointerstitial injury and fibrosis, and by smooth muscle cells and cells in the adventitia of injured arteries in the angiotensin II model. The antiproliferative properties of SPARC might contribute to the resolution of interstitial fibroblast proliferation in the passive Heyman nephritis model.

► A multiplicity of factors have been implicated in the development of interstitial injury that accomplanies most chronic renal disease. SPARC is another of those factors. The protein is expressed by those fibroblasts that have become "myofibroblasts" and are also expressing the smooth muscle actin. Because this protein is said to affect cellular interactions with various interstitial factors, the role of SPARC may be to quell the interstitial response. However, whether this expression is entirely good in limiting fibrosis or bad in occasionally promoting it is not entirely clear. Thus, until specific drugs or, in the present era, animals with knockouts to the expression of SPARC are studied, we will not know whether this is an instigator or mitigator of progressive renal injury. In any case, it would be of interest to determine whether SPARC, like the myofibroblasts themselves, is indicative of progressive renal injury.

T.H. Hostetter, M.D.

Creation of an In Vivo Cytosensor Using Engineered Mesangial Cells: Automatic Sensing of Glomerular Inflammation Controls Transgene Activity

Kitamura M, Kawachi H (Univ College London; Niigata Univ, Japan)
J Clin Invest 100:1394–1399, 1997 4–30

Introduction.—For site-selective, long-term, and high levels of transgene expression, ideal gene transfer systems should be competent. A previous in vivo gene transfer approach targeted the glomerulus of the kidney using the glomerular mesangial cells as a vector for gene delivery. Modifiable expression of transgenes is required for gene transfer approaches in some experimental and clinical settings. Tighter control of transgene may be essential in the gene transfer-based therapies of inflammatory disorders. In response to inflammation, exogenous anti-inflammatory molecules should be elaborated and then should be switched off after recovery from disease. In pathologic situations only, α-smooth muscle actin is known to be expressed in glomerular mesangial cells. A cytosensor that perceives local inflammatory states and regulates foreign gene expression was created. Using glomerulonephritis as a disease model, the mesangial cell vector was combined with an α-smooth muscle actin promoter to explore this idea.

Methods.—For glomerular inflammation, CarG box element, the crucial regulatory sequence of the α-smooth muscle actin promoter, was used as a sensor. An expression plasmid that introduces a β-galactosidase gene under the control of CarG box elements was used to stably transfect rat mesangial cells. Serum-stimulated or unstimulated cells were transferred into normal rat glomeruli or glomeruli subjected to anti–Thy 1 glomerulonephritis to examine whether the cells are able to automatically control transgene activity in vivo.

Results.—After stimulation with serum, the established cells expressed β-galactosidase exclusively in vitro. β-Galactosidase expression was switched off in vivo within 3 days when stimulated cells were transferred into the normal glomeruli. Transgene expression was substantially induced, however, when unstimulated cells were transferred into the nephritic glomeruli.

Conclusions.—The CarG box element can be used as a molecular sensor for glomerular injury. For automatic regulation of local transgene expression where the transgene is required to be activated during inflammation and deactivated when the inflammation has subsided, this approach provides a novel concept in the context of advanced forms of gene therapy.

► The use of mesangial cells as vectors for renal expression of specific genes was pioneered by these authors and their colleagues. This study provides a very ingenious method of switching on genes in the environment of injury. Specifically, the authors take advantage of the known expression of α-smooth muscle actin in injured mesangial cells (above we reviewed papers describing this expression in fibroblasts of the interstitium as they transform to myofibroblasts). This ability of the mesangial cell to form a "smart" gene factory could give obvious benefit in inflammatory circumstances. In those circumstances, the promoter for α-smooth muscle actin would be engaged and the genetically engineered downstream gene expressed, perhaps one that reduced fibrotic consequences such as a protease that might degrade excess matrix accumulation. Obviously, outsmarting endogenous inflammatory regulators is a daunting prospect, but this is a very clever approach.

T.H. Hostetter, M.D.

Cystic Disease

Microtubule Active Taxanes Inhibit Polycystic Kidney Disease Progression in *cpk* Mice

Woo DDL, Tabancay AP Jr, Wang CJN (Univ of California, Los Angeles)

Kidney Int 51:1613–1618, 1997 4–31

Introduction.—Characterized by the presence of bilaterally enlarged kidneys with fibrotic tissues and thousands of fluid-filled cysts, the polycystic kidney diseases are a group of systemic disorders. End-stage renal disease is often caused by polycystic kidney disease. Polycystic *cpk/cpk* mice, which have had kidney abnormalities and disease progression studied in detail, die by 35 days of age. A new antineoplastic drug that acts by stabilizing microtubules is paclitaxel, which has inhibited the progression of polycystic kidney disease of polycystic *cpk/cpk* mice, enabling them to survive to 6 months of age. Paclitaxel binds to microtubules to promote the spontaneous in vitro polymerization of tubulin subunits into microtubules. In polycystic *cpk/cpk* mice, the ability of taxanes with differing ability to promote spontaneous in vitro assembly of tubulin dimers into microtubules was tested for their ability to inhibit the progression of polycystic kidney disease.

Methods.—After 7 days of birth, the *cpk/cpk* mice were given treatment with 5μL of paclitaxel, cephalomannine, 10-deactyl-taxol, or baccatin-III. All polycystic mice were treated for the duration of their life and untreated animals were used as controls. Histologic and determination of renal function were performed.

Results.—Compared with the survival of control animals, the survival of polycystic *cpk/cpk* mice was increased significantly longer by taxanes that are active in promoting microtubule assembly, including paclitaxel, 10-deactyl-taxol, and cephalomannine. The progression of renal failure in *cpk/cpk* mice was not affected by the microtubule-inactive taxane baccatin-III.

Conclusions.—For paclitaxel and related taxanes to modulate the progression of polycystic kidney progression in *cpk/cpk* mice, the ability to promote microtubule assembly may be necessary. Further research is needed to determine the effects of these taxanes on the progression of polycystic disease.

The Effect of Paclitaxel on the Progression of Polycystic Kidney Disease in Rodents

Martinez JR, Cowley BD Jr, Gattone VH II, et al (Univ of Kansas, Kansas City; Hokkaido College of Pharmacy, Japan; Fujita Health Univ, Aichi, Japan)

Am J Kidney Dis 29:435–444, 1997 4–32

Introduction.—Innumerable fluid-filled cysts derived from renal tubules characterize polycystic kidney diseases. A previous study found that paclitaxel prolonged the median survival of *cpk/cpk* mice with a rapidly progressive form of polycystic kidney disease. These mice usually have kidneys that enlarge to more than 10 times their normal size, and the mice die from renal failure within the first 4 weeks of life. It was not known whether paclitaxel would have an effect on other forms of polycystic kidney disease. Using rodents, it was determined whether paclitaxel could alter the progression of other forms of hereditary polycystic kidney diseases.

Methods.—Mice and rats with rapidly progressive polycystic kidney disease and mice and rats with slowly progressive polycystic kidney disease were given paclitaxel by intraperitoneal injection.

Results.—*Cpk/cpk* mice had increased survival from 24.5 days to more than 65 days with paclitaxel treatment (150 μg/wk), and had decreased kidney weight relative to body weight from 16.5%, at 21 days to 8.2% at more than 65 days of age. There was a 12% mortality rate with paclitaxel. No effect on the course of disease was seen with paclitaxel administered to rats with rapidly progressive polycystic kidney disease. In fact, these rats had severe side effects and premature death from paclitaxel. In rats with slowly progressive kidney disease, their body weight gain was reduced, and kidney weight relative to body weight was inconsistently affected by paclitaxel. Their serum urea nitrogen concentration was not affected by paclitaxel. The mice with slowly progressive polycystic kidney disease had slowly progressive renal enlargement and azotemia. Paclitaxel treatment had no effect on the increase in kidney weight or on the level of serum urea nitrogen in comparison with untreated cystic animals.

Conclusions.—*Cpk*/*cpk* mice with a rapidly progressive form of polycystic kidney disease had a diminished rate of renal enlargement and an increased life span with paclitaxel, but the drug had no effect on the other animals. In the treatment of polycystic kidney disease, it seems that paclitaxel has limited potential usefulness.

► Several years ago Woo and colleagues (Abstract 4–31) reported that Taxol (also known as paclitaxel and which is in the general class of taxanes) dramatically improves survival in a mouse model of polycystic kidney disease (*cpk*). Martinez et al. (Abstract 4–32) attempt to determine the pharmacology of this effect in greater detail an they find that those taxanes which interact with the cytoskeleton are most likely to inhibit progression or renal disease in this strain of the mouse. Apparently, there are taxanes other than Taxol that are even more effective at interacting with the microtubular cytoskeleton, and these might be particularly efficacious.

The other study by a group investigating various other types of cystic kidney disease in rodents is somewhat less encouraging. These investigators surveyed 4 different models of genetic cystic diseases in rodents and found that, indeed, it was only in the specific strain studied by Woo and colleagues (*cpk*) that Taxol was useful. Obviously, the key issue is which cystic disease is most reminiscent of human cystic disease. Because the primary gene defect in human cystic disease does not seem to be caused by a cytoskeletal protein, Taxol seems even less promising. However, the cellular pathophysiology of human cystic disease is probably complex. Perhaps more basic understanding will guide the decision whether to test Taxol in clinical trials.

T.H. Hostetter, M.D.

Identification and Localization of Polycystin, the *PKD1* Gene Product

Geng L, Segal Y, Peissel B, et al (Harvard Med School; Millennium Inc, Boston; Univ of Toronto; et al)

J Clin Invest 98:2674–2682, 1996 4–33

Introduction.—A common monogenic disease that affects about 1 in 1,000 individuals, autosomal dominant polycystic kidney disease is manifested by cystic replacement of renal tissue and leads to progressive renal failure. Hepatic and pancreatic cysts are also common in autosomal dominant polycystic kidney disease. Mutations in at least 3 genes cause this disease. Immunobiochemical and immunohistochemical analyses of polycystin expression were performed to elucidate the pathogenesis of autosomal dominant polycystic kidney disease. Polycystin is the cardinal member of a novel class of proteins in this disease.

Methods.—Three types of information were collected to determine the function of polycystin and the pathogenesis of autosomal dominant polycystic kidney disease: the spatial and temporal distribution of the protein within normal tissues, the subcellular location of polycystin, and the effects of autosomal dominant polycystin kidney disease mutations on the patterns of expression in affected tissues. Antisera was directed against a synthetic peptide and 2 recombinant proteins of different domains of polycystin in normal fetal and adult kidneys, as well as in kidneys with autosomal dominant polycystic disease. Immunohistologic studies and electron microscopy were performed.

Results.—An approximately 400-kD protein (polycystin) was found in the membrane fractions of normal fetal and adult kidneys, and kidneys with autosomal dominant polycystic kidney disease. Polycystin was localized to renal tubular epithelia, pancreatic ducts, hepatic bile ductules, and all sites of cystic changes in autosomal dominant polycystic kidney disease, as well as in some tissues not known to be affected by autosomal dominant polycystic kidney disease such as the skin. Plasma membranes were predominantly associated with polycystin. In adults, polycystin was significantly less abundant than in fetal epithelia. In most but not all renal cysts in autosomal dominant polycystic kidney disease, polycystin was overexpressed.

Conclusions.—The first biochemical and ultrastructural evidence that polycystin is a membrane-associated approximately 400-kD molecule is provided. Polycystin is expressed in the tubules where it is found on apical and basolateral domains of the plasma membranes of polarized epithelia in the kidney. To further understand the function of polycystin and the pathogenesis of this disease, identification of the ligands will be a key step.

Vascular Expression of Polycystin

Griffin MD, Torres VE, Grande JP, et al (Mayo Clinic and Mayo Found, Rochester, Minn)

J Am Soc Nephrol 8:616–626, 1997 4–34

Introduction.—Patients with autosomal dominant polycystic kidney disease (ADPKD) are at increased risk for a variety of vascular abnormalities, but it has not been determined whether these vascular manifestations result directly from the genetic defect responsible for ADPKD. Tissue specimens from patients with ADPKD and controls were examined for the expression of polycystin, a large protein of unknown function encoded by the gene *PKD1*, which is responsible for most cases of ADPKD.

Methods.—Tissue specimens obtained at autopsy included control abdominal and thoracic aorta, iliac, renal, mesenteric, and cervicocephalic arteries from 8 individuals who had died in accidents, and sections of intracranial aneurysms from 10 patients with ADPKD and from 13 age-

and gender-matched patients without ADPKD. Additional sections were obtained from 2 patients with ADPKD who had thoracic aortic dissections and from 1 patient with dolichoectatic basilar, vertebral, and internal carotid arteries.

Results.—All control arteries showed moderate-to-weak immunostaining for polycystin, the staining pattern was greatly enhanced by partial digestion of tissue slices with the nonspecific proteases trypsin and pronase. Similar enhancement was seen with specific elastase digestion, but digestion with elastase did not enhance the staining for smooth muscle actin. Specimens of intracranial aneurysms, aortic dissections, and dolichoectatic arteries from patients with ADPKD showed immunostaining of variable intensity for polycystin in arterial smooth muscle cells and myofibroblasts, together with disruption of elastic laminae. Staining patterns were not significantly altered by further elastase digestion. Non-ADPKD intracranial aneurysms also showed a variable degree of immunostaining with polycystin antisera in the same distribution.

Conclusions.—Polycystin is expressed in the vascular smooth muscle of the elastic and large distributive arteries, and may play a role in maintaining the normal functional synergy between arterial smooth muscle cells and adjacent elastic tissue. Findings suggest that vascular complications in ADPKD are not secondary but are directly linked to the underlying genetic defect.

▶ Since the identification of the gene responsible for *PKD1*, the most common type of ADPKD, considerable effort has gone into examining the mechanism whereby defects in this gene lead to cyst formation. The first of the above studies (Abstract 4–33) is something of an atlas of polycystin's (the gene product) expression in fetal and adult tissues. Several notable findings arise. The apical location of polycystin in the kidney is somewhat surprising, because most speculation has been that this protein functions as some sort of cell-matrix connection. This analysis, however, was mostly conducted in fetal tissue and therefore may not represent its final distribution in the mature kidney. A second notable finding of this study was the appearance of polycystin in tissues such as the skin, with no known phenotype in patients with ADPKD. Both of these findings perhaps point out even more clearly that we still know too little about how the molecule works normally. However, the presence of polycystin in most of the cysts in patients with cystic disease certainly indicate that simple failure of expression is not a mechanism of cystogenesis.

More straightforwardly, Griffin and colleagues (Abstract 4–34) report that polycystin can be demonstrated in vascular tissue. This, of course, accords with the well-known clinical findings that cerebral aneurysms and other vascular abnormalities of the aorta occur in patients with ADPKD. As with cysts, polycystin protein is demonstrable in the specimens of intracranial aneurysm, again indicating that failure to produce the protein is not the primary defect. Their precise localization of polycystin to smooth muscle cells leads the authors to speculate that polycystin functions as a connection between these cells and the elastic layer. The loss of this connection or some functional abnormality in it may predispose to aneurysms.

T.H. Hostetter, M.D.

The Molecular Basis of Focal Cyst Formation in Human Autosomal Dominant Polycystic Kidney Disease Type I

Qian F, Watnick TJ, Onuchic LF, et al (Johns Hopkins Univ, Baltimore, Md)
Cell 87:979–987, 1996 4–35

Purpose.—A common inherited condition, autosomal dominant polycystic kidney disease (ADPKD), is a major cause of renal failure. The manifestations of ADPKD, both renal and extrarenal, vary considerably. Genetic variability probably explains at least part of the difference. There is evidence to suggest that cyst formation is a focal process, with an inherited mutation at an ADPKD gene locus being necessary but, by itself, insufficient, for cystogenesis. The molecular basis of focal cyst formation in ADPKD was investigated.

Methods and Results.—The study used a new method of isolating epithelial cells from renal cysts, with minimal contamination by other cells. Clonality studies showed that individual renal cysts were monoclonal. Further analysis revealed loss of heterozygosity within individual cysts for 2 closely linked polymorphic markers within the *PKD1* gene. The normal haplotype was lost in somatic tissues, according to genetic analysis.

Conclusion.—The clinical variability and focal renal cyst formation of ADPKD probably results from random inactivation of the normal *PKD1* allele in somatic tissue, these results suggest. The large number of cysts observed in the population would require a high rate of "second hits," suggesting that the *PKD1* gene has unique features responsible for its mutability. The molecular mechanism of disease appears to be recessive. These findings suggest that polycystin replacement treatments may be useful in preventing cyst formation and end-stage renal disease.

▶ This article represents the greatest advance in understanding ADPKD of the *PKD1* variety, the most common type of ADPKD, since the identification of the gene at fault.[1] Using several sophisticated molecular and cell biological techniques, these authors have demonstrated that an individual cyst represents the combination of the inherited defect in the polycystin gene and a local intrarenal mutation in the initially normal polycystin gene from the other parent. Thus, this "double hit" leads to an individual cell that is homozygous for the defect and the initiation of the cyst formation. Hence, each individual cyst represents a clonal second mutation at the somatic or kidney level giving rise to local homozygosity and pathology.

This general principle was suggested many years ago for tumors such as retinoblastoma and now seems to be the case for polycystic kidney disease. The studies do not answer the question as to how cysts eventually develop, nor do they answer the question as to why mutations in the normal gene seem to be so frequent. It would have been of interest to know whether mutations in the normal gene also commonly occur in other tissues and, thereby, whether the gene in its structural makeup is prone to sporadic mutations or whether there is something about the environment of the tubular epithelial cells that enhances this process.

If the general concept is borne out, an additional field of investigation, with great practical consequences, will be what factors, genetic or environmental, predispose to the second or somatic mutation. If they could be prevented, then the disease itself would be abrogated, even despite persistence of the heterozygote abnormality.

T.H. Hostetter, M.D.

Reference

1. The European Polycystic Kidney Disease Consortium: The polycystic kidney disease gene encodes a 14 kb transcript and lies within a duplicated region on chromosome 16. *Cell* 77:881–894, 1994.

Diabetes

Low Birth Weight—Is it Associated With Few and Small Glomeruli in Normal Subjects and NIDDM Patients?

Nyengaard JR, Bendtsen TF, Mogensen CE (Aarhus Univ, Denmark; Aarhus Kommunehospital, Denmark)

Diabetologia 39:1634–1637, 1996 4–36

Background.—Previous studies suggest that low birth weight may be related to the development of non–insulin-dependent diabetes mellitus (NIDDM) and high blood pressure. The tendency toward hypertension may be more pronounced in subjects born with a reduced number of glomeruli, and therefore with a low glomerular filtration surface area. Kidneys from normal and NIDDM subjects were studied to assess possible associations between low birth weight, low kidney weight, and few or small glomeruli.

Methods.—The study included 79 kidneys taken at autopsy from control subjects and patients with NIDDM. Renal weight was known in all kidneys, in which previous study had established the glomerular number and volume. Information on birth weight was available for 26 NIDDM patients and 19 controls.

Results.—The 2 groups were similar in age, sex, kidney weight, number of glomeruli, glomerular volume, and birth weight. Birth weight was not significantly related to glomerular number or volume, kidney weight, or NIDDM.

Conclusions.—The findings do not support the hypothesis that low birth weight is related to the development of NIDDM, smaller kidneys, or small glomerular size and/or number. However, the study included a limited population and cannot exclude the possibility that very-low-birth-weight infants may have fewer and/or smaller glomeruli.

Glomerular Hyperfiltration in the Prediction of Nephropathy in IDDM: A 10-Year Follow-up Study

Yip JW, Jones SL, Wiseman MJ, et al (Guy's Hosp, London)
Diabetes 45:1729–1733, 1996 4–37

Introduction.—Nephropathy occurs in more than one third of patients with insulin-dependent diabetes mellitus (IDDM). Although microalbuminuria predicts clinical albuminuria, such patients already have significant pathologic changes of the glomeruli. Glomerular hyperfiltration may be an independent risk factor for diabetic nephropathy in patients with IDDM. The renal outcomes of a group of patients with IDDM and glomerular hyperfiltration were studied.

Methods.—The prospective, 10-year, case-controlled study included 25 patients with IDDM and glomerular hyperfiltration, defined as a glomerular filtration rate (GFR) of greater than 135 mL·min^{-1}. Mean age at baseline was 29 years. These cases were matched for age, sex, and duration of diabetes to 25 patients with IDDM and a normal GFR of 85 to 135 mL ·min^{-1}. Mean age in the control group was 30 years. In both groups, measurements of GFR, urinary albumin excretion rate (AER), blood pressure, and glycated hemoglobin were made at baseline and repeated at 5, 8, and 10 years. The 5-year findings were previously reported; the 10-year results are updated here.

Results.—Baseline measurements indicated no significant differences in blood pressure, AER, or glycated hemoglobin. Through 10 years' follow-up, the 2 groups maintained a similar level of metabolic control. The last measured GFR was 122 mL·min^{-1} in the hyperfiltration group versus 103 mL·min^{-1} in the normofiltration group. The rate of decrease in GFR was nonsignificantly higher in the hyperfiltration group, 2.54 versus 1.50 mL·min^{-1}. There was no difference in the risk of progression to microalbuminuria, macroalbuminuria, or hypertension. However, by final follow-up, geometric mean AER was 18.9 in the hyperfiltration group versus 11.0 in the control group. Glomerular filtration rate at baseline was independently associated with blood pressure at the end of the study. Baseline AER and blood pressure were the best predictors of the same values at the end of the study.

Conclusions.—In patients with IDDM, the factors most strongly related to renal outcome are AER and blood pressure. Glomerular hyperfiltration is an independent, but weaker, risk factor. Longer follow-up is needed to confirm that these relationships are clinically significant.

Glomerular Hyperfiltration in Microalbuminuric NIDDM Patients

Vedel P, Obel J, Nielsen FS, et al (Steno Diabetes Ctr, Gentofte, Denmark; County Central Hosp, Næstved, Denmark)

Diabetologia 39:1584–1589, 1996 4–38

Objective.—For patients with insulin-dependent diabetes, glomerular hyperfiltration and microalbuminuria are both risk factors for diabetic nephropathy. However, little is known about the significance of glomerular hyperfiltration in patients with non–insulin-dependent diabetes mellitus (NIDDM) and microalbuminuria. Glomerular filtration rate (GFR) was compared in NIDDM patients at high risk of diabetic nephropathy versus normoalbuminuric patients with NIDDM and nondiabetic controls.

Methods.—The cross-sectional study included 158 patients with microalbuminuria and NIDDM, 39 normoalbuminuric patients with NIDDM, and 20 nondiabetic controls. The 3 groups were comparable in sex, age, and body mass index. All underwent measurement of GFR with injection of a single IV bolus of ^{51}Cr-EDTA and 4-hour measurement of plasma clearance.

Results.—Uncorrected GFR was 139 mL/min in the microalbuminuric NIDDM group, compared with 115 mL/min in the normoalbuminuric NIDDM group and 111 mL/min in the normal controls. Adjusted GFR was 117, 99, and 98 $mL \cdot min^{-1} \cdot 1.73\ m^{-2}$, respectively. Among subjects who had not received treatment for hypertension, GFR was 119 $mL \cdot min^{-1} \cdot 1.73\ m^{-2}$ in the microalbuminuric NIDDM group, 100 $mL \cdot min^{-1} \cdot 1.73\ m^{-2}$ in the normoalbuminuric NIDDM group, and 98 $mL \cdot min^{-1} \cdot 1.73\ m^{-2}$ in the control group. Twenty-three percent of microalbuminuric NIDDM patients had glomerular hyperfiltration, defined as an elevation above the mean GFR plus 2 standard deviations in normoalbuminuric NIDDM patients. Factors significantly correlated with GFR in microalbuminuric NIDDM patients on multiple regression analysis were HbA_{1c}, 24 hr urinary sodium excretion, age, and duration of diabetes.

Conclusions.—Glomerular hyperfiltration is common among microalbuminuric NIDDM patients at high risk of diabetic nephropathy, this cross-sectional study suggests. Glomerular hyperfiltration may be an additional risk factor for progressive nephropathy. The authors are performing a longitudinal study of glomerular function among the microalbuminuric patients from this study.

Risk Factors for Development of Incipient and Overt Diabetic Nephropathy in Patients With Non-insulin Dependent Diabetes Mellitus: Prospective, Observational Study

Gall M-A, Hougaard P, Borch-Johnsen K, et al (Steno Diabetes Ctr, Gentofte, Denmark; Glostrup Univ, Denmark)

BMJ 314:783–788, 1997 4–39

Introduction.—Compared to normoalbuminuric diabetic patients, those with microalbuminuria (i.e., urinary albumin excretion rate between 30 and 299 mg/24 hours) have an increased risk of premature death. The risk for development of diabetic nephropathy among diabetic patients who have persistent microalbuminuria—incipient diabetic nephropathy—is 20-fold. Studies have been conducted to identify risk factors for nephropathy for patients with insulin-dependent diabetes, but little is known about risk factors for nephropathy in patients with non–insulin-dependent diabetes.

Methods.—There were 176 white patients younger than 66 years with non–insulin-dependent diabetes who participated in a prospective, observational study (median follow-up 5.8 years). At baseline, they had normoalbuminuria with a urinary albumin excretion rate of less than 30 mg/24 hours.

Results.—Persistent microalbuminuria developed in 36 of 176 patients. Persistent macroalbuminuria developed in 5 patients. There was a 23% 5-year incidence of incipient diabetic nephropathy. The development of incipient or overt diabetic nephropathy could be predicted by the following risk factors: male sex, increased baseline log urinary albumin excretion rate, increased serum cholesterol concentration, presence of retinopathy, hemoglobin A_1 concentration, and age. The following were not identified as risk factors: history of smoking, preexisting coronary heart disease, serum creatinine concentration, body mass index, arterial blood pressure, or known duration of diabetes.

Conclusion.—The development of incipient and overt diabetic nephropathy in normoalbuminuric patients with non–insulin-dependent diabetes can be predicted by several potentially modifiable risk factors.

► These articles (Abstracts 4–36 through 4–39) concern aspects of risk factor analysis in patients with non–insulin-dependent diabetes mellitus (NIDDM) and, in one instance, patients with IDDM. Predicting which patients with diabetes will have nephropathy is potentially of great use, because only a minority do so. Presumably, understanding those risk factors would illuminate the basic pathophysiology of the disease as well as provide clinically useful data for targeting specific patients for more intensive therapy. The first of these articles (Abstract 4–36) challenges the recent hypothesis that small birth weight and, in consequence, small numbers of glomeruli predispose to renal complications. The study population is quite limited in number of patients and the study focuses on NIDDM. Furthermore, its source within the Danish population raises questions about its general applicability in other more heterogeneous groups.

Two articles dealing with hyperfiltration, one in patients with IDDM, another in patients with NIDDM (Abstract 4–38), continue to demonstrate that hyperfiltration is associated with later evidence of diabetic glomerulopathy. Thus, this hemodynamic stress still seems to be one of the constellation of risks or physiologic stresses culminating in overt diabetic nephropathy and for both metabolic types of diabetes.

Lastly, the article from Gall's group (Abstract 4–39) assesses risk factors in NIDDM. Three features of the results are worthy of mention. First, the role of glycemic control is again confirmed as lower hemoglobin A1cs were associated with reduced risks of nephropathy. Second, hypercholesterolemia is not clearly distinguished as an independent risk factor in these patients, that is, independent of diabetes control or proteinuria. Nevertheless, control of cholesterol is warranted if only to prevent extrarenal vascular disease. Third, the absence of a relation to hypertension seems startling. On examining the data more closely, the relationship was of near statistical difference ($p = 0.06$) for systolic hypertension as a risk factor, but perhaps more important, the patients were treated for hypertension during the course of the study so any effects of hypertension might be successfully blunted or obliterated. In any case, this group had previously shown effects of hypertension on the course of NIDDM nephropathy to be significant. Thus, blood sugar, blood pressure, and probably cholesterol control remain the mainstays in averting this complication.

T.H. Hostetter, M.D.

Podocyte Loss and Progressive Glomerular Injury in Type II Diabetes

Pagtalunan ME, Miller PL, Jumping-Eagle S, et al (VA Palo Alto Healthcare System, Stanford, Calif; Stanford Univ, Calif; Natl Inst of Diabetes and Digestive and Kidney Diseases, Phoenix. Ariz; et al)

J Clin Invest 99:342–348, 1997 4–40

Purpose.—Little is known about the glomerular structural changes leading to renal failure in patients with type II diabetes. This topic is difficult to study, largely because type II diabetes usually develops later in life. Such older patients may also have atherosclerotic vascular disease and hypertension, and their renal disease does not always result from diabetes. In contrast, Pima Indians develop type II diabetes at a young age, without the other changes attributable to age. Changes in glomerular structure were studied among Pima Indians with type II diabetes.

Methods.—The study used renal biopsy specimens from 51 Pima Indians with type II diabetes. Ten had early diabetes; 17 had microalbuminuria; 12 had normoalbuminuria, even though their duration of diabetes was comparable to that of the microalbuminuric group; and 12 had clinical nephropathy. The mean age of these groups ranged from 40 to 47 years. The pattern of mesangial expansion in the renal biopsy specimens was studied. The role of visceral epithelial cell injury in the progression of diabetic glomerulopathy was studied as well, including assessment of podocyte number.

Results.—Glomerular and mesangial volume were moderately increased in the microalbuminuric group compared with the early diabetes group, but not significantly different from the long-term normoalbuminuria group. Findings in the clinical nephropathy group included global glomerular sclerosis and marked structural abnormalities in nonsclerosed glomeruli. As mesangial expansion increased, so did total glomerular volume. Though glomerular capillary surface area was unchanged, the glomerular basement membrane grew thicker and the podocyte foot processes broader. Along with the latter change came a reduction in number of podocytes per glomerulus and an increase in the surface area covered by the remaining podocytes.

Conclusions.—The pathologic mechanism of glomerular injury appears to be the same in types I and II diabetes, this study of Pima Indians finds. In patients with clinical nephropathy, reduced glomerular filtration rate appears to result from loss of glomeruli to sclerosis and changes of capillary wall structure in the glomeruli that remain open. Loss of podocytes appears to be an important factor in the progression of diabetic nephropathy.

► Loss of glomerular epithelial cells (podocytes) has often been proposed as a key step in progressive glomerular injury. These detailed morphometric studies from the Pima Indian population (a group prone to adult onset diabetes and renal injury) demonstrate in extraordinary detail this loss of podocytes as diabetic nephropathy appears. This approach was not designed to examine why these podocytes decline in number in advanced renal disease. However, the authors raise the possibilities that sustained mechanical stresses of glomerular growth and capillary hypertension may be damaging and/or some cellular exhaustion of podocytes enwrapped over large surface areas may cause metabolic compromise. In addition, one wonders whether proteinuria may visit additional toxic effects on these cells. Finally, the studies point out that the Pima, even with very early diabetes and no detectable functional abnormalities, have far larger glomeruli but no more podocytes per glomerulus than nondiabetic subjects of European ancestry. The authors offer the interesting speculation that this relative podocyte deficiency may be an underlying predisposing factor for renal disease within this ethnic group.

T.H. Hostetter, M.D.

Salt Restriction Reduces Hyperfiltration, Renal Enlargement, and Albuminuria in Experimental Diabetes

Allen TJ, Waldron MJ, Casley D, et al (Austin and Repatriation Med Ctr, Heidelberg, Australia)

Diabetes 46:119–124, 1997 4–41

Background.—There is ongoing debate over the role of glomerular hyperfiltration in the development of diabetic nephropathy in insulin-dependent diabetes mellitus (IDDM). Experimental studies suggest that early changes of diabetes could be related to changes in the renin-angiotensin system (RAS). Chronic stimulation of the RAS with a low-salt diet reduces hyperfiltration in diabetic rats, but the long-term effects of salt restriction on glomerular filtration rate (GFR) are unknown. Rats with streptozocin-induced diabetes were studied to determine the effects of a restricted-salt diet on the RAS, GFR, renal size, and albuminuria.

Methods.—Streptozocin was used to induce diabetes in Sprague-Dawley rats. In the first of 2 studies, diabetic and nondiabetic rats were assigned to receive a diet containing very low salt levels (0.005% NaCl) or a normal salt level (0.4% NaCl) for 4 weeks. The short-term effects of severe salt restriction on GFR, kidney size, and plasma angiotensin I and II levels were thereby studied. In the second study, rats assigned to salt restriction diet followed a 0.05% NaCl diet for 24 weeks. Repeated measurements of albuminuria and GFR were performed.

Results.—In the short-term study, the diabetic rats showed a 49% increase in GFR, a 34% increase in renal weight, and an 85% reduction in plasma angiotensin II. Diabetic rats on the very low sodium diet had a reduced GFR, a normal plasma angiotensin II level, and slowing of kidney growth. In this study, there was a negative correlation between GFR and plasma angiotensin II, and a positive correlation between GFR and kidney weight.

In the long-term study, albuminuria got progressively greater over time in the diabetic rats, compared with nondiabetic rats. Diabetic rats on the salt-restricted diet had a lesser increase in albuminuria. They also showed reduced blood pressure and kidney weight, compared with diabetic rats on a normal-salt diet.

Conclusions.—Short-term dietary sodium restriction in diabetic rats results in a reduced GFR and kidney weight. In the longer term, sodium restriction is associated with reduced albuminuria, kidney weight, and blood pressure. The experimental results suggest that salt restriction could be clinically useful for the prevention and treatment of diabetic nephropathy. A low-sodium diet might be clinically acceptable to patients, and could have the added benefit of reducing blood pressure.

Urinary Albumin Excretion Rate During Angiotensin II Infusion in Microalbuminuric Patients With Insulin and Non-Insulin-Dependent Diabetes Mellitus

Spooren PFMJ, Gans ROB, Adèr HJ, et al (Free Univ, Amsterdam)
Nephrol Dial Transplant 12:281–285, 1997 4–42

Introduction.—In both insulin-dependent and non–insulin-dependent diabetes mellitus (IDDM and NIDDM), microalbuminuria predicts later clinical diabetic nephropathy. It has been suggested that glomerular hyperfiltration may lead to proteinuria. Treatment with angiotensin-converting enzyme (ACE) inhibitors has been shown to reduce glomerular protein loss. Patients with IDDM and NIDDM were studied to see if increasing the glomerular transcapillary hydraulic pressure difference with exogenous angiotensin II would increase microalbuminuria.

Methods.—The study included 22 diabetic patients with microalbuminuria, i.e., an albumin excretion rate of 30 to 300 mg albumin/24 hr. Eleven had IDDM and 11 had NIDDM. The patients' acute responses to progressive doses of angiotensin II—1, 3, and 6 mg/kg/min IV—were evaluated.

Results.—Mean arterial pressure increased from 100 mm Hg at baseline to 105, 111, and 116 mm Hg, respectively, at the increasing doses of angiotensin II. Effective renal plasma flow increased from 542 to 478, 429, and 382 mL/min, while filtration fraction increased from 20.2% to 23.1%, 27.1%, and 29.8%. Total renal vascular resistance increased from 9,454 dyne s cm^{-5} at baseline to 11,158, 13,310, and 15,538 dyne s cm^{-5} with angiotensin II treatment. Angiotensin II had no significant effect on glomerular filtration or albumin excretion rate.

Conclusions.—In diabetic patients with microalbuminuria, exogenous angiotensin II leads to decreased effective renal plasma flow and increased filtration fraction and total renal vascular resistance. However, there is no change in microalbuminuria or glomerular filtration rate—thus there is no rise in albumin excretion in response to angiotensin II-induced increased capillary pressure. During manipulation of the renin-angiotensin system in IDDM and NIDDM, glomerular transcapillary hydraulic pressure does not appear to be the factor responsible for determining degree of urinary albumin loss.

▶ Salt restriction is often advised in patients with renal disease, usually in the general hope that it will lower blood pressure. Indeed, some diminution of pressure was obtained in the rats with experimental diabetes studied by Allen et al. (Abstract 4–41). However, in other studies in experimental models of progression, dietary salt restriction has also had beneficial effects on endpoints such as albuminuria without even lowering blood pressure. In any case, low-salt diets certainly raise renin and presumably angiotensin II levels within the kidney, and given the current general view that angiotensin is damaging by hemodynamic and nonhemodynamic effects it is difficult to entirely understand how salt restriction achieves its beneficial effects. Likewise in the paper by Spooren et al. (Abstract 4–42), the infusion of exogenous angiotensin II at levels sufficient to raise arterial pressure still caused no further augmentation of urine albumin excretion in microalbuminuric patients with diabetes. Thus, elevating angiotensin II seems to have little effect, at least in the short term, on this marker of glomerular injury. Although the levels of angiotensin II in the kidney are perhaps 10–to-100 fold higher than plasma, this study and the other with salt restriction again highlight our ignorance as to how angiotensin II may be injuring the kidney. Clearly, the simplistic view that angiotensin II is damaging requires considerable modification.

T.H. Hostetter, M.D.

Orally Absorbed Reactive Glycation Products (Glycotoxins): An Environmental Risk Factor in Diabetic Nephropathy

Koschinsky T, He C-J, Mitsuhashi T, et al (Picower Inst for Med Research, Manhasset, NY; Diabetes Research Inst, Dusseldorf, Germany)

Proc Natl Acad Sci U S A 94:6474–6479, 1997 4–43

Background.—Patients with diabetic or nondiabetic kidney disease (KD) have an impairment in the renal excretion of the catabolic products of endogenous advanced glycation end products (AGEs). The oral absorption and renal clearance kinetics of food AGEs in patients with diabetes mellitus (DM) and kidney disease were studied, and the presence of active glycotoxins in circulating diet-derived AGEs was determined.

Methods.—Thirty-eight diabetic patients with or without kidney disease and 5 healthy persons were given a single meal of egg white, cooked with or without fructose (comprising an AGE or CL diet, respectively). Serum and urine samples were collected for 48 hours and monitored for AGE immunoreactivity based on complex formation with ^{125}I-labeled fibronectin.

Findings.—Only the AGE diet distinctly increased serum AGE levels in direct proportion to the amount ingested. The area under the curve for serum was correlated directly with the severity of kidney disease. Renal excretion of dietary AGE, though normally incomplete, was inversely correlated with the degree of albuminuria in diabetic patients and directly with creatinine clearance, decreased to less than 5% in diabetic patients with renal failure. Serum obtained after the AGE meal showed increased age-crosslinking activity, which was inhibited by aminoguanidine.

Conclusions.—The renal excretion of orally absorbed AGEs is markedly suppressed in patients with diabetic nephropathy. The daily influx of dietary AGEs includes glycotoxins that may represent an additional chronic risk for renal-vascular injury in patients with diabetes. Dietary restriction of AGE food intake may substantially decrease the burden of AGEs in diabetic patients and may improve prognosis.

► This provocative article suggests that the potentially toxic AGE compounds may come not only from internal metabolism but in the food we eat. The presence of AGE proteins in cooked foods was examined even before their recognition as potential metabolic toxins in diabetes was proposed. Indeed, the initial chemical descriptions of the process ("browning") leading to their production appeared in the food science literature. However, these authors have pioneered much of our understanding of the metabolically derived AGEs and now suggest that the additional exogenous load from foodstuffs may have toxic effects. They suggest an analogy to the pro-atherogenic components of lipid oxidation products in foods. Whether ingested AGEs actually increase the risk for vascular complications in diabetic or even nondiabetic individuals remains to be proved. However, will we soon see roasted duck skin, soy sauce, and Classic Coca Cola (foods with high AGE content) restricted because of their metabolic risk?

T.H. Hostetter, M.D.

Glycosaminoglycans Delay the Progression of Nephropathy in NIDDM

Solini A, Ricci F, Vergnani L, et al (Univ of Ferrara, Italy; Univ of Padova, Italy)

Diabetes Care 20:819–823, 1997 4–44

Background.—Many investigators consider increased urinary albumin excretion to be an early marker of progression of diabetic nephropathy lesions. The effect of the oral administration of glycosaminoglycans on metabolic control and albumin excretion rate (AER) in patients with non–insulin-dependent diabetes mellitus (NIDDM) and increased urinary albumin excretion was determined.

Methods.—Twelve hypertensive patients with NIDDM aged a mean 52 years were enrolled in the double-blind, placebo-controlled trial. All patients were taking antihypertensive therapy. The patients were given placebo or sulodexide, 100 mg/day, for 4 months, at which time a crossover was performed. Routine biochemical parameters along with AER and coagulative function were assessed every 2 months.

Findings.—Compared to placebo, glycosaminoglycan treatment significantly reduced plasma fibrinogen and AER, from a mean 4.15 to 2.77 mmol/L and from a mean 128.3 to 39.6 μg/min, respectively. Blood pressure control was also ameliorated in the absence of any treatment variation (Fig 1).

Conclusions.—Glycosaminoglycan treatment appears to prevent the progression of diabetic nephropathy in patients with NIDDM. This effect probably occurs in association with satisfactory control of blood pressure values.

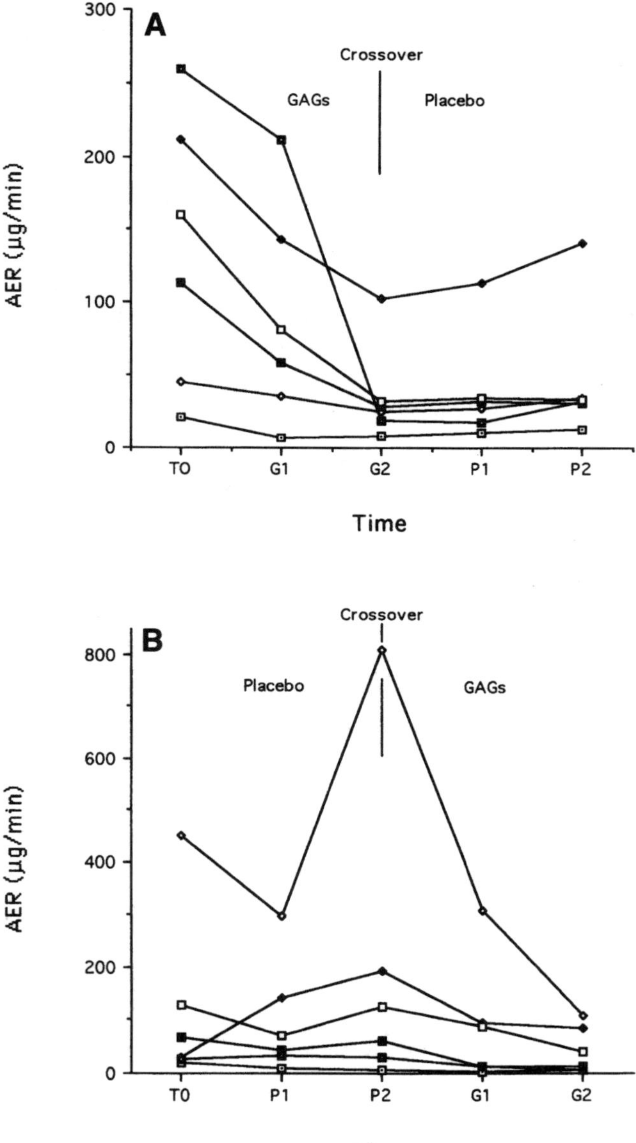

FIGURE 1.—Albumin excretion rate (µg/min) in the 6 patients with non–insulin-dependent diabetes mellitus who started the study with glycosaminoglycans (**A**) and in those who started with placebo (**B**) during the 8 months of the protocol. *Abbreviation*: *AER*, albumin excretion rate. (Courtesy of Solini A, Ricci F, Vergnani L, et al: Glycosaminoglycans delay the progression of nephropathy in NIDDM. *Diabetes Care* 20:819–823, 1997.)

Danaparoid Sodium Lowers Proteinuria in Diabetic Nephropathy

van der Pijl JW, van der Woude FJ, Geelhoed-Duijvestijn PHLM, et al (Leiden Univ, The Netherlands)

J Am Soc Nephrol 8:456–462, 1997 4–45

Background.—Diabetic nephropathy is a progressive illness characterized histologically by thickening of the glomerular basement membrane and mesangial expansion and proliferation. The glycosaminoglycan side chains of heparan sulfate proteoglycan, an important constituent of the glomerular basement membrane, are reduced proportionally to the degree of proteinuria in patients with diabetic nephropathy. The effect of danaparoid sodium, a mixture of sulfated glycosaminoglycans consisting mainly of heparan sulfate, on proteinuria in patients with diabetic nephropathy was investigated.

Methods.—Nine patients completed the randomized, placebo-controlled, crossover study without major side effects. The crossover design included 2 6-week periods of treatment with placebo or 750 anti-Xa units of danaparoid sodium given subcutaneously once a day.

Findings.—Danaparoid sodium resulted in significant declines in albuminuria and proteinuria. After such treatment, the albumin excretion ratio standardized for urinary creatinine declined by 17%, compared to a 23% increase after placebo. At 8 weeks, there was a significant between-treatment difference in the percentage change of urinary protein excretion corrected for urinary creatinine. Treatments did not differ in hematologic, hemostasis, or biochemical safety parameters or in fundus photography.

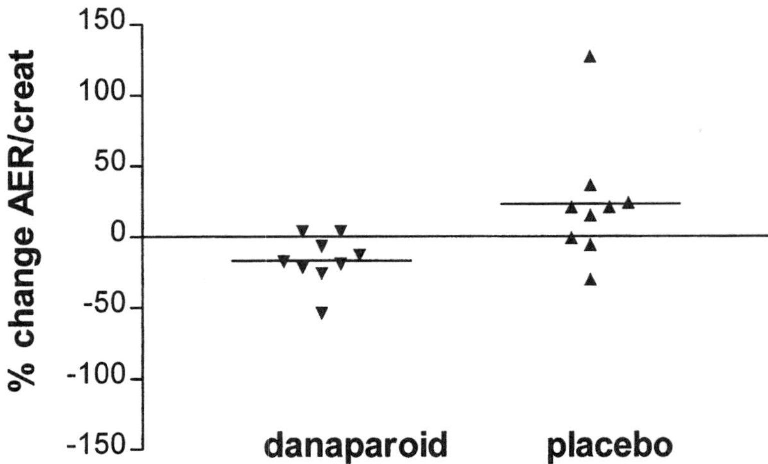

FIGURE 1.—A scatter diagram showing the percentage difference (δ) of the albumin excretion rate (*AER*) standardized for the urinary creatinine excretion comparing 8-weeks with baseline in both treatment arms. Percentage difference (δ) urinary protein excretion rate values for AER/creat and creat were calculated as follows: $(y - x/x)*100\% = \delta$, where y is the 8-week value for AER/creat and x is the 0-week value. The difference is significant ($P < 0.03$). (Courtesy of van der Pijl JW, van der Woulde FJ, Geelhoed-Duijvestijn PHLM, et al: Danaparoid sodium lowers proteinuria in diabetic nephropathy. *J Am Soc Nephrol* 8[3]:456–462, 1997.)

Two patients had minor skin hematomas at the danaproid sodium injection site (Fig 1).

Conclusions.—Danaparoid sodium treatment appears to decrease proteinuria safely in patients with diabetic nephropathy. Further research is needed to determine whether danaparoid sodium can not only reduce proteinuria but also stop the progression of renal disease.

► Several previous observations in animals and humans have suggested that heparin, or even its subunits the disaccharides, glycosaminoglycan, may be beneficial in lessening glomerular injury. These studies follow on those observations with Solini (Abstract 4–44) demonstrating that oral administration of what seems to be a relatively small amount (100 mg/day) of a glycosaminoglycan could reduce albuminuria substantially. However, blood pressure was also reduced in this trial during the period of experimental therapy, and one wonders if the compound was achieving its effect through direct actions of the glycosaminoglycans in the glomerulus, which to me seems rather unlikely given the amounts ingested, or through a hemodynamic action. Indeed, glycosaminoglycans can influence various vasoactive substances not the least of which may be aldosterone.

The study from the Netherlands (Abstract 4–45) using danaparoid proceed generally from the same background and also demonstrate a modestly significant reduction in protein excretion in diabetic patients with proteinuria. Because the danaparoid was administered subcutaneously, the clear preference could be for the oral method. One wonders whether glycosaminoglycans, as part of natural food stuffs, are ever digested as intact units and, if so, whether they would constitute a protective dietary substance.

T.H. Hostetter, M.D.

Increased Renal Production of Transforming Growth Factor-β_1 In Patients With Type II Diabetes

Sharma K, Ziyadeh FN, Alzahabi B, et al (Thomas Jefferson Univ, Philadelphia; Univ of Pennsylvania, Philadelphia; UMDNJ, Camden, NJ)

Diabetes 46:854–859, 1997 4–46

Purpose.—Patients with type I or type II diabetes are at risk of diabetic nephropathy. In this common complication, metabolic and vascular factors may produce chronic accumulation of glomerular mesangial matrix. These processes may involve both transforming growth factor-β (TGF-β) and endothelin. Renal production of TGF-β and endothelin was assessed in patients with type II diabetes.

Methods.—Fourteen patients with type II diabetes and 11 nondiabetic patients, all of whom were undergoing elective cardiac catheterization, were studied. Both groups underwent measurement of TGF-β and endothelin levels in the aortic and renal vein blood and in urine. Net mass balance across the kidney was calculated by measurement of renal blood flow.

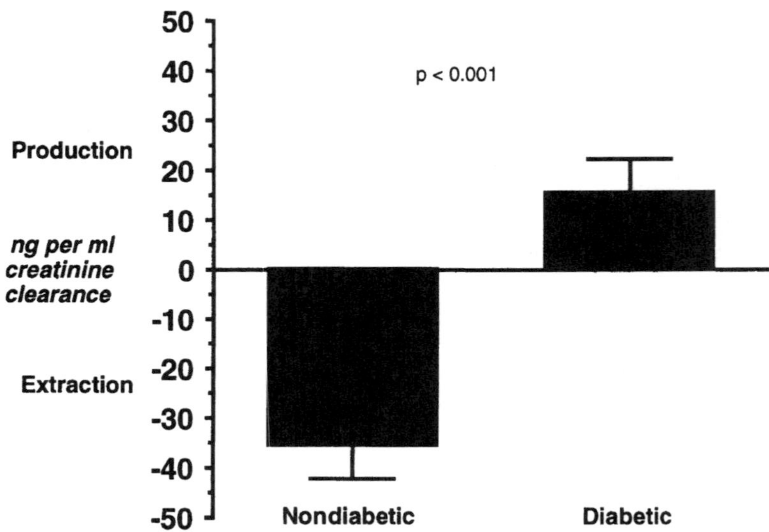

FIGURE 2.—Net renal transforming growth factor-β_1 mass values factored per creatinine clearance (mL · min^{-1} · 1.73 m^{-2} in nondiabetic and diabetic patients. Data are means ± SE. (Courtesy of Sharma K, Ziyadeh FN, Alzahabi B, et al: Increased renal production of transforming growth factor-β_1 in patients with type II diabetes. *Diabetes* 46:854–859, 1997.)

Results.—The results showed net production of immunoreactive TGF-β_1 by the kidneys in patients with diabetes, at a mean rate of 830 ng/min. However, patients without diabetes had net renal extraction of circulating TGF-β_1, at a mean rate of −3,479 ng/min. Mean bioassayable levels of TGF-β in urine were 2.435 ng/mg creatinine in diabetic patients and 0.569 ng/mg in nondiabetic patients. The diabetic patients had a mean renal production value of 15.2 ng and the nondiabetic patients had a mean renal extraction value of −35.5 ng, when the renal TGF-β_1 mass balance was factored per milliliter of creatinine clearance (Fig 2). There was no significant difference between groups in renal production of immunoreactive endothelin.

Conclusions.—Patients with type II diabetes have enhanced net renal production of TGF-β_1, whereas nondiabetic controls show net renal extraction of this cytokine. Elevated production of TGF-β by the kidney may play an important role in the development of diabetic nephropathy. Longitudinal studies are recommended to see whether renal TGF-β production is a useful marker of risk and/or progression of diabetic nephropathy.

Urinary Transforming Growth Factor-β in Patients with Glomerular Diseases

Murakami K, Takemura T, Hino S, et al (Kinki Univ, Osaka, Japan)

Pediatr Nephrol 11:334–336, 1997 4–47

Introduction.—Transforming growth factor-β is a fibrogenic cytokine that increases collagen, proteoglycan, and fibronectin production, upregulates the cellular expression of extracellular matrix receptor, and decreases matrix turnover. Transforming growth factor-β is secreted by various types of cells. In various glomerular diseases, extracellular matrix progressively accumulates. Previous studies of experimental nephritis and human glomerulonephritis demonstrated a causal role of transforming growth factor-β in the overproduction of extracellular matrix by glomerular cells. In the process of mesangial expansion, glomerular sclerosis, and interstitial fibrosis, it appears that transforming growth factor-β plays a central role. In human glomerular diseases, the local expression of transforming growth factor-β was demonstrated.

Methods.—In 12 healthy controls and 42 patients with various glomerular diseases, including mesangial proliferative and nonproliferative types, the urinary levels of active transforming growth factor-β were measured using enzyme-linked immunosorbent assay. The diseases that the patients had included IgA nephritis, Henoch-Schönlein purpura nephritis, IgA-negative mesangial proliferative glomerulonephritis, minimal change nephrotic syndrome, and focal glomerulosclerosis.

Results.—In patients with IgA nephritis and focal glomerulosclerosis, as compared with patients with other types of glomerular diseases and healthy controls, urinary transforming growth factor-β, expressed as a ratio to urinary creatinine (ng/mg creatinine), was significantly elevated. The grade of interstitial fibrosis was significantly correlated to urinary transforming growth factor-β levels. Transforming growth factor-β was significantly correlated with the grade of mesangial matrix increase and the magnitude of proteinuria among patients with proliferative-type disease. There was no significant relationship between urinary transforming growth factor-β levels and the immunostaining intensity of transforming growth factor-β .

Conclusions.—In glomerular diseases, urinary transforming growth factor-β reflects the grade of interstitial fibrosis. In proliferative-type glomerulonephritis, it also reflects the mesangial matrix increase. When monitoring patients with some types of glomerular disease, measuring transforming growth factor-β levels in the urine might be helpful.

► As noted in reviews of several other current articles in this edition of the YEAR BOOK, transforming growth factor-β (TGF-β) has clearly become a focal point for investigations of progressive renal disease. However, its use as a predictive marker is yet to be established at least in any clinically useful way. These studies (Abstracts 4–46 and 4–47) provide both further evidence for its physiologic role and a beginning suggestion of a means of assessing human renal disease. The demonstration of increased production rate in diabetic patients is a truly first-rate piece of applied human physiology. The studies of urinary excretion in various glomerular diseases suggest that the relationship of TGF-β to fibrosis is an important one. The authors call attention to the relation between urinary TGF-β and mesangial matrix increase, but they also note that there is a clear relationship to interstitial fibrosis. The latter pathology so dominates in the chronically injured kidney that one would guess that physiologically, TGF-β may be more related to it than mesangial pathology. In any case, the relation to progression and to therapy will be an interesting next chapter in studying TGF-β dynamics in human renal disease.

T.H. Hostetter, M.D.

Genetics of Diabetic Nephropathy

Parving H-H, Tarnow L, Rossing P (Steno Diabetes Ctr, Gentofte, Denmark)
J Am Soc Nephrol 7:2509–2517, 1996 4–48

Introduction.—Diabetic nephropathy is characterized by persistent albuminuria, a relentless decline in glomerular filtration rate, and higher relative mortality for cardiovascular diseases. It is the leading cause of end-stage renal failure. The pathogenesis of diabetic nephropathy is multifactorial and includes metabolic abnormalities, hemodynamic alterations, and several growth and genetic factors. Genetic susceptibility to diabetic nephropathy is reviewed.

Epidemiologic and Family Risk Factors.—Only a subset of patients have diabetic nephropathy. Familial clustering is seen, and ethnicity contributes to the risk of having this complication. Short stature and low birth weight have been linked to an increased risk of having diabetic nephropathy.

Phenotypic Risk Factors.—Trials evaluating phenotypic markers, such as parenteral hypertension and systemic blood pressure elevation, have produced conflicting findings. Elevated blood pressure is not an important factor in the development of diabetic nephropathy. Most trials have revealed increased sodium–lithium countertransport activity in patients with insulin-dependent diabetes mellitus with nephropathy. Trials evaluating this marker in parents of patients with and without nephropathy have produced conflicting results.

Genetic Markers.—Several trials evaluating DNA markers that involve the regulation of blood pressure and levels of cardiovascular risk factors have shown that the deletion polymorphism in the angiotensin-I–converting enzyme (ACE) is a risk factor for cardiovascular disease in patients with diabetes. Other trials have conflicting findings. Trials assessing diabetic and nondiabetic glomerulopathies have clearly established a deleterious effect of the deletion polymorphism in the ACE on the progression of kidney dysfunction.

Conclusion.—Screening for genetic predisposition to accelerated loss of kidney function should be considered in patients with diabetic and nondiabetic glomerulopathies.

Contribution of Genetic Polymorphism in the Renin-Angiotensin System to the Development of Renal Complications in Insulin-Dependent Diabetes

Marre M, for the Génétique de la Néphropathie Diabétique (GENEDIAB) Study Group (Univ Hosp, Angers, France)

J Clin Invest 7:1585–1595, 1997 4–49

Introduction.—Most of the reduced life expectancy of patients with insulin-dependent diabetes results from diabetic nephropathy. Not all patients with insulin-dependent diabetes will have diabetic nephropathy, which suggests the presence of nonglycemic factors that influence the risk of renal complications. Some studies have suggested that diabetic nephropathy may be associated with polymorphism of the angiotensin I converting enzyme (ACE) gene; although other reports have disputed this association. A multicenter study of patients with insulin-dependent diabetes at risk of renal complications was performed to test the possible effect of genetic factors.

Methods.—The cross-sectional study included 494 patients with insulin-dependent diabetes and past or present proliferative diabetic retinopathy. The patients were drawn from 17 French and Belgian centers. The presence of retinal complications meant that the patients had had long-term exposure to hyperglycemia, placing them at risk of renal complications. The patients' degree of renal involvement was assessed and classified according to the presence of genetic polymorphisms of the renin-angiotensin system: ACE; angiotensinogen (AGT); and angiotensin II, subtype I receptor.

Results.—Assessment of renal involvement showed no nephropathy in 32% of patients; incipient nephropathy, i.e., microalbuminuria, in 21%; established nephropathy, i.e., proteinuria, in 25%; and advanced involvement, i.e., plasma creatinine of 150 µmol/L or greater or renal replacement therapy, in 22%. The presence of an ACE insertion/deletion polymorphism was linked to the severity of renal involvement, the adjusted odds ratio attributable to the D allele was 1.89, with a 95% confidence interval of 1.21–2.95. Other polymorphisms had no direct influence on renal involvement. However, there was a significant interaction between the ACE insertion/deletion and AGT M235T polymorphisms. When the ACE ID and DD genotypes were present, the risk of renal involvement increased from the AGT MM to TT genotypes.

Conclusions.—In patients with insulin-dependent diabetes at risk of diabetic nephropathy, genetic factors affecting production of renal angiotensin II and kinin are risk factors for progression of glomerular disease. As suggested by previous studies, the ACE II genotype appears to reduce the risk of diabetic nephropathy in these patients. Prospective studies are needed to confirm these findings and to test the effects of other candidate genes or acquired factors.

► The review by Parving et al. (Abstract 4–48) is the most comprehensive available discussion of genetic predispositions to diabetic nephropathy. This is a tangled field that began several years ago with the observations or familial clustering of nephropathy and associations with sodium-lithium counter transport and moved, in recent years, to molecular genetic tests, largely of polymorphisms within the renin-angiotensin system.

Multiple conflicting data have appeared in the literature, particularly regarding the polymorphisms, but the most recent finding has been that polymorphisms of ACE are related to progression of kidney disease, if not to a risk for development of kidney disease and diabetes. Specifically, the homozygous DD polymorphism—which represents deletion in each gene copy of sections of the introns to the gene—is associated with both more rapid progression and higher levels of enzyme activity in plasma. Thus, this makes simple, intuitive sense. There is more enzyme, more angiotensin II might be generated, and whatever angiotensin II's deleterious effects on progression are, they would be exaggerated. It might not be this simple.

The study by Marre et al. (Abstract 4–49) is the largest original contribution regarding genetic polymorphisms within the renin-angiotensin system among patients with diabetic nephropathy. These studies, in general, confirm the conclusions of the review article in that the DD polymorphism is associated with progression of disease in this group. The authors also find an interaction between this polymorphism and those of the AGT gene which is associated with higher levels of circulating AGT. Again, this makes some intuitive sense in that higher levels of enzyme and higher levels of the initial source of angiotensin I, namely AGT, should drive production of angiotensin II and amplify the system.

We have clearly entered a phase of examination of the molecular detail of the risk factors for diabetic nephropathy and its progression. However, we still lack strong molecular predictors for the appearance of diabetic nephropathy. Quite likely, the genes outside of the renin-angiotensin cascade are also acting, or perhaps interacting, with that cascade at some physiologic or molecular level.

T.H. Hostetter, M.D.

Randomised Placebo-controlled Trial of Lisinopril in Normotensive Patients With Insulin-dependent Diabetes and Normoalbuminuria or Microalbuminuria

Chaturvedi N, and the EUCLID Study Group (Univ College, London)

Lancet 349:1787–1792, 1997 4–50

Background.—People with insulin-dependent diabetes mellitus (IDDM) have higher rates of morbidity and mortality than the general population.

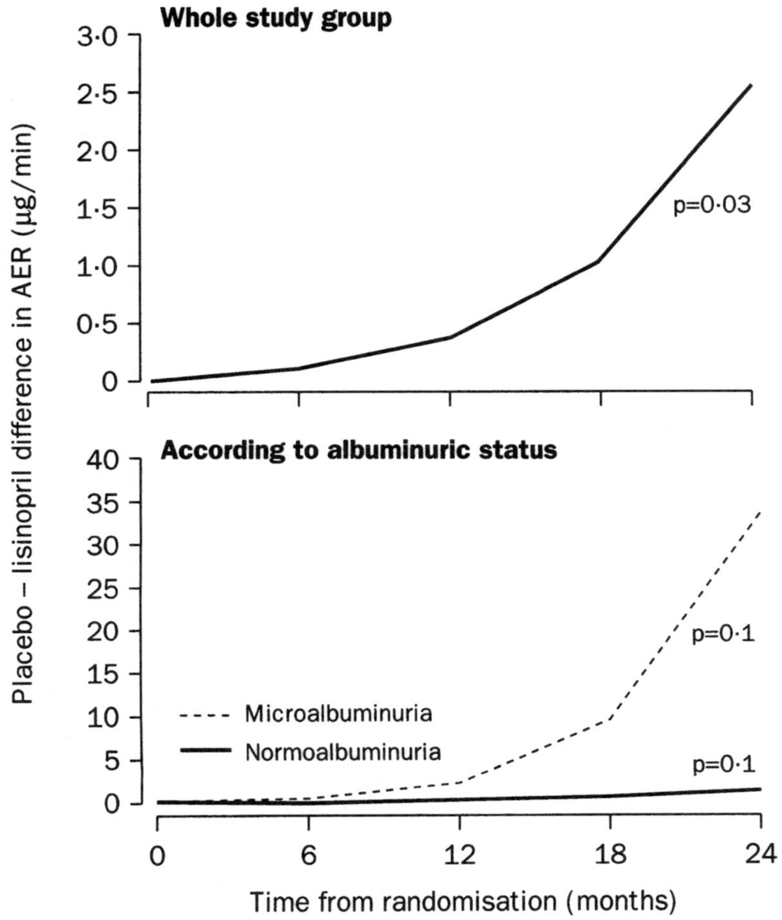

FIGURE 3.—Absolute treatment difference (placebo-lisinopril) in AER (μg/min) adjusted for baseline AER and center and according to albuminuric status. (Courtesy of Chaturvedi N and the EUCLID Study Group: Randomised placebo-controlled trial of lisinopril in normotensive patients with insulin-dependent diabetes mellitus and normoalbuminuria or microalbuminuria. *Lancet* 349:1787–1792, copyright by The Lancet Ltd., 1997.)

Some of this increased risk is the result of renal and cardiovascular complications of insulin-dependent diabetes mellitus (IDDM). A prognostic factor for these complications is the appearance of protein, mostly albumin, in the urine. Elevated blood pressure is a modifiable risk factor for renal disease progression. Inhibitors of angiotensin-converting enzyme (ACE) appear to be especially effective in controlling renal-disease progression in those with IDDM and macroalbuminuria. To determine its effects in IDDM patients with microalbuminuria or normoalbuminuria, a 2-year, randomized, placebo-controlled, clinical trial with the ACE-inhibitor lisinopril was performed.

Study Design.—EUCLID, the EURODIAB controlled trial of lisinopril in IDDM was a double-blind, randomised, parallel-design clinical trial of lisinopril and placebo conducted at 18 European centers. Men and women aged 20–59 years with IDDM were recruited for this study, if their resting blood pressure was at least 75 and no more than 90 mm Hg diastolic and no more than 155 mm Hg systolic. At their initial visit, participants had blood pressure readings to determine eligibility and were issued 1 month's supply of placebo to determine compliance. One month later at the randomization visit, blood pressure was re-assessed and 530 patients were stratified by center and albuminuric status. Patients were re-examined at 1, 3, 6, 12, 18, and 24 months.

Results.—There were no significant differences in baseline characteristics of the participants by treatment group. Intention-to-treat analysis at 2 years demonstrated that albumin excretion rate (AER) was 2.2 µg/min lower in the treatment than in the placebo group (Fig 3). This was equivalent to an 18.8% difference between these two groups. Among the patients with microalbuminuria, the AER difference was 34.2 µg/min. For those who completed the full 2 years of this trial, the difference was 38.5 µg/min in those with microalbuminuria and 0.23 µg/min in those with normoalbuminuria at baseline. There was no difference in hypoglycemic events or in metabolic control between the two treatment groups.

Conclusions.—The ACE inhibitor lisinopril was of clinical benefit to a large group of IDDM patients with early signs of renal disease, but without hypertension. A much greater effect was observed in microalbuminuric than in normoalbuminuric patients, but the exact threshold where therapy should begin could not be determined. Long-term follow-up is required to determine the full impact of lisinopril therapy on outcome. Care guidelines for those with IDDM should include treatment of early stage renal disease with ACE inhibitors.

► Prior smaller studies have suggested that ACE inhibition may slow the appearance of overt proteinuria in patients who are normotensive and only microalbuminuric. This study, conducted as a collaboration among 18 European centers, demonstrates emphatically that patients with IDDM who are microalbuminuric but normotensive have less microalbuminuria that persists for at least 2 years of this study when treated with an ACE inhibitor. The target diastolic pressure of less than 75 mm was reached in the treated group with the ultimate differences being 74 mm Hg (treated) vs. 77 mm Hg. It would have been of interest to know whether lower blood pressures or greater blood pressure reductions were associated with more beneficial results in terms of microalbuminuria; however, this analysis was not provided. Thus, we are still left with the question of the dose we should use in patients whose blood pressure is already normal. Nevertheless, it seems clear that this therapy is beneficial and patients at least with IDDM should be screened for microalbuminuria and if positive begun on an ACE inhibitor. Whether such is the case for NIDDM is less certain.

T.H. Hostetter, M.D.

Acute Renal Failure

Parenteral Ketorolac: The Risk for Acute Renal Failure
Feldman HI, Kinman JL, Berlin JA, et al (Univ of Pennsylvania, Philadelphia; Univ of Medicine and Dentistry of New Jersey, New Brunswick)
Ann Intern Med 126:193–199, 1997 4–51

Background.—Parenteral administration of ketorolac tromethamine has been associated with acute renal failure, but the risk of this complication has not been quantified. The risk for acute renal failure associated with ketorolac was compared with that associated with opioid use.

Methods.—Thirty-five hospitals in the Philadelphia area participated in the retrospective cohort study. Data on 10,219 courses of parenteral ketorolac and on 10,145 courses of parenteral opioids were analyzed. Acute renal failure was defined by a 50% or more increase in serum creatinine concentration and either an absolute increase of 44.2 µmol/L or more for levels less than 132.6 µmol/L at baseline or an absolute increase of 88.4 µmol/L or more for levels 132.6 µmol/L or more at baseline. A secondary definition required a physician's diagnosis.

Findings.—The overall incidence of acute renal failure after either ketorolac or opioid administration was 1.1%. Multivariate-adjusted rate ratios comparing ketorolac with opioids were 1.09 overall, 1.00 for less than 5 days of treatment, and 2.08 for more than 5 days of treatment. Findings were similar when the secondary definition of acute renal failure was used.

Conclusions.—Overall, acute renal failure was not common in this cohort. The rate of renal failure after 5 days or less of ketorolac was not greater than after opioid administration. However, the rate of acute renal failure associated with ketorolac may be increased among patients receiving analgesics for more than 5 days.

► Multiple small series and case reports have identified ketorolac as a nephrotoxin, perhaps through the same mechanisms as conventional oral nonsteroidal anti-inflammatory drugs (NSAIDs). This study has the advantage of size and formal statistical analysis over that earlier data. Although the authors report a more than doubling of risk for acute renal failure with more than 5 days of therapy, they surprisingly found no risk short of this protracted period of therapy. Perhaps even more interesting, they found no interaction with risk factors believed to precipitate acute failure with other NSAIDs such as cirrhosis or congestive heart failure. It would have been of interest to have had parallel information on conventional NSAIDs in this large study population to determine whether ketorolac was more or less nephrotoxic than the standard oral members of this group. Nevertheless, there seems to be some nephrotoxic potential and the smaller initial series are unlikely to have been directionally in error. As is often the case when larger populations are examined, the risks are somewhat less than when reported as smaller series representing perhaps "the tips of an iceberg."

T.H. Hostetter, M.D.

Poison On Line—Acute Renal Failure Caused by Oil of Wormwood Purchased Through the Internet

Weisbord SD, Soule JB, Kimmel PL (George Washington Univ, Washington, DC)

N Engl J Med 337:825–827, 1997 4–52

Introduction.—Rhabdomyolysis, which has a variety of causes, can lead to acute renal failure. There have been no previous reports of rhabdomyolysis caused by drinking absinthe, a liqueur derived from oil of wormwood. A patient with acute renal failure caused by drinking essential oil of wormwood—which he purchased over the Internet—is reported.

Case.—Man, 31, was brought to the emergency department with agitation, disorientation, tonic and clonic seizures with decorticate posturing. Haloperidol treatment was followed by improvement in the man's mental status. He reported consuming about 10 mL of essential oil of wormwood, thinking it was absinthe. He had obtained the wormwood oil from an aromatherapy provider over the Internet. On laboratory tests, the patient was found to have hypernatremia, hypokalemia, and hypobicarbonatemia. The next day, the patient reported moderate soreness of the muscles in both legs, with a sharp increase in serum creatine kinase concentration. Treatment consisted of IV sodium bicarbonate and saline. Congestive heart failure occurred, necessitating treatment with diuretics, sodium restriction, and discontinuation of alkalinization. The patient's serum creatinine concentration peaked at 4.4 mg/dL on day 2, declining thereafter. There was no oliguria, hypocalcemia, or hypophosphatemia. The muscle soreness resolved quickly, and the electrolyte, creatine kinase, and creatinine concentrations normalized by day 17.

Discussion.—This patient had seizures, apparently caused by drinking essential oil of wormwood, and followed by rhabdomyolysis and acute renal failure. The mechanism of this effect is unknown. Absinthe is illegal in the United States and most European countries, but wormwood and the other ingredients are readily available—in this case, over the Internet.

► Not only do patients and their families scrutinize our care through disease-related web sites, but potential patients apparently become so by surfing the net. In addition to raising our anxiety about mayhem on the electronic highway, this brief report does emphasize 2 points. First, oil of wormwood (the active ingredient of absinthe) is still a nephrotoxin probably due to its propensity to cause seizures and rhabdomyolysis. Second, the need to pursue a careful history for nephrotoxins seems even greater today, given the availability of rather rare ingestants. For example and discussed in last year's YEAR BOOK, the Chinese diet herbs, some of which caused acute renal failure, still are advertised on the Internet.

T.H. Hostetter, M.D.

Outcomes and Cost-effectiveness of Initiating Dialysis and Continuing Aggressive Care in Seriously Ill Hospitalized Adults

Hamel MB, Phillips RS, Davis RB, et al (Beth Israel Deaconess Med Ctr, Boston; Univ of Tennessee, Chattanooga; Univ of Virginia, Charlottesville; et al)

Ann Intern Med 127:195–202, 1997 4–53

Introduction.—Patients who require dialysis for renal failure during the course of a serious illness have a poor prognosis. The question of whether to initiate dialysis and continue aggressive care is a difficult one for patients, their families, and physicians. The clinical outcome and cost-effectiveness of initiating dialysis and providing aggressive care for patients in whom renal failure developed during hospitalization for serious illness were examined prospectively.

Methods.—Study participants were drawn from 5 geographically diverse teaching hospitals and enrolled in the Study to Understand Prognoses and Preferences for Outcomes and Risks of Treatments (SUPPORT). All had renal failure after enrollment and were treated with hemodialysis or peritoneal dialysis. Data collected by chart abstraction and interview included diagnoses, comorbid conditions, resource utilization, patients' functional status 2 weeks before and 6 months after study entry, and quality of life. Estimates were obtained for hospital costs, outpatient costs of long-term dialysis, and life expectancy.

Results.—Of the 9,105 patients enrolled in SUPPORT, 490 had dialysis initiated during the study period. The median age of these patients was 61 years; 69% had acute respiratory failure or multiorgan system failure with sepsis. Median survival after the initiation of dialysis was 32 days, and only 27% of patients were alive 6 months later. Among survivors, 62% rated their quality of life as "good" or better. Survivors had a median of 1 dependency in activities of daily living. The SUPPORT patients had been assigned to 5 prognostic groups defined by survival estimates. Among those who began dialysis, actual survival closely approximated predicted survival. Overall estimated costs per quality-adjusted life-year saved with dialysis and aggressive care vs. withholding dialysis was $128,200; cost estimates ranged from $61,900 for the best prognostic category to $274,100 for the worst prognostic category.

Conclusion.—The few patients who survived after undergoing dialysis for renal failure that developed during the course of a serious illness had a fairly good quality of life and functional status. For the majority of patients, however, the cost of this decision far exceeded the commonly cited upper limit for cost-effective care ($50,000 per quality-adjusted life-year).

► This study develops some of the most rigorous cost-effective data regarding dialysis outcomes in acutely ill patients. Although costs alone are clearly important, they are rarely deciding criteria. Not many will be dissuaded from dialysis by even a 6-figure cost for a year of quality life. However, these studies tend to emphasize, from the cost angle, the frequent futility of dialysis in this setting. Although issues of rationing are (as the authors conclude in their discussion), complex and devolve quickly on who will do the rationing, one implication of this study would be to place hemodialysis as a nodal point for decision making in such cases. That is, initial denial of dialysis may rarely be acceptable simply because of the projected long-term outcome. However, its use should probably be more explicitly temporary and contingent on the assessment of the patient. Once the threat of imminent renal death is removed, reversible conditions can be sought and the family's considered decisions made in light of this sort of data. Thus, this information and their personal experience may lead nephrologists to more often withdraw therapy in circumstances of high risk to the patient.

T.H. Hostetter, M.D.

Anaritide in Acute Tubular Necrosis

Allgren RL, for the Auriculin Anaritide Acute Renal Failure Study Group (Scios, Inc, Mountain View, Calif et al)

N Engl J Med 336:828–834, 1997 4–54

Purpose.—The hormone atrial natriuretic peptide (ANP) dilates afferent arterioles while constricting efferent arterioles, thus increasing glomerular filtration rate and glomerular hydrostatic pressure. Animal models of acute renal dysfunction have shown that ANP can improve renal function. The effects of anaritide, a 25-amino acid synthetic form of ANP, were studied in patients with acute tubular necrosis.

Methods.—The multicenter, randomized, double-blind, placebo-controlled trial included 504 adults with acute tubular necrosis caused by recent ischemic or nephrotoxic insults. Patients with other causes of acute renal dysfunction were excluded, as were those who had already had dialysis for their current episode of acute tubular necrosis. They were randomly assigned to receive IV placebo or anaritide. Anaritide was given at an initial dose of 0.05 µg/kg/min, which was escalated to 0.20 µg/kg/min over 90 minutes, then continued at that level for the rest of the 24-hour treatment period. The 2 groups were compared on such measurements as urinary output and creatinine clearance, serum creatinine concentration, need for dialysis, and mortality. The patients received full supportive care, including low-dose dopamine or diuretics, as indicated.

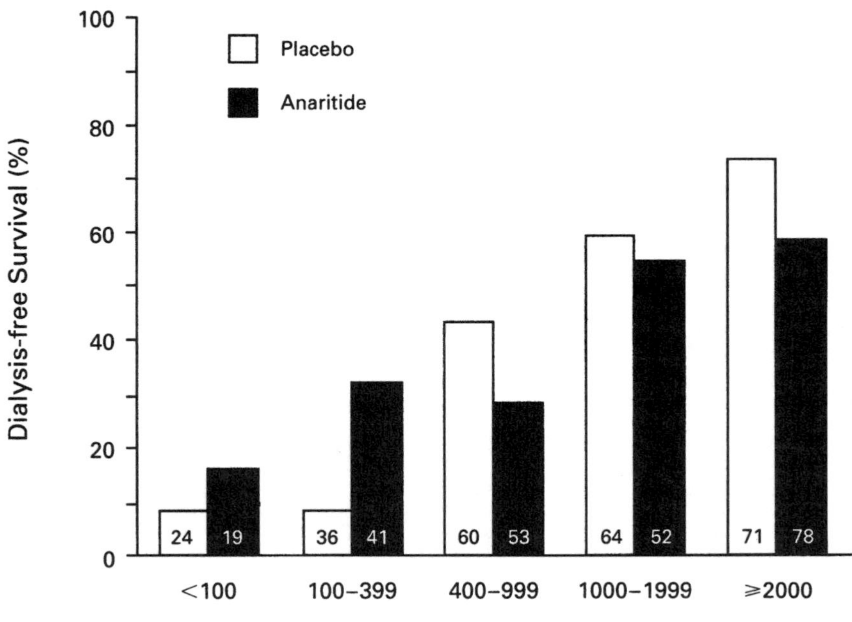

FIGURE 1.—Dialysis-free survival at 21 days in the anaritide and placebo groups, according to baseline urinary output. The *numbers* inside the *bars* indicate the number of patients in each subgroup. (Reprinted by permission of *The New England Journal of Medicine*, from Allgren RL, for the Auriculin Anaritide Acute Renal Failure Study Group: Anaritide in acute tubular necrosis. *N Engl J Med* 336:828–834. Copyright 1997, Massachusetts Medical Society. All rights reserved.)

Results.—The 21-day dialysis-free survival was 43% in the anaritide group and 47% in the placebo group. Among patients with prospectively defined oliguria (urinary output less than 400 mL/day), dialysis-free survival rate was 27% with anaritide vs. 8% with placebo. The benefits of anaritide were greatest for patients in the oliguric group who no longer had oliguria after treatment. For patients without oliguria, the dialysis-free survival rate was 48% with anaritide vs. 59% with placebo (Fig 1).

Conclusions.—In a large group of critically ill patients with acute tubular necrosis, anaritide treatment does not improve dialysis-free survival rates. However, it may improve survival rates for patients with initial oliguria, and may worsen survival for those who are not oliguric. Future studies should stratify patients according to their urinary output.

▶ This large multicenter study sought to determine whether the multiple animal studies and smaller scale clinical studies suggesting that ANP was beneficial for acute renal failure could be borne out. The results are mixed. There was some proven extension of dialysis-free time in oliguric patients, but actually some diminution in patients with sufficient urine output before the drug was given. Unfortunately, shortly after this publication, further studies investigating the drug were discontinued. We may never know whether this particular agent has a place in the therapy of acute renal failure. This is an area in which demonstration of efficacy is extraordinarily difficult given the severity of illness and its complexity in these patients. One almost wonders whether penicillin could have been proven effective in such a population.

T.H. Hostetter, M.D.

5 Electrolyte Abnormalities

Introduction

This year's offerings include a number of interesting observations concerning molecular aspects of fluid and electrolyte metabolism. In addition, several clinical observations have been elucidated with the use of various animal models. The chapter has been divided into three sections. The first is concerned with molecular aspects of renal epithelial water transport. The second section reviews experimental and clinical observations regarding the acute postoperative hyponatremic syndromes. The third section discusses recently discovered aspects of the molecular abnormalities which produce Bartter's syndrome and its various subtypes.

Michael Emmett, M.D.

Molecular Aspects of Renal Epithelial Water Transport

INTRODUCTION

Recent studies have improved our knowledge of the physiology and pathophysiology of renal water transport. We understand more precisely how water crosses epithelial membranes and how the water permeability of certain membranes is regulated. The water permeability of an epithelial membrane is a function of the cellular permeability together with that of the intercellular spaces. We now understand that the permeability of the apical and basolateral cell membranes is determined by a family of specific water-carrying channels called aquaporins (AQP).

Certain AQPs are constitutively expressed in a variety of cell membranes, whereas the membrane density of other AQPs is regulated by various factors, such as vasopressin. M.D. Lee et al. provide a good general review and update of this fast-changing subject (Abstract 5–1). The water permeability of the apical surface of renal collecting duct cells is determined by AQP2 channel density in the apical membrane and this is regulated by vasopressin. AQP1 is the water channel responsible for the constitutive high water permeability of renal proximal tubule cells, red blood cells, and other cell membranes. The water permeability of the basolateral membranes of renal tubule epithelial cells is imparted by AQP3 and or AQP4. The function of AQP0, AQP5, and other AQP1–4 locations are described in the Figure 1 of this abstract.

The first AQP protein to be characterized (although it was not initially recognized as an AQP) was AQP0, which is the major protein component of the ocular lens. It was initially named the major intrinsic protein of the lens, or *MIP*. The designation *AQP0* is indicative of the protein's identification as a lens molecule decades before its characterization as a water-transporting protein.

AQP2, the water channel in the apical membrane of principal cells lining the renal collecting ducts, is presently of greatest interest to the nephrologists. This is the channel regulated by vasopressin. When vasopressin levels are low. Synthesis of this AQP slows and the protein is located primarily within cytoplasmic vesicular clusters. When vasopressin is released from the posterior pituitary, it is transported to the kidney where it binds to and activates the V_2 receptors located on the basolateral membranes of collecting duct principal cells. V_2 receptor activation initiates a series of reactions that result in the movement of these vesicles to a subapical location followed by the exocytic insertion of AQP2 molecules into the apical membranes. High AQP2 membrane density markedly increases collecting duct cell water permeability. The high vasopressin levels also increase the AQP2 synthetic rate. When vasopressin activity again decreases, the AQP2 channels are removed from the apical membrane by means of an endocytotic process and returned to cytoplasmic vesicles. AQP2 synthesis slows, and water permeability decreases.

A variety of osmotic or nonosmotic signals initiate a cascade of events which results in the modulation of urine osmolality. This cascade includes osmotic sensors which control the release of vasopressin (AVP) from posterior pituitary into the circulation, the transport of this hormone to the basolateral surface of renal collecting duct cells where it is bound by, and activates, V_2 receptors; and finally G-protein signal linkage which causes insertion of functional AQP-2 water channels into the apical membrane of these cells. Each step in this cascade can be affected by multiple inherited or acquired defects. The removal of channels from the membrane can also be accelerated or slowed abnormally. For example, nephrogenic diabetes insipidus may be caused by: (1) the synthesis of an abnormal V_2 receptor, (2) abnormal signal linkage from this receptor to the AQP2-containing vesicles, (3) a decreased AQP2 synthetic rate, (4) production of intrinsically defective AQP2 water channels, or (5) abnormally rapid removal or degradation of functional water channels.

Most cases of hereditary nephrogenic diabetes insipidus are caused by a defect in the *V_2 receptor gene*, which is located on the X chromosome. Phenotypic expression of this form of the disease follows a classic X-linked recessive inheritance pattern, i.e., relatively asymptomatic mothers carry the trait and transmit the full-blown disease to 50% (on a statistical basis) of their sons. However, in some families, the transmission of hereditary nephrogenic diabetes insipidus follows an autosomal recessive pattern. This form of hereditary nephrogenic diabetes insipidus is much less common than the sex-linked type.

In 1994, Deen et al. showed that some patients with autosomal recessive nephrogenic diabetes insipidus had inherited two defective AQP2 genes.[1] These homozygous mutations resulted in the synthesis of nonfunctional AQPs. More recently, the same group showed that other AQP2 mutations resulted in functional water channels that become defective because they are misrouted to an incorrect cell membrane or incorrectly inserted into the apical membranes (Abstract 5–2).

Ecelbarger et al. working with Joseph Verbalis at Georgetown and Mark Knepper at the National Institutes of Health use techniques of molecular physiology to explain several clinical observations (Abstract 5–3). Individuals with persistent and "inappropriate" hormone secretion (or deficiency), must adapt to their abnormal hormonal environment to survive. For example, patients with the syndrome of chronic inappropriate antidiuretic hormone secretion (SIADH) eventually reestablish water balance at a low sodium concentration. If this did not occur, inexorable water retention would be fatal. The adaptive response to chronic vasopressin stimulation includes multiple counter-regulatory neural and hormonal mechanisms. AQP2 expression was measured in the renal collecting ducts of rats which had been exposed to persistent vasopressin stimulation. The adaptive response includes a fall in AQP2 expression despite persistent high vasopressin levels. As described, AQP2 water channels shuttle plasma vesicles and the apical membrane. Therefore, reduced AQP2 membrane expression could be the result of decreased AQP2 synthesis, a decreased rate of insertion into the apical membrane, increased AQP2 removal from the membrane, or increased metabolic degradation of the channels.

The study showed that water-loaded rates with SIADH adapt by reducing the synthetic rate of AQP2. This type of chronic regulation of membrane water permeability in animals with SIADH and hyponatremia oppose the acute effects of vasopressin to increase AQP2 apical membrane density and water permeability.

Congestive heart failure (CHF) is a common disorder which is associated with persistent nonosmotic antidiuretic hormone stimulation. Several recent papers demonstrate that experimental CHF increases AQP2 expression in the collecting duct (Abstracts 5–4 and 5–5). It is likely that with time the markedly increased AQP2 expression associated with CHF also decreases via the adaptive mechanisms described above. This would allow stabilization of hyponatremia and reestablishment of water balance in patients with CHF.

Michael Emmett, M.D.

Reference

1. Deen PM, Muldens SM, Kansen SM, et al: Aquaporins and ion conductance. *Science* 264:92–95, 1997.

The Aquaporin Family of Water Channel Proteins in Clinical Medicine

Lee MD, King LS, Agre P (Johns Hopkins Univ, Baltimore, Md)
Medicine 76:141–156, 1997 5–1

Introduction.—The aquaporins are a family of membrane channel proteins. They function as selective water pores across the plasma membrane of many human tissues and cells. The structure and function of the aquaporins, with emphasis on clinical implications are discussed.

Identification.—Aquaporin-1 (AQP1) was the first protein to be identified as a functional water channel. Hydropathy analysis suggests that AQP1 has 6 transmembrane domains with intracellular amino and carboxy termini. Subsequently, 5 other mammalian aquaporins have been identified. This includes AQP0, which is the major intrinsic protein (MIP) of the lens. (MIP was recognized as a lens protein decades before its possible role as water channel protein was recognized.) (Fig 1).

Distribution.—Each of the 6 mammalian aquaporins which have been identified has a unique pattern of tissue expression. These proteins have a particularly important role at sites where rapid water transit occurs in response to transepithelial osmotic gradients or electrolyte transport. For example, AQP1–4 are expressed at a number of different sites in the kidney. AQP1 is also found in red cell membranes; AQP3 and 4 in the brain, and AQPO, 1, 3, 4, and 5 in various ocular structures. AQP2 (found in the renal collecting duct) is the water channel which is regulated by

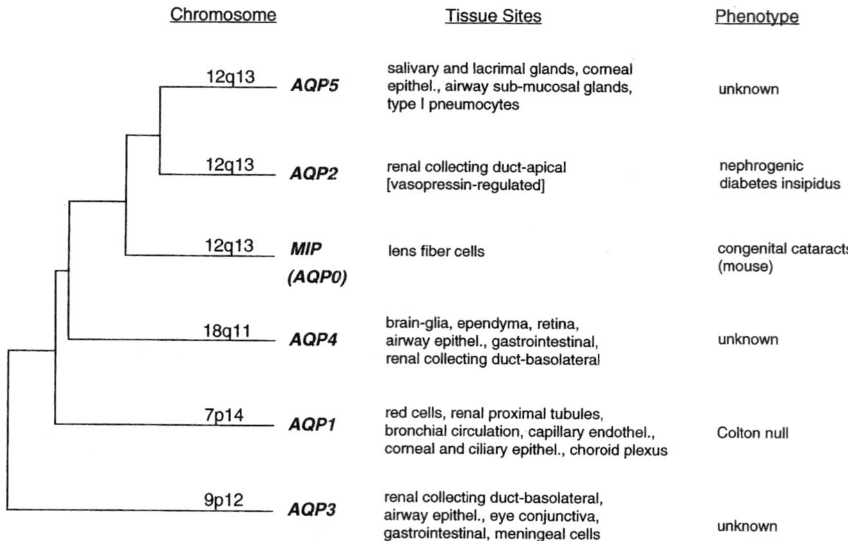

FIGURE 1.—Phylogenetic tree of the mammalian aquaporins. Indicated are the sites on human chromosomes, the predominant tissue sites of expression, and the known mutant phenotypes. *Abbreviations: AQP*, aquaporin; *MIP*, major intrinsic protein. (Courtesy of Lee MD, King LS, Agre P: The aquaporin family of water channel proteins in clinical medicine. *Medicine* 76[3]:141–156, 1997.)

vasopressin. Defects in AQP2 may produce nephrogenic diabetes insipidus. Mutated AQPO (MIP of lens) can produce congenital cataracts. AQP1 mutations have not been associated with any severe clinical abnormalities.

Conclusions.—The aquaporins are a family of membrane channel proteins that function as water transporting pores through the hydrophobic membranes of tissues and cells. These proteins participate in virtually all physiologic processes that involve water movement. Mutations of these proteins produce various disease processes, including nephrogenic diabetes insipidus (AQP2). (However, the more common x-linked form of hereditary nephrogenic diabetes insipidus is caused by a V_2 receptor defect rather than a AQP2 mutatation.) Aquaporins may also play a secondary role in many clinical disorders.

New Mutations in the AQP2 Gene in Nephrogenic Diabetes Insipidus Resulting in Functional but Misrouted Water Channels

Mulders SM, Knoers NVAM, Van Lieburg AF, et al (Univ of Nijmegen, The Netherlands; Universitäts-Kinderklinik Zurich, Swizterland; Univ of Heidelberg, Germany; et al)

J Am Soc Nephrol 8:242–248, 1997 5–2

Background.—Previous studies have shown that abnormal aquaporin-2 (AQP2) proteins cause some forms of the autosomal recessive nephrogenic diabetes insipides (NDI). Three patients with NDI were shown to have unique homozygous mutations in the *AQP2* gene.

Methods.—Three children with signs and symptoms of NDI were studied. They were members of 3 families of different ethnic origins. The inheritance patterns observed in these families were autosomal recessive. The genetic mutations responsible for these *AQP2* abnormalities were determined.

Results.—Three entirely different missense mutations of the *AQP2* gene were identified. Each patient was found to be homozygous for each respective mutation. In patient 1, a G533A transition in exon 2 caused an alanine substitution for a threonine (A147T). A methionine was substituted for threonine in patient 2 as a result of a C471T transition in exon 2 (T126M). The third patient had an asparagine substituted for serine (N68S) as a result of an A297G transition in exon 1. Oocyte expression studies showed that the abnormal AQP2 molecules produced by the first 2 patients were functional water channels, whereas that from the third patient (N68S) was not. Additional immunoblotting and immunochemical analysis showed that the defective renal water transport in the first 2 patients was primarily caused by misrouted AQP2 channels, i.e., they were not correctly inserted in the apical membranes. In contrast, a nonfunctional water channel was the cause of diabetes insipidus in the third patient.

Conclusion.—Three patients with severe NDI were each found to have a unique and different homozygous mutation in the *AQP2* gene. Two of these mutations led to synthesis of channels with reduced but measurable water transport functions, while the third produced a nonfunctional protein. The first 2 mutations caused water channels to be misrouted, and this was responsible for NDI.

Role of Renal Aquaporins in Escape From Vasopressin-induced Antidiuresis in Rat

Ecelbarger CA, Nielsen S, Olson BR, et al (NIH, Bethesda, Md; Univ of Aarhus, Denmark; Waterbury Hosp, Conn; et al)

J Clin Invest 99:1852–1863, 1997 5–3

Background.—Vasopressin is the chief regulator of renal water excretion. Inappropriately high plasma vasopressin levels produce water retention and hyponatremia. The severity of these abnormalities is limited by the vasopressin escape phenomenon. Vasopressin escape increases water excretion and stabilizes serum sodium levels, despite continued high levels of vasopressin. A rat model of persistent vasopressin stimulation and vasopressin escape was used to determine whether aquaporin water channels are involved in this phenomenon.

Methods.—Adult male rats received 5 ng/hr of 1-deamino-[8-D-arginine]-vasopressin (dDAVP) for 4 days. Rats were then randomly assigned to continue receiving dDAVP only or dDAVP plus excess water. The urine volume, osmolality and sodium concentration were measured. Rats from both groups were sacrificed 1, 2, 3 and 7 days after starting water loading. Plasma was collected and kidneys were harvested to provide samples for immunoblotting, Northern blotting, and immunocytochemistry analysis.

Results.—By day 2 of water loading, a significant increase in urine volume was detected. This indicated the onset of vasopressin escape and coincided with a significant decrease in renal aquaporin-2 (AQP2) protein, as assessed by semiquantitative immunoblotting. By the third day, AQP2 levels had decreased to 17% of the control levels. There was no decrease in the renal levels of aquaporins 1, 3, or 4. The suppression of renal AQP2 expression was accompanied by a fall in renal AQP2 mRNA levels, as assessed by Northern blotting.

Conclusions.—A rat model of persistent vasopressin stimulation with water loading was used to determine whether vasopressin escape from antidiuresis was associated with altered regulation of the renal aquaporin water channels. The increase in renal water excretion associated with vasopressin escape is related to a significant and selective disease in the renal AQP2 expression. Further studies will be required to elucidate the mechanism of AQP2 downregulation. This knowledge will improve our understanding of the vasopressin-mediated hyponatremic syndromes.

Upregulation of Aquaporin-2 Water Channel Expression in Chronic Heart Failure Rat

Xu D-L, Martin P-Y, Ohara M, et al (Univ of Colorado, Denver)

J Clin Invest 99:1500–1505, 1997 5–4

Introduction.—Patients with advanced congestive heart failure (CHF) characteristically retain free water and deveop hyponatremia. The recently cloned aquaporin-2 (AQP2) water channel, which is regulated by vasopressin, is responsible for mediating collecting duct water permeability. The possibility that the water retention of CHF is caused by upregulation of the AQP2 water channel was examined in a rat model.

Methods.—Rats underwent ligation of the left coronary artery to induce CHF. Control animals received sham surgery. About 1 month after the surgery, mean arterial pressure and cardiac output were measured. The following day animals were sacrificed and *AQP2* gene expression was measured. In parallel experiments, the effects of a nonpeptide V_2 vasopressin receptor antagonist, OPC 31260, were studied.

Results.—Compared with sham-operated controls, rats with experimental CHF had significantly reduced cardiac output and plasma osmolality. Plasma vasopressin levels were increased. The CHF rats also had significantly increased kidney AQP2 messenger RNA (mRNA) and AQP2 protein. Oral OPC 31260 produced a diuresis, and reduced urinary osmolality, which caused an increase in plasma osmolality. Levels of AQP2 mRNA and protein in both the renal cortex and inner medulla decreased significantly in OPC 31260–treated rats.

Conclusion.—Upregulation of AQP2 is an early feature of CHF in this rat model and is blocked by a V_2 receptor antagonist. Therefore, vasopressin plays an important role in the upregulation of AQP2 water channels and the water retention and hyponatremia of CHF.

Congestive Heart Failure in Rats Is Associated With Increased Expression and Targeting of Aquaporin-2 Water Channel in Collecting Duct

Nielsen S, Terris J, Andersen D, et al (Univ of Aarhus, Denmark; NIH, Bethesda, Md; Univ of Copenhagen; et al)

Proc Natl Acad Sci U S A 94:5450–5455, 1997 5–5

Background.—Severe congestive heart failure (CHF) produces defective renal processing of water and electrolytes, leading to extracellular fluid expansion and hyponatremia. Persistent vasopressin secretion plays an important role in the development of these abnormalities. However, the specific renal mechanisms involved are not well defined. The role played by renal aquaporins (AQPs) in CHF syndrome was analyzed.

Methods.—An adult rat CHF model was produced by ligation of the left coronary artery. A control group received a sham operation. Three weeks after surgery, arterial and left ventricular end-diastolic pressure (LVEDP) were assessed and arterial blood samples were obtained. The kidneys were then harvested and membrane fractionation was performed. Expression of AQP subtypes 1, 2, and 3 were measured by quantitative immunoblotting. Immunocytochemistry and immunoelectron microscopy were used to localize intracellular AQP2.

Results.—Compared with the sham-operated animals, coronary ligated rats developed severe heart failure with elevated LVEDP, and their plasma sodium concentration fell. Quantitative immunoblot analysis of total kidney membrane fractions demonstrated a significantly and selectively increased AQP2 expression in CHF rats, while AQPs 1 and 3 showed no change. Immunocytochemical and immunoelectron microscopic analysis revealed abundant AQP2 in the apical plasma membranes and much less in the intracellular vesicles of collecting duct cells from CHF rats. These findings are consistent with increased trafficking of AQP2 from cytoplasm into the apical membranes.

Conclusions.—A rat model of severe CHF demonstrates that significant and selective upregulation of the AQP2 water channel in the renal collecting duct develops in animals with this condition. The resulting increase in collecting duct water absorption partially explains the excessive free-water retention and hyponatremia associated with severe CHF.

Acute Postoperative Hyponatremic Syndromes

INTRODUCTION

Severe acute postoperative hyponatremia is a very rare and catastrophic disorder. The victims are often otherwise normal, relatively young women who have just completed an elective surgical procedure. This form of severe hyponatremia is often associated with brain edema, seizures, and death. The disorder has been attributed to the combination of persistent antidiuretic hormone (ADH) secretion (produced by pain, nausea, surgery, anesthesia, or analgesics) and perioperative hypotonic fluid infusion. The high ADH levels prevent renal excretion of the infused water load. Surgeons and anesthesiologists have been warned to avoid the routine use of perioperative hypotonic fluids in an effort to prevent this catastrophe. However, infusion of isotonic fluid together with ADH can also generate progressive hyponatremia. Under such conditions, hyponatremia develops because the infused sodium (and endogenous potassium) is excreted at high concentration in a relatively small volume of urine. In other words, a desalination process occurs.

Two recent articles from Mitchell Halpern's Toronto group address these issues. The first is a study by Gowrishankar et al. (Abstract 5–6) of a rat model exhibiting inappropriate ADH. An infusion of normal saline, together with ADH, reduced the average plasma sodium concentration of these rats from 140 to 127 mmol/L. The hyponatremia developed because sodium and potassium were excreted in a very small volume of urine. This is not a new observation. What is new is the observation that hyponatremia did not develop if the animals were pretreated with a low electrolyte diet. Under those conditions they did not become hyponatremic because the salt deficit caused retention of sodium together with the water (because of the ADH). The take-home messages: (1) Switching from perioperative hypotonic to isotonic IV fluids may not prevent catastrophic postoperative hyponatremia syndrome. (2) The development of this syndrome may be influenced by the patient's antecedent salt intake, sodium balance, volume status, and renal salt avidity.

The study by Steele et al. (Abstract 5–7) extends these observations in rodents to man (or more correctly, woman). The charts of five women who died as a result of acute postoperative hyponatremia syndrome were reviewed. Their fluid and electrolyte balance records indicated that retention of administered hypotonic fluid could not alone account for the fall in sodium concentration. Their kidneys must have also generated a large quantity of electrolyte-free water which was retained (i.e., they excreted electrolyte rich, hypertonic urine). The investigators then prospectively studied 22 women undergoing elective gynecologic procedures. Although each of these patients received only isotonic IV fluids, normal saline or Ringer's lactate, their plasma sodium concentrations fell. The mean fall was only 4 mmol/L. However, in two patients the sodium concentration fell to 131 mmol/L. No patient developed symptomatic hyponatremia.

This study emphasizes that a switch to isotonic IV fluids may not always prevent this complication. Indeed, isotonic fluid infusions may be dangerous under certain conditions (for example, when high ADH levels coexist with and expanded extracellular fluid volume).

Fluid and electrolyte replacement should be individualized and never administered on the basis of generic formulae. Further, although surgeons and consultants are often pleased to see their patients produce large volumes of urine following surgery, this observation should actually raise concern. Large urine volumes may indicate appropriate mobilization and excretion of retained or administered fluid. However, it could also indicate the development of diabetes insipidus or diabetes mellitus, or rarely, could be a sign of a desalination process. Consequently, large urine outputs should raise as much concern as low urine output, and measurement of serum electrolytes, urine tonicity, or urine osmolality and electrolytes should be considered.

Michael Emmett, M.D.

Hyponatremia in the Rat in the Absence of Positive Water Balance

Gowrishankar M, Chen C-B, Cheema-Dhadli S, et al (Univ of Toronto)

J Am Soc Nephrol 8:524–529, 1997 5–6

Background.—The development of hyponatremia is generally assumed to be caused by exogenously administered free water which is inappropriately retained. The water retention is caused by high levels of antidiuretic hormone (ADH), renal insufficiency, or both. This study demonstrates that the kidney can also generate free water sufficient to produce hyponatremia when only isotonic fluid has been administered. The impact of renal salt avidity on this water-generating response is also examined.

TABLE 3.—Effect of a Saline Infusion on the Development of Hyponatremia in Rats on a Regular or Low Electrolyte Diet for 3 Days

Diet	Time (h)	Plasma [Na] (mM) None	DDAVP	Saline	Saline + DDAVP
Normal	0	140 ± 0.3	143 ± 0.3	142 ± 0.1	140 ± 1.0
Normal	24	142 ± 1.0	144 ± 0.4	143 ± 1.0	127 ± 2.0*
Lowsalt	0	139 ± 1.0	139 ± 2	138 ± 1.0	139 ± 1
Lowsalt	24	144 ± 1.0	144 ± 1	141 ± 1.0	140 ± 1

Note: Rats were fed their regular diet until the day of the experiment. The number of rats was 8 in each group; results are presented as the mean ± SE.

$P < 0.01$ for paired observations.

Abbreviation: DDAVP, desmopressin acetate.

(Courtesy of Gowrishankar M, Chen C-B, Cheema-Dhadli S, et al: Hyponatremia in the rat in the absence of positive water balance. *J Am Soc Nephrol* 8:524–529, 1997.)

Methods.—Rats were given intraperitoneal isotonic sodium chloride with or without ADH. Food and water were then withheld for 24 hours and electrolyte levels were measured. Another group of rats was first pretreated with a low electrolyte diet for 3 days before undergoing a similar protocol. Appropriate control groups were studied. Plasma and urine urea, osmolality, and sodium (Na), potassium (K), and chlorine content were measured (Table 3). Electrolyte and water balance were also measured.

Results.—Rats which ingested a normal diet before the study developed hyponatremia despite a slightly negative total water balance. The hyponatremia developed as a result of markedly negative Na and K balance. Rats pretreated with a low electrolyte diet developed only slight negative K balance and positive Na balance (because of avid renal sodium retention) and did not become hyponatremic. Their kidneys retained both water (because of the ADH) and electrolytes (because of their volume contraction.)

Conclusion.—The development of hyponatremia in this model requires renal generation and retention of electrolyte-free water. This occurs when the kidneys excrete a large quantity of Na and K at high urine concentrations. Increased renal salt avidity (produced by prior electrolyte depletion) prevents the development of this form of hyponatremia.

Postoperative Hyponatremia Despite Near-Isotonic Saline Infusion: A Phenomenon of Desalination

Steele A, Gowrishankar M, Abrahamson S, et al (Univ of Toronto)
Ann Intern Med 126:20–25, 1997 5–7

Background.—Severe postoperative hyponatremia is a potentially fatal but preventable disorder which occurrs primarily in young women. The pathophysiologic explanation which is generally invoked is the infusion of excessive amounts of electrolyte-free water combined with persistent antidiuretic hormone secretion which prevents its excretion into the urine.

TABLE 1.—Summary of Water Balance in Five Patients With Fatal Hyponatremia

Patient	Age	Surgery	Sodium Level			Weight	Electrolyte-Free Water Required*	Fluid Given		"Missing" Electrolyte-Free Water
			Before Surgery†	After Surgery	Corrected‡			Total	Electrolyte-Free Water	
	y		← *mmol/L* →			*kg*	← *L* →			
1	29	Cholecystectomy	NA	124	126	80	4.4	4.3	2.9	1.5
2	29	Gynecologic	NA	117	124	45	2.9	3.2	2.3	0.6
3	24	Gynecologic	NA	126	127	60	3.1	5.5	1.2	1.9
4	49	Gynecologic	142	114	118	65	6.1	10.0	4.8	1.3
5	33	Gynecologic	NA	115	122	55	4.1	3.0	1.3	2.8

Note: Data from 5 female patients with fatal postoperative hyponatremia are summarized.
*Amount of electrolyte-free water necessary to produce the degree of hyponatremia in each patient, calculated on the basis of total body water.
†Initial plasma sodium level was assumed to be 140 mmol/L when data were not available.
‡Corrected for hyperglycemia.
Abbreviation: NA, not available.
(Courtesy of Steele A, Gowrishankar M, Abrahamson S, et al: Postoperative hyponatremia despite near-isotonic saline infusion: A phenomenon of desalination. *Ann Intern Med* 126:20–25, 1997.)

However, clinical and experimental observations suggest that this mechanism may not always underlie these disorders.

Methods.—This study is divided into 2 parts. First, a retrospective analysis of 5 women who died as a result of the acute postoperative hyponatremia syndrome was carried out. Their records were carefully examined with regard to fluid and electrolyte balance, although the data were generally incomplete. The second part of the article is a prospective cohort study of 22 randomly selected, otherwise normal women who underwent uterine surgery under general anesthesia. None of these patients were receiving diuretics. All perioperative IV fluids were near isotonic (either isotonic saline or Ringer's lactate solution). Water and electrolyte balances were carefully measured for 24 hours starting at the time of anesthesia induction. Plasma electrolytes were measured before and 24 hours after anesthesia.

Results.—The retrospective fluid and electrolyte balance analysis of the 5 fatal patients indicated that retention of exogenously administered free water could not alone account for the degree of hyponatremia which developed. The kidneys of these women must also have generated a large volume of electrolyte-free water by excreting electrolytes in the urine at very high concentration (Table 1). The prospectively studied women experienced an average decrease in sodium concentration of 4.2 mmol/L. The lowest observed sodium concentration was 131 mmol/L (in 2 patients). The average volume of near isotonic fluid infused over 24 hours was 5.3 liters. Average urine output was 2.5 liters. Urine remained persistently hypertonic in every patient for at least 16 hours following induction of anesthesia.

Conclusion.—Postoperative hyponatremia can occur even in the absence of hypotonic fluid infusion. Desalinization of the infused isotonic fluid causes renal generation and retention of free water. Desalination probably also contributes to the development of severe hyponatremia when hypotonic fluids are infused.

Molecular Aspects of Bartter's and Gitelman's Syndromes

INTRODUCTION

Drs. Frederick Bartter and John Gill, and their associates first described the syndrome bearing Bartter's name in the early 1960s. Bartter's syndrome (BS) is characterized by marked hypokalemia, metabolic alkalosis, high plasma levels of renin and aldosterone, juxtaglomerular apparatus hyperplasia, and normal to low blood pressure. Subsequently, Drs. Gitelman and Welt described a variant of BS associated with marked hypomagnesemia and hypocalciuria. In contrast, most patients with classic BS are hypercalciuric, often develop nephrocalcinosis and may progress to renal failure. The Gitelman's syndrome (GS) variant is much more common than classic BS.

Over the ensuing years, it was recognized that many patients thought to have BS or GS were individuals who secretly vomited or abused diuretics. Some of these patients were incorrectly reported in the medical literature as examples of "BS." Nephrologists now recognize that "barfer's syndrome" is far more common than BS. The urine chloride concentration can be an important differential clue. A spot urine chloride concentration of less than 15 mEq/L strongly suggests the patient (usually a woman) has been chronically vomiting. A high urine chloride concentration is consistent with BS or GS. However, surreptitious ingestion of loop or thiazide diuretics can mimic BS or GS in almost every respect, including a persistently high urine chloride concentration. Indeed, for years I have taught that virtually every clinical and chemical feature of these two syndromes can be remembered if one considers the consequences of a continuous endogenous infusion of a loop or thiazide diuretic. Therefore, it has been fascinating to read the exciting series of articles by Simon and his coworkers in Richard Lifton's laboratory at Yale, which elucidate a series of molecular defects responsible for some forms of these disorders. They have shown that defects in the code for the Na-K-2C1 co-transporter (*NKCC2*) are the cause of some forms of familial BS (Abstract 5–8). This is the transporter which is inhibited by loop diuretics. The resulting transporter malfunction causes natriuresis, hypercalcuria, volume contraction, hypokalemic alkalosis, and high renin and aldosterone levels, which together characterize this disorder. Additional work by the same group (Abstract 5–9) shows that some cases of familial GS result from defects in the gene which codes for the thiazide-sensitive Na–C1 co-transporter (*TSC*). This defect explains the hypomagnesemia, volume contraction, high renin and aldosterone levels, hypokalemic metabolic alkalosis and—distinct from BS—hypocalciuria (i.e., similar to the effects of chronic thiazide therapy). These 2 genetic defects each segregate as autosomal recessive traits. The *NKCC2* or BS gene has been localized to the long arm of chromosome 15 and the *TSC* or GS gene is on the long arm of chromosome 16.

Heterozygous patients with a single defective gene have not been carefully studied but probably express subtle transport defects. These defects could be potentially beneficial—they might reduce blood pressure, reduce urine calcium excretion, etc. It has also been suggested that heterozygotes may be especially sensitive to side effects of diuretics such as hypokalemic metabolic alkalosis.

These articles characterize one genetic explanation for each of these disorders. It remains to be determined whether sporadic cases of BS or GS are caused by similar genetic or acquired defects. In addition, the biochemical and clinical abnormalities produced by abnormal *NKCC2* (BS) or *TSC* (GS) genes can be mimicked by defects in other renal epithelial ion transporting or energy generating systems. Probably a number of congenital or acquired defects can produce similar or identical clinical syndromes. Simon et al. have already reported that a defective potassium channel in the renal tubule thick ascending limb causes a BS look-alike phenotype.[1]

The article by Colussi et al. (Abstract 5–10) is a renal electrolyte clearance study that demonstrates GS patients have an excretion pattern consistent with defective thiazide-sensitive Na–C1 transporter. Patients with GS had a below normal natriuretic response to thiazide diuretics because their *TSC* transporter activity is already impaired. Furthermore, normal individuals who chronically use thiazide diuretics develop hypertrophy of other sodium transporting sites including the *NKCC2* pumps in the thick ascending limb. These individuals become hypersensitive to the natriuretic effect of loop diuretics. Similar tubule and transporter hypertrophy and heightened sensitivity to loop diuretics would be expected in patients with GS, and Colussi et al. show that loop diuretics do cause supranormal sodium clearance in GS patients.

Michael Emmett, M.D.

Reference

1. Simon DB, Kanet FE, Rodriguez-Soniano J, et al: Genetic heterogenicity of Bartter's syndrome revealed by mutations in the K^+ channel, ROMK. *Nat Genet* 14:152–156, 1996.

Bartter's Syndrome, Hypokalaemic Alkalosis With Hypercalciuria, Is Caused by Mutations in the Na-K-2Cl Cotransporter *NKCC2*

Simon DB, Karet FE, Hamdan JM, et al (Yale Univ, New Haven, Conn; Dharan Health Ctr, Saudi Arabia; Ospedale A Cardarelli, Napoli, Italy; et al)

Nature Genet 13:183–188, 1996 5–8

Background.—A number of physiologic clearance studies have localized the defect in Bartter's syndrome to the loop of Henle or the distal tubule. However, the exact site and specific molecular transport defect or defects have not been previously identified. This study describes the genetic defect which produces classic Bartter's syndrome (the form associated with hypercalciuria, nephrocalcinosis, and occasionally renal failure).

Methods.—Five families with Bartter's syndrome were genotyped for markers surrounding the Na-K-2Cl (NKCC2). Functional mutations in the *NKCC2* gene were then sought. In each family, defects in the NCCT gene (the gene defective in Gitelman's syndrome) were ruled out.

Results.—(Fig 1) Bartter's syndrome was linked to the *NKCC2* cotransporter gene. Both frame shift and non-conservative missense mutations of the *NKCC2* gene co-segregated with the disease.

Conclusion.—The molecular basis for some forms of Bartter's syndrome was identified by this study. The affected site codes for the transporter that is inhibited in normal individuals by loop diuretics. The potential clinical impact of the heterozygous carrier state of a *NKCC2* mutation is also discussed. Heterozygotes may have lower blood pressures and may also be especially susceptible to the actions and the side effects of diuretics.

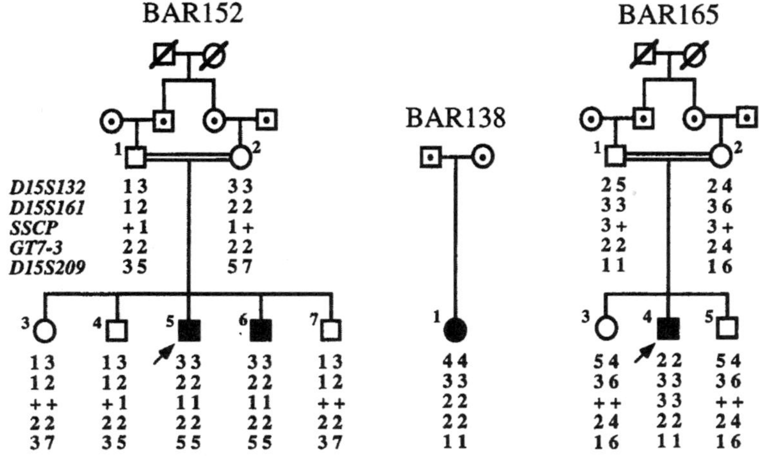

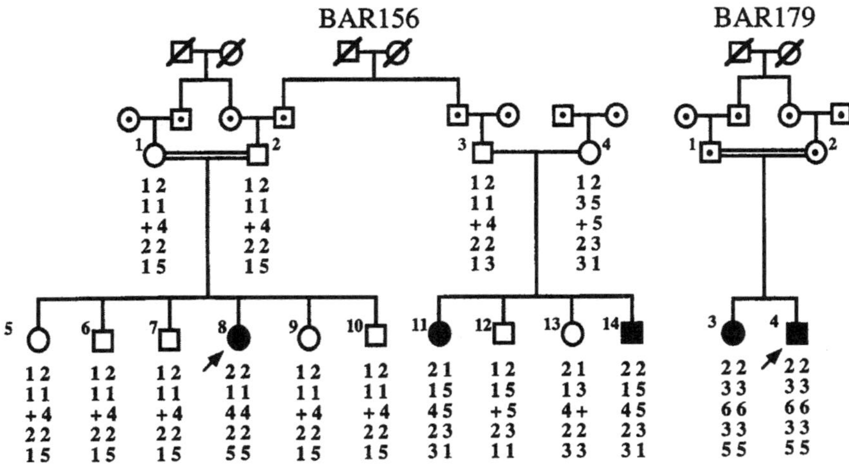

FIGURE 1.—Bartter's syndrome kindreds. Family relationships are shown; affected subjects, unaffected subjects, living unsampled subjects, and deceased subjects are indicated by *filled symbols*, *open symbols*, *dotted symbols*, and *diagonal lines*, respectively. Index cases are indicated by an *arrow*. Genotypes of loci tightly linked to *NKCC2* are indicated and are arranged in their chromosomal order; loci are identified to the left of kindred BAR152. Novel SSCP variants detected in *NKCC2* in each kindred are numbered, with the wild-typed SSCP variant denoted by a plus sign. Affected offspring of consanguineous union are seen to be homozygous for all loci linked to *NKCC2*, and are homozygous for novel SSCP variants. *Abbreviation: SSCP*, single strand conformational polymorphism. (Courtesy of Simon DB, Karet FE, Hamdan JM, et al: Bartter's syndrome, hypokalaemic alkalosis with hypercalciuria, is caused by mutations in the Na-K-2Cl cotransporter *NKCC2*. *Nature Genet* 13:183–188, 1996.)

Gitelman's Variant of Bartter's Syndrome, Inherited Hypokalaemic Alkalosis, Is Caused by Mutations in the Thiazide-sensitive Na–Cl Cotransporter

Simon DB, Nelson-Williams C, Bia MJ, et al (Yale Univ, New Haven, Conn; Hosp Son Dureta, Palma de Mallorca, Spain; County Hosp of Växjö, Sweden; et al)

Nature Genet 12:24–30, 1996 5–9

Background.—Bartter's syndrome has been subdivided into several discrete subtypes. Gitleman's syndrome (GS) is a well characterized subtype which is distinguished from the classic form of Bartter's syndrome by the presence of marked hypocalciuria and hypomagnesemia. This study identified the molecular basis of GS by linkage and mutational analysis.

Methods.—The test subjects were 30 patients from 12 unrelated families with features typical of GS. Markers for the thiazide-sensitive sodium–chloride cotransporter (*TSC*) were identified, and complete linkage of GS with chromosome 16 was demonstrated (Fig 1). Mutations in the *TSC* gene were then sought in these patients.

Results.—The trait for GS was shown to be genetically homogenous and to have an autosomal recessive inheritance pattern. A number of different *TSC* gene mutations were identified in the test patients.

Conclusion.—Linkage and mutational analysis show that genetic abnormalities in the *TSC* gene are responsible for the type of functional loss in sodium–chloride reabsorption which is clinically characterized as GS. This defect explains why these patients develop hypovolemia, metabolic alkalosis, and high renin and aldosterone levels. Although it remains uncertain how this defect causes hypocalciuria and hypomagnesemia, these abnormalities also occur in patients taking thiazide diuretics. The potential impact of the heterozygous state is also discussed. Such individuals may be protected from the development of hypertension. They may also be extremely sensitive to the actions and side effects of diuretic agents.

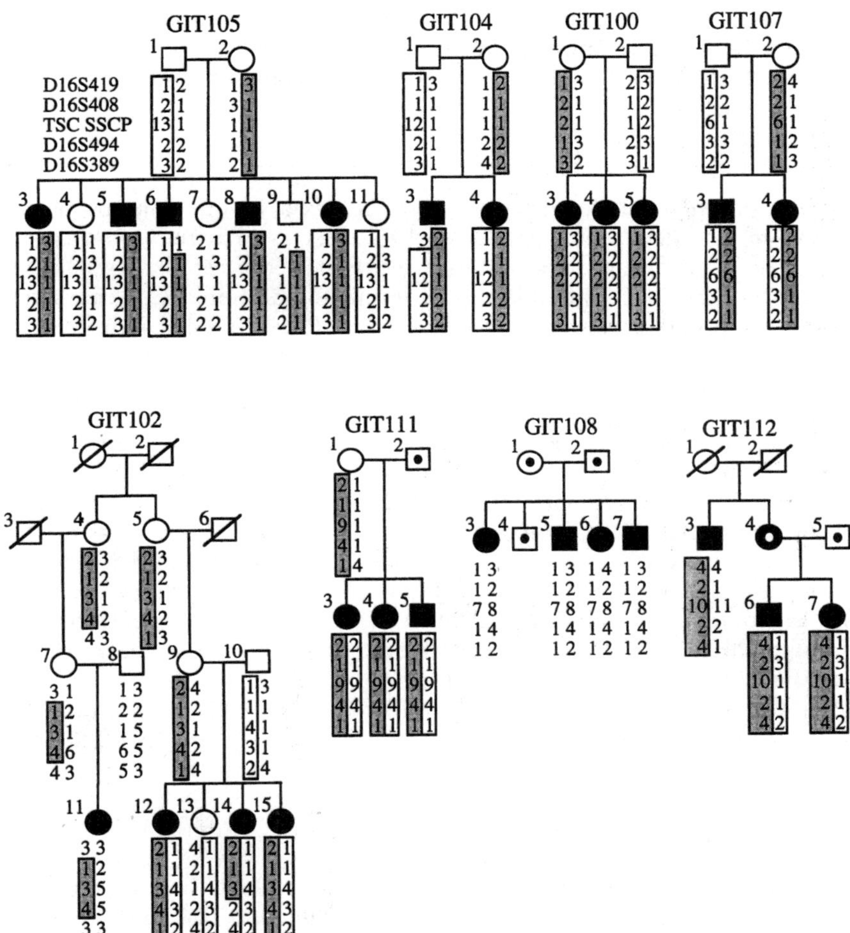

FIGURE 1.—Gitelman's syndrome kindreds used for linkage studies. Individuals with GS are indicated by *filled symbols*; unaffected individuals are indicated by *open symbols*; deceased individuals are indicated by a *diagonal line*. Individuals not sampled for genetic studies are indicated by a *dot* within the symbol. Each kindred is given a unique kindred number, and each individual within the kindred is numbered **above** and to the **left** of the symbol. **Below** each symbol, genotypes at loci on chromosome 16 are shown in their map order. In descending order, loci shown are *D16S419, D16S408, TSC SSCP, D16S494*, and *D16S389. TSC SSCP* refers to variants identified in *TSC*; different variants are given different allele numbers. *SSCP allele 1* represents the wild-type SSCP variant. Inferred haplotypes cosegregating with GS are enclosed by *boxes*, with maternal and paternal haplotypes distinguished by *shaded* or *open boxes*. respectively. (Courtesy of Simon DB, Nelson-Williams C, Bia MJ, et al: Gitelman's variant of Bartter's syndrome, inherited hypokalaemic alkalosis, is caused by mutations in the thiazide-sensitive Na–Cl cotransporter. *Nature Genet* 12:24–30, 1996.)

Abnormal Reabsorption of Na^+/Cl^- by the Thiazide-inhibitable Transporter of the Distal Convoluted Tubule in Gitelman's Syndrome

Colussi G, Rombolà G, Brunati C, et al (Ospedale Niguarda-Ca' Granda, Milano, Italy)

Am J Nephrol 17:103–111, 1997 5–10

Background.—Gitelman's syndrome (GS) is a unique subtype of the group of disorders previously lumped together as "Bartter's syndrome." All of these syndromes have chloride-resistant metabolic alkalosis associated with high renin and aldosterone levels. In addition, GS is characterized by hypocalciuria and hypomagnesemia. Recent studies indicate that defects in the gene coding for the thiazide-sensitive symporter cause GS. This study indirectly demonstrates this defect by an analysis of the response of GS patients to thiazide and loop diuretics.

Methods.—Eleven adult patients with GS and 23 healthy controls were studied. Before the study all medications were withheld for 10 days, and patients ingested a regular diet. Then each test subject was given hydrochlorothiazide (HCT) or furosemide (FUR). After a period of at least 7 days the other diuretic was administered. All GS patients and 17 control subjects were given FUR; 6 GS patients and 6 control subjects also received HCT. Following administration of each diuretic, the concentration of sodium (Na), chloride (Cl), and potassium in blood and urine and their renal excretion rates were determined.

Results.—HCT produced significantly lower renal excretion rates of Na and Cl in the 6 GS patients than the 6 controls (Fig 3). This finding is consistent with reduced basal NaCl reabsorption by the thiazide-sensitive Na–Cl symporter in the distal convoluted tubule of GS patients. FUR produced slightly higher renal excretion of Na and Cl in the 11 GS patients than the 17 controls. This result is consistent with reduced NaCl reabsorption in the tubular sites beyond the loop of Henle (i.e., the thiazide sensitive site), increased NaCl reabsorption in the loop itself, or both. Each alteration may develop in response to chronic inhibition of the thiazide-sensitive site.

Conclusion.—Patients with GS exhibit blunted natriuresis and chloruresis following HCT yet have a slightly exaggerated response to the administration of FUR. These findings are consistent with defective renal thiazide-sensitive Na–Cl cotransporter gene function in GS patients. The differential response to these diuretic agents could be the basis of a diagnostic tool for GS.

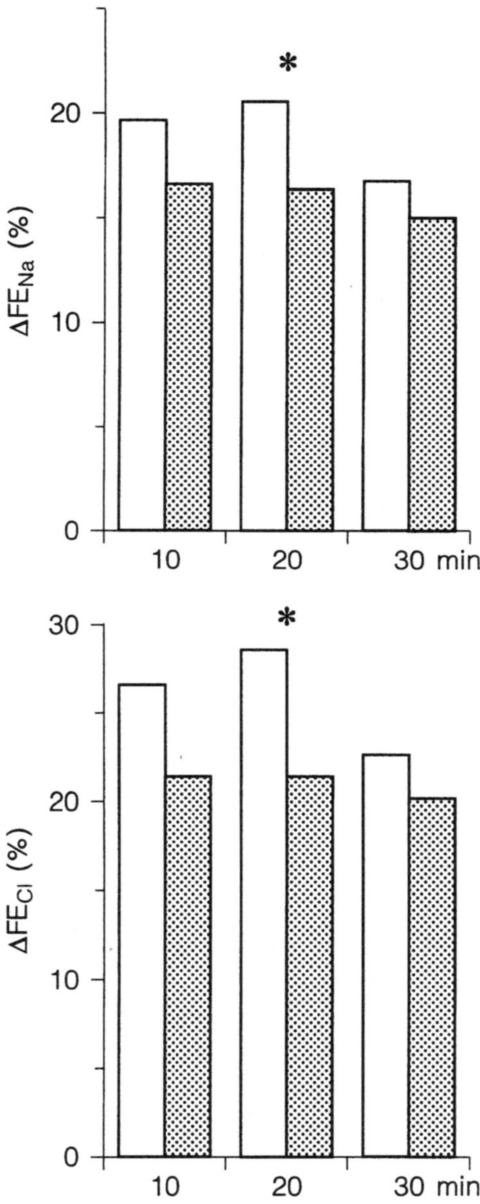

FIGURE 3.—Furosemide-induced mean absolute changes above basal levels (mean of 3 basal clearance) of Na and Cl fractional excretions at different times after diuretic administration in patients with GS (*open columns*) and controls (*filled columns*). *Asterisks* indicate a significant difference at $P < 0.05$. (Courtesy of Colussi G, Rombolà G, Brunati C, et al: Abnormal reabsorption of Na^+/Cl^- by the thiazide-inhibitable transporter of the distal convoluted tubule in Gitelman's syndrome. *Am J Nephrol* 17:103–111, 1997. Reproduced with permission of S. Karger AG, Basel, publisher.)

6 Minerals, Bones, and Metabolism

Introduction

This year's selections on calcium, phosphorus, parathyroid hormone, and metabolic bone disease are heavily weighted in favor scientific investigations. Multiple novel investigations, seeking to understand the basic genetics and pathobiology of bone disease, have emerged. Some of these, such as Abstract 6–1, involve new techniques for attempting to understand what happens when using bone explants or cultured cells. Others deal with genetic abnormalities or with basic cellular and subcellular pathways that may influence bone development and maturation (Abstracts 6–5 through 6–12).

Four clinical studies are spotlighted. Abstract 6–13 deals with the possible future role of androgens in the treatment of osteoporosis. Abstract 6–14 studies the role of selective estrogen receptor modulators in the treatment of osteoporosis. Abstract 6–15 deals with the value of androgens in the relatively rare condition of osteoporosis in men. Abstract 6–16 looks at bone loss after transplantation and evaluates the role of three potential immunosuppressive strategies in the amelioration of bone loss.

Rajiv Kumar, M.B.B.S.

In Situ Microdialysis in Bone Tissue

Thorsen K, Kristoffersson AO, Lerner UH, et al (Univ of Umeå, Sweden)
J Clin Invest 98:2446–2449, 1996 6–1

Introduction.—Bone can adapt to the load applied to it, but it is unknown how bone detects and converts mechanical load into a biologic response. Osteocytes are important mechanosensors in bone. Prostaglandin (PG)E_2 may be involved in the recruitment of mesenchymal (osteoblastic) precursor cells and osteoclastic cells in bone marrow. The microdialysis technique was used to examine release of PGE_2 in the proximal tibia metaphysis after mechanical loading.

Methods.—There were 9 healthy adult female subjects. A standard microdialysis catheter was inserted into the tibia metaphyseal bone. High-impact heel-drops were done for 5 minutes by the 6 subjects in the loading group. The 3 subjects in the control group performed no exercise. Samples of dialysate were taken every 15 minutes.

Results.—There was a 2.5-fold to 3.5-fold increase in release of PGE_2 after mechanical loading. This increase was significant 1 hour after mechanical loading and persisted for the remainder of the experiment. There were no major changes in the control group.

Discussion.—A rapid and significant increase in PGE_2 occurred after mechanical loading in these subjects. In situ microdialysis is useful for investigating the production of PGE_2 in human bone.

► Bone biology is frequently studied by using bone explants or cultured cells. These techniques do not always give a true picture of what is occurring in vivo. The microdialysis technique described by these authors is an ingenious way in which to sample the chemical milieu in bone. The method can also be applied to determine changes that occur within bone after a given perturbation. In the article, the authors examined the effect of impact on the release of prostaglandin E_2. Stay tuned for further results using this method for the study of bone biology.

R. Kumar, M.B.B.S.

Hereditary Vitamin D Resistant Rickets Caused by a Novel Mutation in the Vitamin D Receptor That Results in Decreased Affinity for Hormone and Cellular Hyporesponsiveness

Malloy PJ, Eccleshall TR, Gross C, et al (Stanford Univ, CA Institut de Pathologie et de Géretique, Loverval, Belgium; Katholieke Univ, Leuven, Belgium)

J Clin Invest 99:297–304, 1997 6–2

Background.—Mutations in the vitamin D receptor cause organ resistance to the active form of vitamin D (1α,25-dihydroxyvitamin D) in hereditary 1,25-dihydroxyvitamin D–resistant rickets. The vitamin D receptor was studied in a patient with hereditary 1,25-dihydroxyvitamin D–resistant rickets, congenital total lipodystrophy, and persistent müllerian duct syndrome.

Results.—After treatment with very high dose calcitriol (12.5 μg/day), the patient's serum calcium normalized, and his rickets improved. The patient had a normal amount of vitamin D receptor with slightly lower binding affinity compared with normal fibroblasts at 0° C. The fibroblasts showed $1,25(OH)_2D_3$-induction of 24-hydroxylase messengerRNA, but the effective dose was 5 times higher than that in control cells. A single point mutation, H305Q, was detected by sequence analysis of the vitamin D receptor gene. After the re-created mutant vitamin D receptor was transfected into COS-7 cells, a 5–10 times lower response to $1,25(OH)_2D_3$ in gene transactivation was observed. An eightfold lower affinity for $[^3H]1,25(OH)_2D_3$ was detected in the mutant vitamin D receptor than in the normal vitamin D receptor at 24° C. Restoration fragment length polymorphism revealed that this patient was homozygous for the mutation and the parents were heterozygous.

Discussion.—A new ligand-binding domain mutation in the vitamin D receptor was described. This mutation causes hereditary 1,25-dihydroxyvitamin D–resistant rickets from lowered affinity for 1,25$(OH)_2D_3$. This can be treated with high doses of hormone.

► The vitamin D receptor associates with 1,25-dihydroxyvitamin D_3 and the receptor-sterol complex mediates many of the functions of the vitamin. The receptor is related to other steroid receptors and is comprised of a portion that binds to DNA in vitamin D–responsive genes and a portion that binds to 1,25-dihydroxyvitamin D_3. The authors describe a patient with hereditary vitamin D–resistant rickets who had a mutation in the receptor gene. Amino acid residue 305, which is normally a histidine residue, was replaced by a glutamine residue. The functional effect of this mutation was to reduce the ability of 1,25-dihydroxyvitamin D_3 to bind to the receptor, thus resulting in vitamin D resistance. Several other types of mutations have been described in the ligand-binding domain and the DNA-binding domain of the receptor. The patient responded to exceptionally high doses of 1,25-dihydroxyvitamin D_3.

R. Kumar, M.B.B.S.

Pex/PEX Tissue Distribution and Evidence for a Deletion in the 3' Region of the _Pex_ Gene in X-Linked Hypophosphatemic Mice

Beck L, Soumounou Y, Martel J, et al (McGill Univ, Montreal)

J Clin Invest 99:1200–1209, 1997 6–3

Background.—Researchers recently identified *PEX*, a phosphate-regulating gene with homology to endopeptidases on the X chromosome, as the candidate gene for X-linked hypophosphatemia. This study was undertaken to advance understanding of *Pex/PEX* function and the mechanisms by which *Pex/PEX* mutations perturb phosphate homeostasis, bone mineralization, and growth.

Methods.—Mouse and human *Pex/PEX* complementary DNAs (cDNAs) encoding part of the 5' untranslated region, the protein coding region, and the entire 3' untranslated region were cloned. The tissue distribution of *Pex/PEX* messenger RNA (mRNA) was determined, and the *Pex* mutation in the murine *Hyp* homologue of the human disease was characterized. The reverse transcriptase–polymerase chain reaction (RT/PCR) and ribonuclease protection assays were used.

Findings.—*Pex/PEX* mRNA was expressed mainly in human fetal and adult mouse calvaria and long bone. With RNA from *Hyp* mouse bone, an RT/PCR product was generated with 5' but not 3' *Pex* primer pairs. A protected *Pex* mRNA fragment was detected with 5' but not 3' *Pex* riboprobes by ribonuclease protection assay. Analysis of the RT/PCR product derived from *Hyp* bone RNA demonstrated an aberrant *Pex* transcript with retention of intron sequence downstream from nucleotide 1302 of the *Pex* cDNA. *Pex* mRNA was not detected on Northern blots of poly (A)+ RNA from *Hyp* bone. By contrast, a low-abundance *Pex* transcript of about 7 kb was observed in normal bone. Southern analysis of genomic DNA from *Hyp* mice showed no hybridizing bands with cDNA probes from the 3' region of the *Pex* cDNA.

Conclusion.—Pex/PEX is a low-abundance transcript expressed predominantly in the bone of mice and humans. A large deletion in the 3' region of the *Pex* gene is present in the murine *Hyp* homologue of X-linked hypophosphatemia.

▶ The *PEX* gene is mutated in humans with X-linked hypophosphatemia. The mutation is thought to allow a phosphatemic factor, "phosphatonin," to function unchecked. Now, these authors show that the mouse homologue of the human disease also has a mutation in the *PEX* gene. This will, undoubtedly, lead to further studies concerning the characterization of phosphatonin.

R. Kumar, M.B.B.S.

Idiopathic Low Molecular Weight Proteinuria Associated With Hypercalciuric Nephrocalcinosis in Japanese Children Is Due to Mutations of the Renal Chloride Channel (CLCN5)

Lloyd SE, Pearce SHS, Günther W, et al (Hammersmith Hosp, London; Universität Hamburg, Germany; Tokyo Metropolitan Children's Hosp; et al)

J Clin Invest 99:967–974, 1997 6–4

Background.—All Japanese children older than the age of 3 years undergo an annual urinary screening. This annual urinary screening has identified a progressive, proximal renal tubular disorder characterized by low molecular weight proteinuria, hypercalciuria, and nephrocalcinosis in this population. This disease usually occurs in males and appears to run in families. The renal proximal tubulopathy is similar to the British Dent's disease, North American XRN, and XLRH of Italian families. All of these disorders are caused by mutations in the renal chloride channel gene, CLCN5. Japanese patients with idiopathic low molecular weight proteinuria, hypercalciuria, and nephrocalcinosis were examined for mutations in the CLCN5 gene to determine whether the Japanese syndrome was related to these other conditions.

Methods.—Twelve members of 4 unrelated affected Japanese families were clinically and biochemically examined for idiopathic low molecular weight proteinuria, hypercalciuria, and nephrocalcinosis. Peripheral blood samples were obtained and used to establish a lymphoblastoid cell line. The RNA from this cell line was used for reverse transcription-polymerase (PCR) to obtain DNA to sequence the CLCN5 gene and identify any mutations. Genomic DNA was also amplified by PCR and used for single-stranded conformational polymorphism (SSCP) analysis as a screen for mutations in the CLCN5 gene. Functional expression was achieved in *Xenopus* oocytes.

Results.—In each of the 4 unrelated affected families, a different mutation in the CLCN5 gene was identified. All mutations were predicted to lead to loss of chloride channel function. Expression of 1 of these mutations in the heterologous *Xenopus* oocyte expression system revealed a 70% reduction in channel function compared with the wild-type channel. Analysis with SSCP could be used to detect 75% of CLCN5 mutations.

Conclusions.—A syndrome in Japanese families characterized by low molecular weight proteinuria, hypercalciuria, and nephrocalcinosis was found to be associated with mutations in the CLCN5, renal chloride channel, gene. Mutations in the CLCN5 gene had previously been associated with Dent's disease, XRN, and XLRH. The mechanism by which a functional loss of the renal chloride channel causes these syndromes remains to described.

► In this manuscript, the authors identify mutations in a chloride channel gene that are associated with proteinuria and hypercalciuric nephrocalcinosis. The exact mechanism by which hypercalcemia and proteinuria occur remains uncertain.

R. Kumar, M.B.B.S.

Removal of Osteoclast Bone Resorption Products by Transcytosis

Salo J, Lehenkari P, Mulari M, et al (Univ of Oulu, Finland)

Science 276:270–273, 1997 6–5

Background.—Bone resorption is essential to bone modeling and remodeling during bone growth and turnover. During resorption, osteoclasts seal tightly to the bone surface, so that the resorption area is isolated from extracellular fluid. Large amounts of inorganic and organic material are released by the bone resorption process, but their removal process has not been well understood. Viral glycoproteins are targeted to a specific membrane area in the middle of the basolateral membrane in resorbing osteoclasts. This article provides evidence that this membrane area is a target for endocytosed membrane vesicles that contain bone degradation products. This area is described as a functional secretory domain.

Methods.—Isolated rat osteoclasts were cultured on bovine bone slices. The presence of an actin ring or of resorption lacunae were used to identify resorbing osteoclasts. The surface of the bovine bone was biotinylated to enable the organic bone degradation products to be traced. The bone was treated with tetracycline to enable inorganic bone degradation products to be traced.

Results.—Fluorescence microscopy of osteoclasts growing on biotinylated bone indicated that 85% of resorbing osteoclasts had a biotin label. Biotin was not detected in non-resorbing cells. Confocal laser scanning microscopy confirmed these results and was then further used to scan 51 resorbing labeled osteoclasts. These osteoclasts had biotin accumulation in the upper part of the cell, correlating with the earlier defined functional secretory membrane domain. Antibodies to bovine osteocalcin and bovine osteonectin revealed a similar distribution of these proteins to the biotin-labeled material. Transmission electron microscopy confirmed these results. In resorbing osteoclasts, the biotin label was contained in small membranous vesicles from the bone-facing ruffled border to the functional secretory membrane domain. In the functional secretory domain, the biotin-labeled material was in vesicles and in extracellular aggregates. A small area of plasma membrane was also labeled. This suggests that transcytotic vesicles containing organic bone degradation products fuse to the plasma membrane and empty into the extracellular space. To determine whether inorganic bone degradation products also follow this pathway during the resorption process, bone was labeled with tetracycline, which binds to bone mineral. Laser scanning confocal microscopy revealed that nonresorbing cells were not labeled. Resorbing osteoclasts were labeled by tetracycline. This tetracycline labeling followed a similar pattern to that detected in biotin labeling experiments. Double labeling experiments demonstrated co-localization of organic and inorganic bone resorption products along the same pathway in bone resorbing osteoclasts.

Conclusions.—Osteoclasts cultured in vitro on labeled bone slices were used to demonstrate that during bone resorption osteoclasts endocytose both organic and inorganic bone degradation products through the ruffled border membrane. These bone degradation products are then transcytosed in membranous vesicles to a newly defined functional secretory membrane domain where their contents are emptied into the extracellular space. These results explain how osteoclasts can simultaneously remove large amounts of bone degradation products during resorption and penetrate into bone.

Trafficking of Matrix Collagens Through Bone-resorbing Osteoclasts

Nesbitt SA, Horton MA (Univ College London)

Science 276:266–269, 1997 6–6

Background.—Osteoclasts are bone cells capable of degrading the extracellular matrix of the skeleton. Cytoskeletal rearrangement creates a tight seal that encloses a specialized secretory membrane, the ruffled border, the site of bone resorption. It has been assumed that degraded bone matrix leaks from the osteoclast without a specific transport pathway. Evidence for a specific transport pathway for degraded bone materials was found.

Methods.—The intracellular trafficking of matrix components was examined by immunostaining and confocal microscopy of cultured human osteoclasts in a bone resorption model with a biotinylated dentine substrate.

Results.—As the osteoclasts tunneled through the dentine, they formed resorption tracks that could be detected by immunostaining and confocal microscopy. Matrix components could be detected within the osteoclast ruffled border. The staining pattern within the osteoclast indicated that released matrix proteins were endocytosed along the ruffled border and transcytosed through the osteoclast to the basolateral membrane facing the extracellular space. When these osteoclasts were examined with an antibody to native type I collagen, it was detected inside the osteoclast cell. This collagen must have been endocytosed, as these cells do not produce type I collagen. Type I collagen was localized throughout the osteoclast cytoplasm, with 2 foci: the resorption surface and the basolateral membrane facing the extracellular space. This pattern was similar to that observed for the labeled dentine matrix proteins. No bone matrix collagens were detected in nonresorbing osteoclast cultures or in cultures where resorption was inhibited.

Conclusions.—These results demonstrate that a transcytotic pathway for degraded bone matrix proteins is present in resorbing osteoclasts. The presence of a specific transport pathway for the products of bone degradation may provide a mechanism that permits these cells to monitor and control proteolytic activity. This pathway may provide an opportunity for pharmacologic intervention in the regulation of tissue breakdown.

▶ These 2 articles (Abstracts 6–5 and 6–6) demonstrate the mechanism by which osteoclasts resorb bone. Previously, it was believed that osteoclasts resorbed bone, after which the products were released into the extracellular fluid when the osteoclast became detached from bone. These 2 articles offer fascinating insights into how the osteoclast actually gets rid of resorbed bone matrix and calcium. The results of both studies show that bone degradation products are endocytosed at the ruffled border membrane, that is, the membrane in direct contact with bone. These products are then transported in vesicles through the cell and are released at the plasma membrane. These articles are important, not only because they describe the mechanism by which osteoclasts resorb bone, but also because they describe potential new mechanisms by which osteoclast activity can be modulated or inhibited. Thus, inhibitors of endocytosis and transcellular movement of vesicles might have a salutary effect on bone diseases characterized by excessive resorption of bone, such as hyperparathyroidism and some forms of osteoporosis.

R. Kumar, M.B.B.S.

Quantification of Vitamin D Receptor mRNA by Competitive Polymerase Chain Reaction in PBMC: Lack of Correspondence With Common Allelic Variants

Mocharla H, Butch AW, Pappas AA, et al (Univ of Arkansas, Little Rock; McClellan VA Med Ctr, Little Rock, Ark)

J Bone Miner Res 12:726–733, 1997 6–7

Introduction.—It has been suggested that polymorphism for the vitamin D receptor (VDR) affects several aspects of calcium and bone metabolism. The abundance of VDR mRNA in peripheral blood mononuclear cells (PBMCs) between varying VDR genotypes was assessed to determine the physiologic plausibility of the aforementioned claims.

Findings.—A quantitative reverse transcribed polymerase chain reaction–based method was used. This approach is based on the coamplification of VDR cDNA and an internal standard of known concentrations of a human VDR cDNA mutated at a Bgl/II restriction site (the interassay coefficient of variation being 11%). This method was validated using earlier receptor binding studies demonstrating that normal human monocytes and activated, but not resting, lymphocytes expressed the VDR. The concentration of the VDR mRNA was 10^{-8} to 10^{-7} g/g of total RNA in cell-sorted monocytes and in in vitro activated lymphocytes. This concentration was only 10^{-12} g/g of total RNA in resting lymphocytes. This suggests that the VDR mRNA determined by this approach in PBMCs occurs because of constitutive expression in monocytes. An initial genotype screening of 85 healthy volunteers was conducted using polymerase chain reaction or restriction fragment length polymorphism analysis. There were 14, 12, and 12 individuals, respectively, selected with the Bb, bb, and BB genotypes. Corrected for the number of monocytes, the concentration of VDR mRNA was similar among the 3 genotypes.

Conclusion.—The VDR polymorphism does not influence the abundance of VDR and mRNA. It is either of no importance or is no more than an inconsistent marker for other genes that may be the real cause of the observed associations.

▶ The authors show that vitamin D receptor polymorphisms do not affect the abundance of vitamin D receptor mRNA in peripheral blood mononuclear cells. There has been considerable controversy in the literature following the initial report concerning the influence of allelic variants of the vitamin D receptor on bone mass and bone cell biochemistry. The importance of the original study lay in the observation that allelic variants were associated with increased or decreased risk of osteoporosis and bone fracture.[1] Subsequently, many studies have appeared supporting or refuting this contention.[2–15] Clearly, the risk of developing osteoporosis as a result of a given vitamin D receptor allele should be correlated with the amount of mRNA present within cells or the amount of vitamin D receptor protein present within cells. This study shows that there does not appear to be any effect of vitamin D receptor polymorphisms on the mRNA for the vitamin D receptor in peripheral blood mononuclear cells. It remains possible that there may be changes in the abundance of vitamin D receptor mRNA in bone cells that are not detected in peripheral blood mononuclear cells. Animals in which one vitamin D receptor gene was knocked out did not show large changes in bone mineral density at birth. It is possible that vitamin D receptor polymorphisms may have an effect on bone mineral density, but the effect, if present, is likely to be small and it is unlikely that this test will gain widespread acceptance as a predictor of bone mineral density.

R. Kumar, M.B.B.S.

References

1. Morrison NA, Qi JC, Tokita A, et al: Prediction of bone density from vitamin D receptor alleles. *Nature* 367:284–287, 1994.
2. Kinyamu HK, Gallagher JC, Knezetic JA, DeLuca HF, Prahl JM, Lanspa SJ: Effect of vitamin D receptor genotypes on calcium absorption, duodenal vitamin D receptor concentration, and serum 1,25-dihydroxyvitamin D levels in normal women. *Calcif Tiss Int* 60:491–495, 1997.
3. Rauch F, Radermacher A, Danz A, et al: Vitamin D receptor genotypes and changes of bone density in physically active german women with calcium intake *Exp Clin Endocrinol Diab* 105:103–108, 1997.
4. Francis RM, Harrington F, Turner E, Papiha SS, Datta HK: Vitamin D receptor gene polymorphism in men and its effect on bone density and calcium absorption. *Clin Endocrinol* 46:83–86, 1997.
5. Uitterlinden AG, Pols HA, Burger H, et al: A large-scale population-based study of the association of vitamin D receptor gene polymorphisms with bone mineral density. *J Bone Min Res* 11:1241–1248, 1996.
6. Salamone LM, Ferrell R, Black DM, et al: The association between vitamin D receptor gene polymorphisms and bone mineral density at the spine, hip and whole-body in premenopausal women. *Osteoporosis Int* 6:63–68, 1996.
7. Spotila LD, Caminis J, Johnston R, et al: Vitamin D receptor genotype is not associated with bone mineral density in three ethnic/region groups. *Calcif Tiss Int* 59:235–237, 1996.
8. Viitanen A, Karkkainen M, Laitinen K, et al: Common polymorphism of the vitamin D receptor gene is associated with variation of peak bone mass in young finns. *Calcif Tiss Int* 59:231–234, 1996.
9. Houston LA, Grant SF, Reid DM, Ralston SH: Vitamin D receptor polymorphism, bone mineral density, and osteoporotic vertebral fracture: Studies in a UK population. *Bone* 18:249–252, 1996.
10. Lim SK, Park YS, Park JM, et al: Lack of association between vitamin D receptor genotypes and osteoporosis in koreans. *J Clin Endocrinol Metab* 80:3677–3681, 1995.
11. Carling T, Kindmark A, Hellman P, et al: Vitamin D receptor genotypes in primary hyperparathyroidism. *Nature Med* 1:1309–1311, 1995.
12. Barger-Lux MJ, Heaney RP, Hayes J, DeLuca HF, Johnson ML, Gong G: Vitamin D receptor gene polymorphism, bone mass, body size, and vitamin D receptor density. *Calcif Tiss Int* 57:161–162, 1995.
13. Garnero P, Borel O, Sornay-Rendu E, Delmas PD: Vitamin D receptor gene polymorphisms do not predict bone turnover and bone mass in healthy premenopausal women. *J Bone Min Res* 10:1283–1288, 1995.
14. Sainz J, Vantornout JM, Loro ML, Sayre J, Roe TF, Gilsanz V: Vitamin D-receptor gene polymorphisms and bone density in prepubertal american girls of mexican descent. *N Engl J Med* 337:77–82, 1997.
15. Riggs BL: Vitamin D-receptor genotypes and bone density. *N Engl J Med* 337:125–126, 1997.

The Presence of a Polymorphism at the Translation Intitiation Site of the Vitamin D Receptor Gene Is Associated With Low Bone Mineral Density in Postmenopausal Mexican-American Women

Gross C, Eccleshall TR, Malloy PJ, et al (Stanford Univ, Calif; Palo Alto Veteran Affairs Med Ctr, Calif)

J Bone Min Res 11:1850–1855, 1996 6–8

Introduction.—Reports conflict regarding an association of vitamin D receptor (VDR) polymorphisms with bone mineral density (BMD). The association between BMD with a VDR polymorphism that causes a change in the predicted protein sequence was analyzed.

Findings.—The polymorphism is caused by a C-to-T transition and generates an initiation codon (ATG) 3 codons proximal to a downstream start site. The polymorphism may be defined by a restriction fragment length polymorphism, using the restriction endonuclease *Fok*I. The presence of a *Fok*I site, designated f, permits protein translation to start from the first ATG. The allele lacking the site (designated F), starts from a second ATG site. Translation products from these alleles are anticipated to differ by 3 amino acids with the f variant elongated. One hundred Mexican-American Caucasian women who were postmenopausal underwent bone densitometry and genotyping. Of these, 15% with the ff genotype had a 12.8% lower BMD at the lumbar spine, compared to 37% of women with FF genotype. Heterozygotes represented 48% of the population and had intermediate BMD. The relationship between BMD and genotype was not observed at the femoral neck of forearm. During 2-year follow-up, women with the ff genotype had a significant decrease in BMD at the femoral neck, compared to the FF genotype (this was not observed at the lumbar spine or forearm). Genotype groups did not differ significantly in 25-hydroxyvitamin D, calcitriol, parathyroid hormone, osteocalcin, or urinary pyridinolines.

Conclusion.—There is a significant correlation between the *Fok*I polymorphism of the VDR gene and decreased BMD at the lumbar spine. Women with the ff genotype experienced an increased rate of bone loss at the hip. These findings must be cautiously scrutinized before this polymorphism may be considered a genetic marker for BMD and osteoporosis risk.

▶ This article shows an association between polymorphisms at the translation initiation site of the vitamin D receptor gene and bone mineral density. Nevertheless, the authors emphasize that the initial data should be interpreted with great caution, and that the utility of polymorphisms of the vitamin D receptor gene require further study.

R. Kumar, M.B.B.S.

Mutations Involving the Transcription Factor CBFA1 Cause Cleidocranial Dysplasia

Mundlos S, Otto F, Mundlos C, et al (Klinikum der Johannes-Gutenberg-Universität, Mainz, Germany; Harvard Med School, Boston; Harvard School of Dental Medicine, Boston; et al)

Cell 89:773–779, 1997 6–9

Introduction.—Cleidocranial dysplasia (CCD) is an autosomal-dominant disorder manifested by hypoplasia/aplasia of the clavicles, patent fontanelles, supernumerary teeth, short stature, and other changes in skeletal patterning and growth. A transcription factor in the *runt*family, *CBFA1*, is needed for osteoblastic differentiation. Inactivation of *1 CBFA1* allele in mice is enough to cause skeletal defects essentially identical to those seen in human CCD. Members of CCD families were evaluated for mutations in the transcription factor *CBFA1*.

Findings.—In some families, the phenotype segregated with deletions, causing a heterozygous loss of *CBFA1*. In other families, insertion, deletion, and missense mutations caused translation stop condons in the DNA binding domain or in the C-terminal transactiviating region. In an affected family, in-frame expansion of a polyalanine stretch segregates with brachydactyly and minor clinical findings of CCD.

Conclusion.—The CBFA1 mutations are responsible for CCD. Heterozygous loss of function is sufficient to cause this condition.

Cbfa1, a Candidate Gene For Cleidocranial Dyplasia Syndrome, Is Essential For Osteoblast Differentiation and Bone Development

Otto F, Thornell AP, Crompton T, et al (Imperial Cancer Research Fund, London; Royal Postgraduate Med School, London; Natl Inst for Med Research, London; et al)

Cell 89:765–771, 1997 6–10

Introduction and Findings.—In *Cbfa1*-deficient mice, homozygous mutants die of respiratory failure soon after birth. There is an absence of osteoblasts and bone in their skeletons. Heterozygotes have distinctive skeletal abnormalities characteristic of cleidocranial dysplasia (CCD), a human heritable skeletal disorder. This article describes defects in a mouse Ccd mutant for this disorder. Examination of embryonic *Cbfa1* expression using a *lacZ* reporter gene showed strong expression at sites of bone formation before earliest stages of ossification.

Conclusion.—The *Cbfa1* gene is necessary for osteoblast differentiation and bone formation. The *Cbfa1* heterozygous mouse may be considered a paradigm for CCD.

Osf2/Cbfa1: A Transcriptional Activator of Osteoblast Differentiation

Ducy P, Zhang R, Geoffroy V, et al (Univ of Texas, Houston)

Cell 89:747–754, 1997 6–11

Introduction.—There are no data on the molecular mechanism of osteoblast-specific gene expression and differentiation. The authors previously reported the presence of an osteoblast-specific *cis*-acting element, designated OSE2, in the *Osteocalcin* promoter. They now report the cloning of the complementary DNA (cDNA) encoding Osf2/Cbfa1, the protein that binds to OSE2.

Methods and Findings.—*Osf2/Cbfa1* was identified by Northern blot analysis using poly(A)$^+$ RNA from mouse thymus and spleen and from primary osteoblasts. In adult mice, *Osf2/Cbfa1* transcripts were detected only in bone and osteoblasts, not in other tissues. When C3H10T1/2 fibroblasts were treated with BMP7, which induces osteoblast differentiation, *Osf2/Cbfa1* expression occurred before expression of any osteoblast-specific gene. In primary mouse osteoblasts, *Osf2/Cbfa1* expression was abolished by treatment with $1{,}25(OH)_2D_3$. Analysis of DNA-binding ability identified a core sequence in which mutations affected His-Osf2/Cbfa1 binding to DNA. A 2-bp mutation in OSE2 abolished binding of His-Osf2/Cbfa1. In mouse embryos, peak expression of *Osf2/Cbfa1* occurred 2 days before the first ossification centers appeared. Study of the ossification centers showed high levels of *Osf2/Cbfa1* expression before the bones had become mineralized. Expression was restricted to the cells of the mesenchymal condensations and of the osteoblast lineage. Studies of the effects of *Osf2/Cbfa1* on expression of genes expressed in osteoblasts suggested that *Osf2/Cbfa1* could induce osteoblast differentiation of nonosteoblastic cells. This was confirmed by studies in calvarial cells committed to the osteoblast lineage and in mouse skin fibroblasts.

Conclusion.—The findings show that *Osf2/Cbfa1* is an osteoblast-specific transcription factor and a regulator of osteoblast differentiation. It plays an essential function during bone development in vivo. Its contribution to osteoblast differentiation, compared with that of other factors, will be clarified when the cDNAs for those factors become available.

Targeted Disruption of *Cbfa1* Results in a Complete Lack of Bone Formation Owing to Maturational Arrest of Osteoblasts

Komori T, Nomura S, Yamaguchi A, et al (Osaka Univ, Japan; Showa Univ, Tokyo; Tufts Univ, Boston; et al)

Cell 89:755–764, 1997 6–12

Introduction.—The transcriptional factor, *Cbfa1*, is expressed restrictively in fetal development and is a member of the *runt*-domain gene family. Mice with a mutated *Cbfa1* locus were generated to determine the function of *Cbfa1*.

Findings.—Mice with a homozygous mutation in Cbfa did not breathe and died after birth. Their skeletons had a complete lack of ossification. Immature osteoblasts expressed alkaline phosphatase weakly and a few immature osteoclasts were observed at the perichondrial region. Osteopontin and osteocalcin were not expressed. There was no vascular or mesenchymal cell invasion in the cartilage.

Conclusion.—Both intramembranous and endochondral ossification were completely blocked because of maturational arrest of osteoblasts in mutant mice, establishing the essential role of *Cbfa1* in osteogenesis.

▶ This is a series of four important articles (Abstracts 6–9 through 6–12) from various groups that identify core-binding factor 1, a transcription factor that belongs to the *runt* domain gene family as a transcription factor critical in osteoblast formation. Two groups, namely that of Komori et al and Otto et al, generated *Cbfa1* deficient mice. In both these experiments, homozygous mice showed complete lack of ossification. Ducy et al cloned the cDNA for *Osf2/Cbfa1* and showed that its expression in the mesenchymal condensations were strictly restricted to cells of the osteoblast lineage. They also showed that this factor was regulated by BMP7 and vitamin D_3. They also showed that forced expression of *Osf2/Cbfa1* in non-osteoblastic cells induced the expression of osteoblast-specific genes. These studies are supported by the studies of Mundlos et al who showed that mutations in the *Cbfa1* gene were associated with cleidocranial dysplasia, an autosomal dominant condition characterized by hypoplasia/aplasia of the clavicles, patent fontanelles, supernumerary teeth, short stature, and other changes in skeletal patterning and growth.

R. Kumar, M.B.B.S.

The Localization of Androgen Receptors in Human Bone

Abu EO, Horner A, Kusec V, et al (Univ of Cambridge, England; Med Research Council Bone Research Lab, Oxford, England)

J Clin Endocrinol Metab 82:3493–3497, 1997 6–13

Introduction.—In the human skeleton of males and females, androgens have important effects. The presence of androgen receptors suggests that androgens have a direct effect on bone. Bone density in aging women is strongly associated with circulating levels of adrenal androgens. The expression of human androgen receptors in normal developing and osteophytic bone of both sexes was investigated by using specific monoclonal antibodies to the human androgen receptor, to provide further evidence for a direct action of androgens on bone via androgen receptors.

Methods.—Three males and two females, ranging in age from 9 to 15 years, had samples of tibial growth plates obtained during surgery for corrective osteotomy. Osteophytes were obtained from patients having shoulder surgery. Immunolocalization was performed, as was cytochemistry, histologic staining, and quantitation.

Results.—In hypertrophic chondrocytes and in osteoblasts at sites of bone formation, androgen receptors were predominantly expressed in the growth plates from the developing bone. Androgen receptors were also seen in mononuclear and endothelial cells of blood vessels within the bone marrow, and in osteocytes in the bone. At sites of endochondral ossification, androgen receptors were widely distributed in proliferating, mature, and hypertrophic chondrocytes in the osteophytes. They were also distributed at sites of bone remodeling in osteoblasts. Within the bone marrow, they were seen in osteocytes and mononuclear cells. In both sexes, the pattern and number of cells expressing the receptor was similar.

Conclusions.—In normal developing human and osteophytic bone in situ, the presence and distribution of androgen receptors were confirmed. This provides further evidence that androgens act directly on cartilage cells and bone.

▶ The authors detected and localized the androgen receptor in human bone from males and females. Androgen receptors were found in osteoblasts at the site of bone formation, in osteocytes, and in mononuclear and endothelial cells of blood vessels within the bone marrow. The results show the presence and distribution of androgen receptors in normal developing human and osteophytic bone, and suggest that androgen may have a direct effect on bone and cartilage cells. The therapeutic potential of androgen analogs in the treatment of osteoporosis will require further exploration.

R. Kumar, M.B.B.S.

Raloxifene and Estrogen: Comparative Bone-remodeling Kinetics

Heaney RP, Draper MW (Creighton Univ, Omaha, Neb; Eli Lilly Co., Indianapolis, Ind)

J Clin Endocrinol Metab 82:3425–3429, 1997 6–14

Introduction.—Raloxifene is a selective estrogen receptor modulator that binds and interacts with the estrogen receptor, but which in certain tissues acts as an estrogen agonist and in others as an estrogen antagonist. Raloxifene does not have estrogen agonist effects on the endometrium and is said to suppress biochemical markers of bone remodeling. The biochemical markers of remodeling have not been calibrated with raloxifene against actual remodeling measured by total body calcium kinetics. The effects of estrogen and raloxifene on the components of bone-remodeling activity in early postmenopausal women were compared to determine whether the pattern of change in remodeling is the same for both agents over time.

Methods.—In 33 early postmenopausal women randomly assigned to receive raloxifene, estrogen, or no treatment, the pattern of changes in human bone remodeling produced by raloxifene, 60 mg/day, was compared to that of estrogen given as hormone replacement therapy. Calcium tracer kinetic methods were used to measure remodeling under a constant diet and full metabolic balance conditions. Studies were performed at baseline, 4 weeks, and 31 weeks of treatment.

Results.—At each treatment measurement point, raloxifene and estrogen produced a significant positive balance shift. At 4 weeks, the calcium balance shift was +74 mg/day with raloxifene and +60 mg/day with estrogen. At 31 weeks, the calcium balance shift was +60 mg/day with raloxifene and +91 mg/day with estrogen. A highly significant decrease in the urinary calcium level and marginal improvement in calcium absorption efficiency were the external causes for this balance change. Bone resorption was significantly reduced. At 4 weeks, it was −64 mg/day with raloxifene and −60 mg/day with estrogen. At 31 weeks, it was −82 mg/day with raloxifene and −162 mg/day with estrogen. At 4 weeks, bone formation was not significantly affected by either drug. At 31 weeks, estrogen had reduced bone formation, but raloxifene did not.

Conclusions.—For the 2 drugs, the general pattern of remodeling was identical at 4 weeks, but remodeling suppression was greater for estrogen at 31 weeks than for raloxifene. The remodeling balance, however, was the same for the 2 drugs. There is a similar effect on bone remodeling with raloxifene and estrogen. Raloxifene acts on bone as an estrogen agonist.

► Selective estrogen receptor modulators (SERM) will be widely used in the treatment of osteoporosis. They have selective effects on bone without effects on the endometrium, and thus the incidence of endometrial cancer is lower than with estrogens. There is some evidence that these agents may also be protective with respect to breast cancer. Heaney and Draper compared the effects of a SERM, raloxifene, and estrogen in early, postmenopausal women randomly assigned to receive raloxifene, estrogen, or no treatment. Raloxifene and estrogen had similar effects on bone. Both agents induced positive calcium balance. It is likely that SERMS will become important agents for the treatment of osteoporosis.

R. Kumar, M.B.B.S.

Androgen Supplementation in Eugonadal Men With Osteoporosis: Effects of Six Months' Treatment on Markers of Bone Formation and Resorption

Anderson FH, Francis RM, Peaston RT, et al (Freeman Hosp, Newcastle upon Tyne, England; Newcastle Gen Hosp, England)

J Bone Miner Res 12:472–478, 1997 6–15

Introduction.—Osteoporosis is a disorder that affects men as well as women, and with an aging population the need for an established treatment becomes more urgent. Osteoporotic vertebral fractures, which lead to increases in both morbidity and mortality, appear to be occurring now at higher rates in men. The efficacy and mode of action of testosterone therapy in eugonadal men with osteoporotic vertebral crush fracture were investigated. Previous studies have found low serum levels of testosterone in 20% of men with vertebral fractures and up to 50% of men with hip fractures.

Methods.—Men eligible for this open study were referred with idiopathic vertebral fractures and met criteria for classification as eugonadal. Twenty-three of 25 consecutive men agreed to participate. Testosterone was given as an IM injection every 2 weeks for 6 months. The injections contained testosterone propionate 30 mg, testosterone phenylpropionate 60 mg, testosterone isohexanoate 60 mg, and testosterone decanoate 100 mg. Calcium and vitamin D supplements were not provided. Bone mineral density (BMD) was measured by dual-energy X-ray absorptiometry at baseline and 6 months. Blood and urine samples obtained at baseline and at 3 and 6 months were analyzed for biochemical markers of bone turnover, testosterone, estradiol, sex hormone binding globulin (SHBG), and gonadotropins.

Results.—Treatment was well tolerated and overall compliance exceeded 95%. There was a 5% increase in mean BMD at the lumbar spine from baseline to 6 months, but changes in BMD at the femoral neck, trochanter, or total hip were not significant. All bone markers decreased, an indication that testosterone treatment suppressed bone turnover. Serum osteocalcin levels fell slightly, but large reductions occurred in urinary deoxypyridinoline and N-telopeptide; these reductions were correlated with the increase in spinal BMD. Other markers including bone-specific alkaline phosphatase and pyridinoline showed a wide scatter of values, making interpretation of findings difficult. There was a 55% increase in serum testosterone and a 45% increase in serum estradiol. A 20% decrease in SHBG led to a 90% rise in free androgen. Changes in spinal BMD were significantly correlated with changes in serum estradiol but not with changes in serum testosterone.

Conclusions.—Testosterone treatment in eugonadal men with idiopathic osteoporosis suppressed bone resorption by a mechanism that may involve estrogen. The sustained rise in serum estradiol in these men led to a significant increase in spinal BMD.

► Osteoporosis in men, although uncommon, frequently results in morbidity. The authors in this study administered androgen supplementation to eugonadal men and examined the effects of this treatment on bone density and on hormone levels. The authors showed an increase in BMD of approximately 5%. They also noticed a reduction in bone turnover. Serum testosterone increased as did serum estradiol. They found that the increase in bone density correlated with estradiol levels but not with testosterone levels. They suggested that this treatment may be of value in the treatment of idiopathic osteoporosis in men. This interesting study is flawed by its rather short duration, although the authors do point out that the findings are consistent with a longer term study they had published earlier. The precise mechanism by which androgen supplementation stabilizes bone mass is uncertain.

R. Kumar, M.B.B.S.

Effects of Three Immunosuppressive Regimens on Vertebral Bone Density in Renal Transplant Recipients

Aroldi A, Tarantino A, Montagnino G, et al (Istituti Clinici di Perfezionamento, Milan, Italy)

Transplantation 63:380–386, 1997 6–16

Background.—Osteoporosis commonly occurs after kidney transplantation and is contributed to by corticosteroids used to prevent rejection. The effects of cyclosporine on bone metabolism are not well known in humans but several studies of animals have reported a negative effect on bone metabolism.

Methods.—Changes in lumbar spine bone mineral density were evaluated every 6 months for 18 months by dual energy x-ray absorptiometry and Z-score in 3 groups of patients after kidney transplantation. The 53 patients were randomly assigned to different immunosuppressive regimens with cyclosporine. The mean patient age was 38 years. Patients in group 1 were given cyclosporine alone, patients in group 2 were given cyclosporine plus steroids, and patients in group 3 were given cyclosporine plus steroids and azathioprine.

Results.—At 18 months, Z-scores had increased significantly in group 1 and decreased significantly in groups 2 and 3. Z-scores decreased less in women who were premenopausal than in men (Fig 2). There was no correlation between Z-score change and steroid dosage. The change in Z-score was high in patients with high basal bone mineral density and was directly correlated with length of dialysis.

Discussion.—These findings show a negative effect of corticosteroids and male gender on bone mineral density after kidney transplantation. In these selected patients, those receiving cyclosporine alone did not develop osteopenia and had improved skeletal mineralization.

► Bone loss frequently occurs after the administration of steroids for immunosuppression. In this article, the authors compared the effects of cyclosporine alone, cyclosporine plus steroids, and cyclosporine plus steroids and azathioprine on loss from the spine. In patients treated with cyclosporine alone, bone mineral density increased significantly by 18 months after transplantation and institution of therapy. On the other hand, regimens associated with steroid administration were associated with reductions in bone mineral density at 18 months. The authors also showed that bone mineral density decreased less in premenopausal women than in men and that the change in bone mineral density was not directly related to the steroid dose. The change in bone mineral density was associated with the duration of dialysis. Interestingly, the addition of azathioprine to steroid therapy did not materially change the rate of bone loss. The number of acute rejection episodes and the number of patients who received intravenous methylprednisolone pulse therapy were not statistically significant among the three groups. However, the authors point out that several of the patients receiving monotherapy were switched to double therapy if they had several

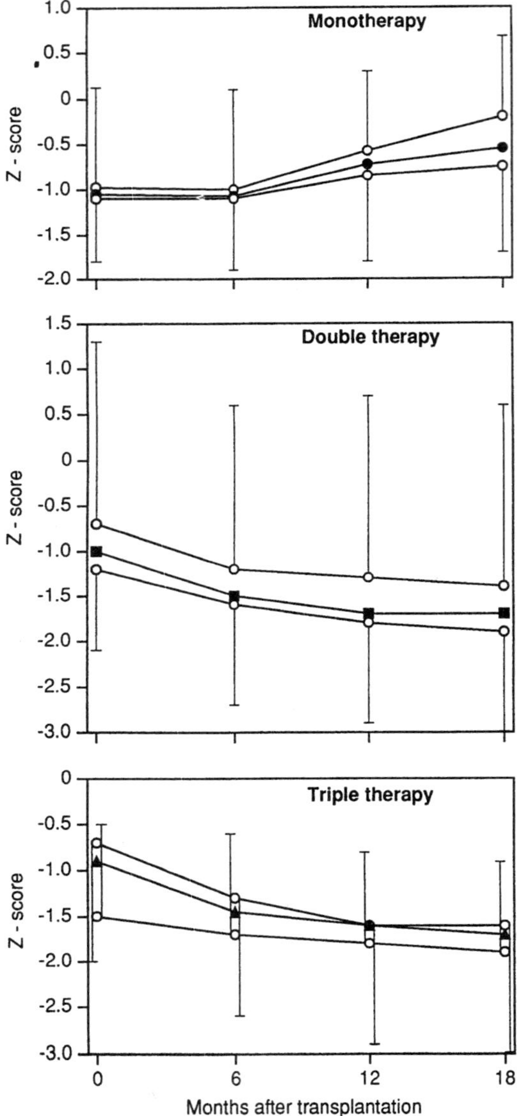

FIGURE 2.—Temporal trend analysis of the Z-scores of the 3 immunosuppressive regimens. In the monotherapy group (top), the Z-score increased significantly with time (P = 0.044) and more in women than in men (P = 0.048). In the double therapy group (middle), the Z-score decreased significantly with time (P = 0.02). In the triple therapy group (bottom), the Z-score decreased significantly with time (P = 0.049) and more in men than in women (P = 0.005). Patients were randomized to monotherapy (filled circles, 13; 8 men, bottom open circles; 5 women, top open circles), double therapy (filled squares, 20; 14 men, bottom open circles; 6 women, top open circles), and triple therapy (filled triangles, 20; 14 men, bottom open circles; 6 women, top open circles). (Courtesy of Aroldi A, Tarantino A, Montagnino G, et al: Effects of three immunosuppressive regimens on vertebral bone density in renal transplant recipients. *Transplantation* 63:[3]380–386, 1997.)

rejection episodes. This study shows that cyclosporine in vivo probably does not have a significant effect on bone mineral density, although experimental studies in animals show that cyclosporine may induce a state of high turnover osteopenia. Because bone loss is a significant complication in transplant recipients who receive steroids, further studies of different immunosuppressive regimens that do not contain steroids are indicated in patients with particularly severe bone loss.

R. Kumar, M.B.B.S.

Subject Index

A

B

C

D

E

F

G

H

L

M

N

O

Q

R

S

T

U

V

W

X

Author Index

A

B

C

D

E

F

G